TOPICS IN THE PREVENTION, TREATMENT AND COMPLICATIONS OF TYPE 2 DIABETES

Edited by **Mark B. Zimering**

Topics in the Prevention, Treatment and Complications of Type 2 Diabetes
Edited by Mark B. Zimering

Published by InTech
Janeza Trdine 9, 51000 Rijeka, Croatia

Publishing Process Manager Mirna Cvijic

Technical Editor Teodora Smiljanic

Cover Designer InTech Design Team

Additional hard copies can be obtained from orders@intechopen.com

Topics in the Prevention, Treatment and Complications of Type 2 Diabetes,
Edited Mark B. Zimering
p. cm.
ISBN 978-953-307-590-7

For EU product safety concerns:
IN TECH d.o.o., Prolaz Marije Krucifikse Kozulić 3, 51000 Rijeka, Croatia,
info@intechopen.com or visit our website at intechopen.com.

Meet the editor

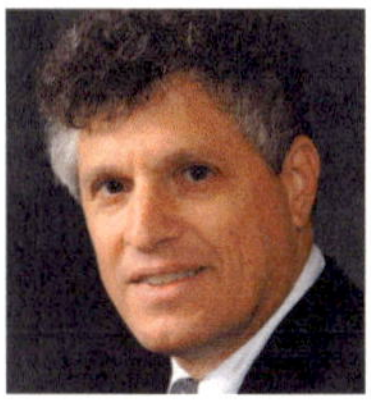

Dr. Mark Zimering is the Chief of Endocrinology at the Department of Veterans Affairs in East Orange, New Jersey and Associate Professor of Medicine Co-Terminous at UMDNJ/Robert Wood Johnson Medical School. Dr. Zimering received his undergraduate training at Harvard College, MD and PhD degrees from the Albert Einstein College of Medicine, and completed an endocrinology fellowship at the NIH. His research has focused on roles for basic fibroblast growth factor (or autoantibodies which mimic or inhibit its effects) in diabetic vascular complications. He reported markedly increased plasma basic fibroblast growth in a subset of obese adult participants from the Veterans Affairs Diabetes Trial having increased coronary heart disease occurrence. His group reported low levels of plasma basic fibroblast growth factor in adult diabetes having a cluster of microvascular complications (macular edema, albuminuria, painful neuropathy) in association with endothelial cell inhibitory autoantibodies which activated the RhoA/Rho kinase signaling pathway in endothelial cells or caused global increases in intracellular calcium in endothelial cells, neurons or cardiomyocytes.

Contents

Preface

Type 2 diabetes is estimated to affect 120 million people worldwide- and according to projections from the World Health Organization this number is expected to double over the next two decades. Novel, cost-effective strategies are needed to reverse the global epidemic of obesity which is driving the increased occurrence of type 2 diabetes and to less the burden of diabetic vascular complications. In the current volume, *Topics in the Prevention, Treatment and Complications of Type 2 Diabetes* experts in biology and medicine from four different continents contribute important information and cutting-edge scientific knowledge on a variety of topics relevant to the management and prevention of diabetes and related illnesses.

In the opening section, *Economic burden and Relation to Alzheimer's Disease,* Atanasijevic-Kunc & Drinovec use mathematical modeling and simulation to forecast the economic burden from type 2 diabetes in the coming decades. Alzheimer's disease has been referred to as 'type 3 diabetes' because of its increased prevalence in populations having obesity, insulin resistance and dyslipidemia. In two excellent chapters- DiCarlo et al present evidence suggesting that type 2 diabetes has manifestations of a protein misfolding disease akin to several well-known neurodegenerative diseases and then Sung Min Son and colleagues argue in favor of mechanistic links underlying an association between insulin resistance and Alzheimer's disease.

The section on *Treatment* starts with a concise review of GLP-1 receptor analogues by Perusicova & Owen. Next, Somsak and colleagues summarize experimental and clinical data supporting the efficacy of new glycomimetic compounds for the treatment of type 2 diabetes in animal models. Ishizuka et al review data showing that the adrenal androgen DHEA can improve glucose sensitivity and protect against the development of diabetes in obese rats. Finally, Cheow Peng Ooi et al summarize the results of clinical trials using various botanical compounds for the treatment of type 2 diabetes.

In a brief section *Prevention,* McLellan et al present the results of their study of lifestyle interventions in preventing type 2 diabetes. Maki and Rains review existing data on how the consumption of dietary fiber can lower the risk for development of type 2 diabetes.

Finally, the closing section on *Complications* offers an in-depth, expert treatment on such diverse topics as vitamin B12 deficiency, the microcirculation, hypertriglyceridemic-waist as a predictor of cardiovascular disease, and psychological aspects of type 2 diabetes, all by notable contributors in each field.

Mark B. Zimering, MD, PhD
Chief, Endocrinology
Veterans Affairs New Jersey Healthcare System
East Orange, New Jersey,
USA
Associate Professor of Medicine
University of Medicine and Dentistry of New Jersey,
Robert Wood Johnson Medical School, New Brunswick, New Jersey,
USA

Part 1

Economic Burden & Relation to Alzheimer's Disease

1

Burden of Diabetes Type 2 Through Modelling and Simulation

Maja Atanasijević-Kunc[1] and Jože Drinovec[2]
[1]*University of Ljubljana, Faculty of Electrical Engineering*
[2]*University of Maribor, Faculty for Medicine*
Slovenia

1. Introduction

Modelling and simulation represent well established approaches when analyzing systems' properties, their behaviour, predicting possible scenarios, or estimating potential results or responses when influencing the observed system (Cellier, 1991; Cassandras & Lafortune, 1999; Cellier & Kofman, 2006; D'Inverno & Luck, 2010). Such **knowledge organization about a given problem** can help in its presentation, understanding, explanation and it is also frequently used through system design (Matko et al., 1992).

Modelling and model usage can be classified and/or chosen as methodology regarding different criteria which can in addition be interdependent due to important activities needed in such situations. Criteria can represent the way of data collecting, their form and degree of confidence, model structure and possibilities of model experimentations, the level of problem abstraction and its aggregation, the selection of time granulation, etc. One of the most important aspect (in spite of the fact that it is often not mentioned) which has to be taken into account, is also ***the goal of modelling*** which should lead the designer through the whole procedure of model development, its interpretation and experimentation. The last two facts are very important also for the user of developed model. This is perhaps also one of important reasons why very different mathematical approaches and descriptions are used, where the disciplines like medicine, pharmacy and the life sciences are no exception (Hoppensteadt & Peskin, 2002; Atanasijević-Kunc et al., 2008a; Stahl, 2008; Belič, 2009; Arnold 2010). This is true even in the cases where the same problem, like certain disease development (diabetes for example) is observed.

Here the following questions can arise:

- Which presented or known model regarding certain problem (disease) is the most important or relevant one?
- Should this model be chosen in all situations?
- Can different modelling structures, descriptions or approaches predict the same or very similar results?
- When there is a need to develop a new approach or problem description?
- Is it possible to benefit from the usage of several different descriptions of the same problem?
- If the answer to the previous question is positive, it can be important also to find out, **how different** descriptions or **models can share their results and/or complement each other**?

The answers to the first questions are not surprising. Process descriptions should be suitably chosen regarding modelling goal(s), modelling phase and other important design factors. As indicated in (Stahl, 2008) the investigators should choose the modelling methods that fit the defined problem. It means that different descriptions can predict similar or complementary results using, for example, *different complexity* (nonlinear or linear descriptions, high or low order descriptions) or *different granularity* (observation of the whole population, observation of an individual patient, observation of dynamical processes on molecular level), *different aggregation* (development of one or several diseases) or perhaps only *different model presentations* are suitable when performing different analysis functions (state space or transfer function description, continuous or discrete time description, time or frequency domain description, ...). Whenever a new point of view of certain problem is under investigation, whenever some new facts or perhaps only different assumptions are taken into account, when modelling results are meant to be used by different groups of people also a new or improved description can be important. All mentioned facts can be verified also when observing different aspects of diabetes mellitus. But, in spite of great diversity of results' description regarding this dangerous chronic disease practically nowhere attention is devoted to the idea of their complementary usage. This viewpoint can become especially interesting when several factors influencing the problem are taken into account.

The literature dealing with different aspects of diabetes has become enormous and very heterogeneous even in the case when searching is limited to mathematical modelling and simulation processes of this disease. Some of them are describing **glucose-insulin dynamics** (Boutayeb & Chetouani 2006; Makroglou et al., 2006; Shianga & Kandeelc 2010), some represent **epidemiological descriptions** of this non communicable disease (Boutayeb et al., 2004; Boutayeb et al., 2006; Atanasijević-Kunc et al., 2008b), while others describe **disease development** (Eddy & Schlessinger, 2003a; 2003b; Kristöfel, et al., 2007) or the **relations to risk factors** which are in correlation with diabetes development (Brock et al., 2009; MMWR 2004; Atanasijević-Kunc et al., 2008c). Diabetes can represent by itself or even more intense in combination with other possible chronic diseases (dislipidemia, hypertension) or life style (smoking, alcohol consumption, inactivity) the risk for developing different cardiovascular diseases (Levenson et al., 2002; Atanasijević-Kunc et al., 2008c; 2011). Additional aspect, important for modelling structure, can represent **social and economical burden** of the discussed disease and/or **treatment efficacy**, which is often interpreted through different **pharmacoeconomical studies** (Boutayeb et al., 2004; Tarride et al., 2010; Arnold, 2010; Atanasijević-Kunc et al., 2011), where cost-effectiveness analysis and cost - utility analysis provide a basic comparison of different treatment policies or drug efficacy. All mentioned situations can be interpreted as **open** or **closed - loop problems (**Atanasijević-Kunc et al., 2008c; 2011; Bellazzi, 2001; Lam, 2002; Makroglou, 2006), where especially in the second case the analysis should take into account stability and sensitivity of system behaviour.

The modelling and simulation approach aims to indicate, use and/or develop mathematical problem presentations which can be used for the evaluation of the burden of diabetes type 2 (D2) mellitus and correlated processes which can contribute to disease development or can represent the source of expenses (direct and/or indirect). This burden is not important only from the economical but also from the social point of view due to the possible severe health complications which usually essentially influence the quality of life.

For the evaluation of mentioned disease burdens regarding certain population it is of most importance first to estimate the number of patients and the treatment expenses. In addition also the treatment efficacy can be taken into account which can compare different treatment strategies and/or their influence to further complications development. In addition, of course, also the reasons which influence D2 development can be taken into account, as usually the prevention offers the most effective positive influence to economical and social situation.

This chapter is organized in the following manner. In the next session some modelling structures are indicated which have been used for modelling purposes of D2 presentation. Special attention is devoted to the possibilities of coexistence of different modelling descriptions. Simulation results are illustrated in session 3, where also some of expenses, related to observed patients are estimated. The work ends with conclusion remarks and some ideas for future investigations. It is also important to mention that all presented results were realized using Matlab (Matlab, 2005) with Simulink (Simulink, 2005).

2. Modelling structures

One of the simplest presentation which is describing the D2 population, two - compartment linear model, is illustrated in Fig. 1 (Boutayeb et al., 2004). Input signal $u(t)$ represents the incidence of D2, while $C(t)$ and $D(t)$ are the numbers of D2 patients with and without complications, respectively. It is expected that patients with D2 are developing complications with $k_1D(t)$ rate, in the compartment $C(t)$ they can recover and therefore return to $D(t)$ compartment (with $k_2C(t)$ rate), they can die due to natural causes (with $c_1C(t)$ rate) or due to severe complications (with $c_2C(t)$ rate), and they can also become seriously disabled (with $c_3C(t)$ rate). The authors have suggested stability analysis with respect to model parameters and numerical problem solving. In this simple description the population in each compartment is observed as a homogeneous set of patients and it is expected that parameters are time - independent. Important aspects as for example patients' age, life style, body mass, simultaneous joint diseases and similar are not presented explicitly, they can only influence (through the identification process) the values of model parameters. Further extension to nonlinear description was proposed in (Boutayeb et al., 2006), but basic viewpoint remains unchanged.

Far more complex dynamical nonlinear model, as schematically presented in Fig. 2, was originally developed and tuned for the USA (Homer et al., 2004) and later on also adapted with some improvements to the population of Austria (Kristöfel et al., 2007). In comparison to the structure in Fig. 1 this one recognises also the patients with pre-diabetes, not only those where D2 is completely developed, while both groups can be diagnosed or not. So additional four compartments are needed, while special attention was devoted also to the transition flows, which are dependent on a great number of important factors and ratios, like population age, obesity, activity and similar. One difference in comparison to model in Fig. 1 is also the interpretation regarding patients with complications, as they can't reach the state without complications anymore.

It is important to mention that authors have in this last case devoted detailed attention to the validation and verification of proposed models using extensive data, which are in general not available for all countries. Due to model complexity sensitivity and stability analysis demanded the introduction of expected range of variables' changes and simulation testing.

When economical burden of disease treatment and/or treatment efficacy is of interest in many cases the so called decision modelling techniques are used (Arnold, 2010). Decision trees have been for more than forty years the most common and simplest formalism, comprising choices, chances, and outcomes. For the similar situation as in previous two presentations the idea is indicated in Fig. 3.

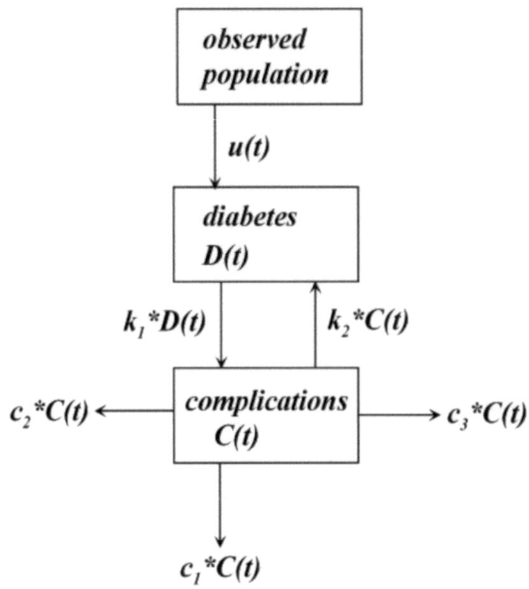

Fig. 1. Two - compartment modelling structure

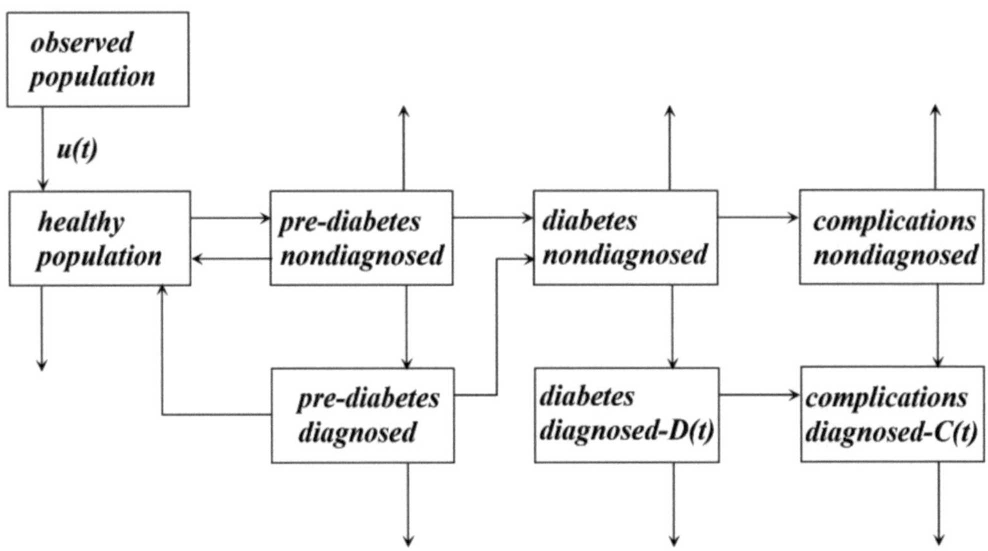

Fig. 2. System dynamics model for the diabetes prevalence

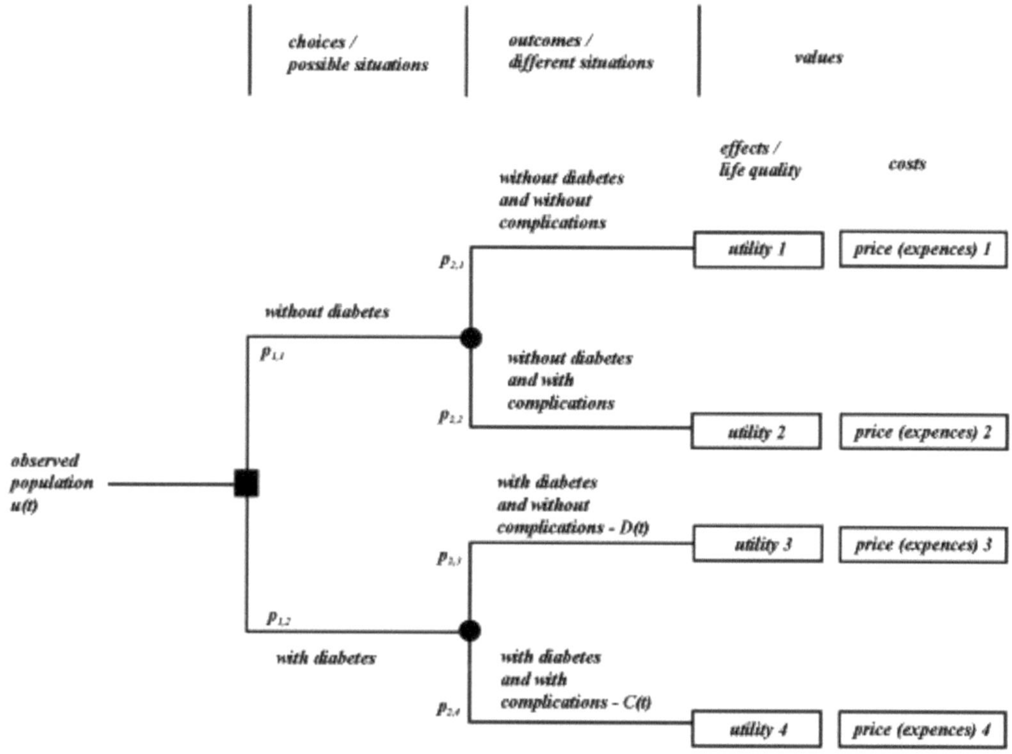

Fig. 3. Decision tree modelling structure

Such problem presentations are static and they don't enable the observation of patients' history, as in the previously mentioned cases. In problems that lead to long - term differences in outcome such presentation can be insufficient. One way to avoid (at least partly) this drawback is to use the description in the form of the so called Markov process (Stahl, 2008; Shih, 2007) or to extend the decision tree to include also Markov processes, for example at the outcome node as illustrated in Fig. 4 (Arnold, 2010). The advantages of such presentations are that they are relatively simple, frequently used and therefore also well accepted as abstract problem presentation. But there are also two main limitations (Stahl, 2008; Arnold, 2010). State transitions can only occur at the end of a cycle, which can create some biases, and Markov cycle time may force the analyst to make simplifying assumptions regarding transition probabilities.

Economical burden regarding the situation inside the observed population was investigated also by (Briggs & Sculpher, 1998; Atanasijević-Kunc et al., 2008b; 2008c; 2011). When summarizing the mentioned results the modelling structure can be presented as illustrated in Fig. 5. The problem presentation and design is separated into three main phases. Through the first phase risk factors and chronic diseases are described in the form of prevalence distribution regarding patients' age, in the second design phase also the prevalence of different complications are added, where among the patients with more problems indicated in the first phase or in the case where chronic diseases were not correspondingly treated, also the development of complications was more frequent. Input signal to the first phase is unity step indicating the start of problem observation, namely at the birth. The results from the first and the second phase are entering the third phase together with input signals $u_2(t)$ and $u_3(t)$. Input signal $u_2(t)$ provides the information regarding the number of people in the observed population with respect to their age, while with $u_3(t)$ also the prices for needed treatment are defined. Combining the signal $u_2(t)$ with calculated prevalence distribution enables the definition of patients' number in the observed population, and using the prices from $u_3(t)$ also the economical burden can be calculated.

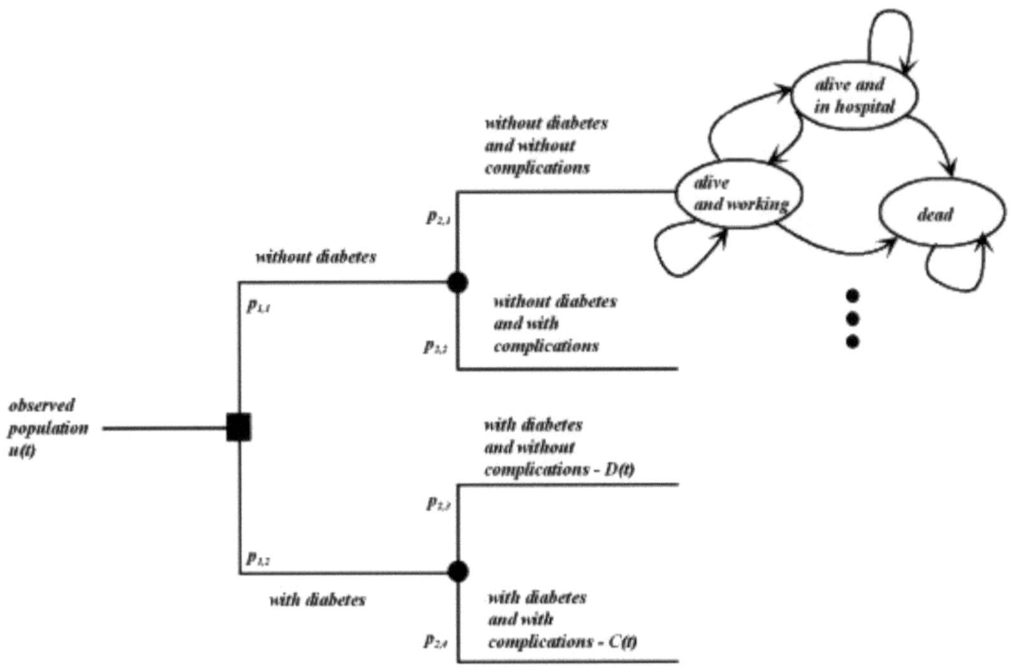

Fig. 4. Usage of Markov processes in decision tree structure

Presented structure gives very good insight how patients are distributed regarding their age and also how this influences the economical burden of observed population. In the case of similar disease distribution only demographic data can be changed and perhaps (if essentially different also) prices and model gives the estimation of patients' number or treatment economical burden for another country or group of people. This approach is therefore especially interesting for the countries or areas for which national diseases registers are not available. But, the drawback of this mathematical presentation is, that it is very difficult to identify the influence on population, which is the result of some actions realized on only one part of the population where also the transient response due to dynamical system properties should be taken into account. To indicate how to overcome this problem let's present only one part of the situation from Fig. 5 and from a slightly different view point. The idea is illustrated in Fig. 6 taking into account also the possibility of coexistence of different dynamical processes descriptions.

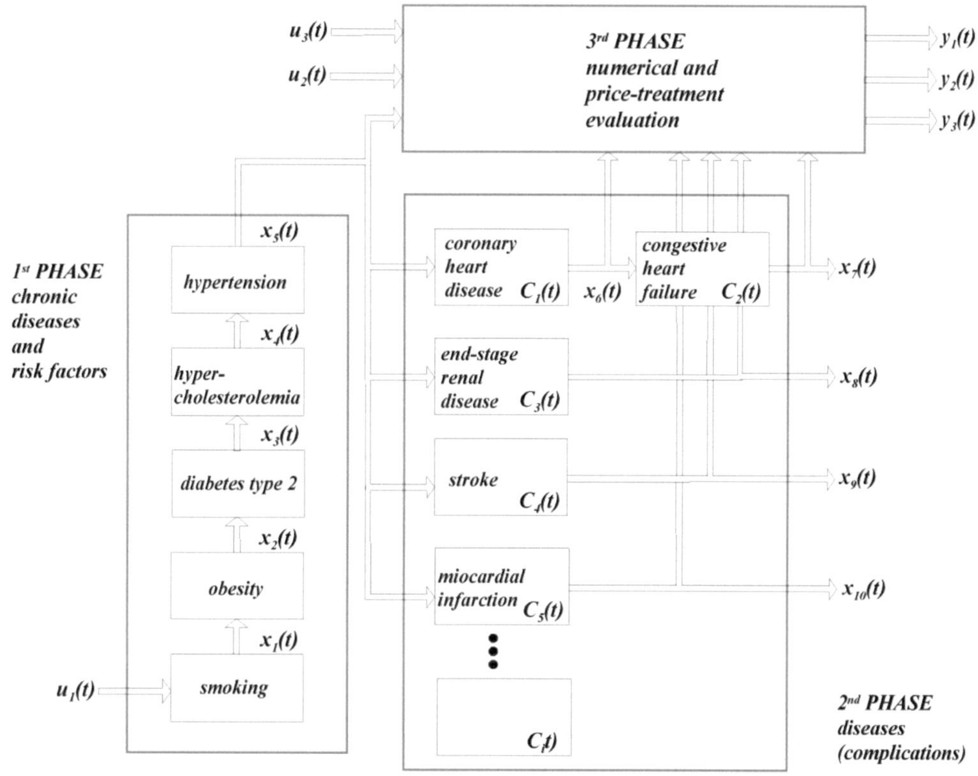

Fig. 5. Diseases prevalence, number of patients and expenses presentation

Here D2 is a disease of the third level due to the fact that on one side risky and/or unhealthy life style (population status observed in the second level of the structure) can influence the development of this chronic disease, but D2, as already mentioned, can also contribute to development of different health complications (presented at the fourth level of the proposed structure). At the second level two important problems, namely activity or inactivity and obesity are taken into account, which are two most important problems leading to D2 (Defay et al., 2001; DPPRSG, 2002; Kriska et al., 2003; Mokdad et al., 2003; ADA, 2007;).

D2 is usually preceded by a pre-diabetes ("a metabolic condition characterised by insulin resistance and primary or secondary beta cell dysfunction which increases the risk of developing type 2 diabetes and cardiovascular disease" (Tuomilehto et al., 2001; Valensi et al., 2005). It is extremely common, especially in elder population (40+). Efficient pharmacological therapies are known, which can be very efficient together with lifestyle interventions in prevention or delayed D2 development.

As mentioned processes are observed regarding certain population, an important influence to overall situation can contribute also demographic changes which are influencing the system's states at the first level.

Expenses are here presented as a static property, but can be in the future extensions reformulated to indicate the results of economical and financial flows.

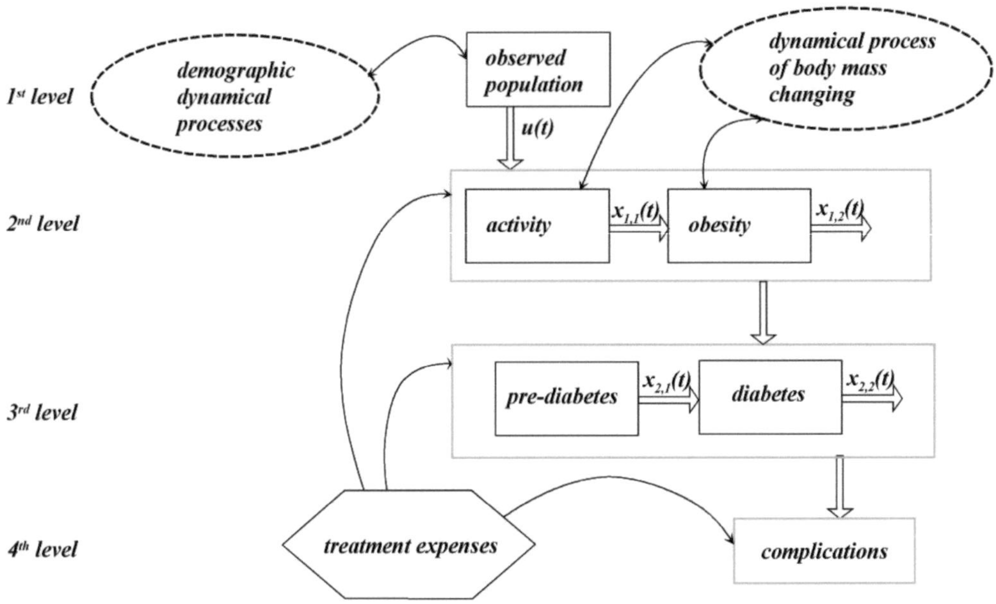

Fig. 6. Limited sub-problem with dynamic processes at different levels

3. Simulation results

Modelling procedure of the structure indicated in Fig. 6 has started by observing the available information regarding the prevalence of population activity/inactivity and obesity as they are closely related to the probability of developing D2. It is important to mention that statistical data differ slightly for different world areas (Berghöfer et al., 2008; WHO, 2011a), but data for larger countries seem to be reliable also for the countries with comparable demographic, economic and social situation.

As very well known, activity has a significant direct influence to body weight and especially to adequate body mass maintainance, but is important also by itself as a prevention regarding the development of D2 (Defay, 2001; Brock, 2009). In adult population to the group of high active are classified those, who are active 30 minutes or more on at least five days a week, medium active are those, who are active 30 minutes or more 1 to 4 days a week, other are low active. In children the following division was adopted: high (recommended): 60 minutes or more on all 7 days per week; medium: 30–59 minutes on all 7 days per week; low: lower level of activity. Usually activity in men and women slightly differ (men and boys are slightly more active), but average data, which were used for modelling purposes, are summarized in Table 1 (British Heart Foundation Statistics Website, 2008).

Overweight and obesity are defined as abnormal or excessive fat accumulation that may impair health. The number of these people is constantly increasing and consequently the World Health Organization (WHO, 2000) has recognized obesity being a disease too and as such it deserves far more attention. It is mainly a consequence of unbalance between energy intake and energy expenditure in each individual.

For adults, overweight and obesity ranges are determined by using weight and height to calculate a number called "body mass index" (BMI). It is defined as the weight in kilograms

divided by the square of the height in meters (kg/m^2). BMI is used because, for most people, it correlates with their amount of body fat. However, it should be considered as a rough guide because it may not correspond to the same degree of fatness in different individuals.
WHO defines "overweight" as a BMI equal to or more than 25, and "obesity" as a BMI equal to or more than 30 (WHO, 2011b). WHO's latest projections indicate that globally in 2005 approximately 1.6 billion adults (age 15+) were overweight and at least 400 million adults were obese. Children were defined as overweight or obese using the 85th and 95th percentiles of the reference curves. At least 20 million children under the age of 5 years were overweight globally in 2005. Once considered a problem only in high-income countries, overweight and obesity are now dramatically rising in low- and middle-income countries, particularly in urban settings. The prevalence of obesity differs from country to country and is also different regarding men and women. An average situation, which can be taken into account for most European countries, is presented in Table 2 (British Heart Foundation Statistics Website, 2010).
From data given in Tables 1 and 2 it is clear that activity or inactivity, as well as overweight and obesity can, regarding the whole observed population, be interpreted as dynamical processes where age of people is represented as independent variable.
In Fig. 7 the model response is illustrated which shows that activity is decreasing through the whole life time and is becoming especially intensive after the age of 40. When activity is defined also the prevalence of inactive are known, as is indicated in Fig. 8. The dynamical structure which gives the responses presented in Figs. 7 and 8 was identified so that good matching was achieved with data in Table 1 (dynamical nonlinear model of 11th order).

age [years]	0	1	2	3	4	5	6	7
average [%]	70	69	68.5	69	70	62	62.5	69
age [years]	8	9	10	11	12	13	14	15
average [%]	68.5	64.5	64.5	64	64.5	64.5	58.5	56.5
age [years]	16-24	25-34	35-44	45-54	55-64	65-74	75+	
average [%]	43	44	40.5	36	31	18.5	6.5	

Table 1. Prevalence of high active population

age [years]	2-15	16-34	35-54	55-74	75+
average prevalence: 25=<BMI<30 [%]	13.5	27	39	41.5	37.5
average prevalence: BMI=>30 [%]	16	19	33.5	31.5	22.5
average prevalence: BMI=>25 [%]	29.5	46	72.5	73	60

Table 2. Prevalence of overweight (25=<BMI<30) and obese population (BMI=>30)

It is important to note that such representation enables the extension of decision tree formalism to comprise also a time component, namely the age of observed people (and/or patients). This time component is of crucial importance also regarding the prevalence of great number of chronic diseases and corresponding consequences. Another advantage is that when certain population is observed these responses can be combined with demographic data to evaluate the number of observed people.

In Fig. 9 the result of the last count of the population in Slovenia in 2003 is illustrated. When combined with the prevalence of activity in Fig. 7 it becomes clear that in Slovenia around 780 000 people or 39% are active, while other 61% do not match this criteria. Distribution of the number of active people regarding their age is presented in Fig. 10.

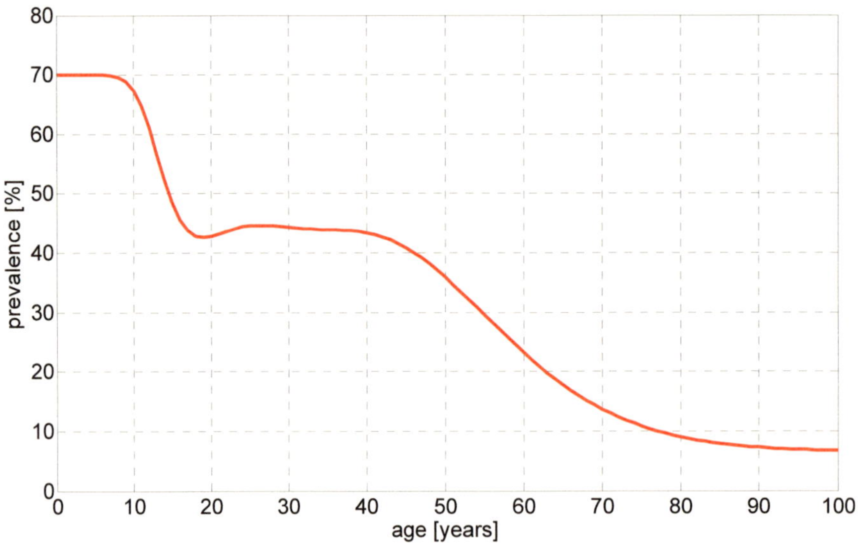

Fig. 7. Prevalence of activity

Two output signals from the block "activity" (see Fig. 6) are entering the block "obesity". For modelling purposes the information from Table 2 was used. It is clear that the ratio between overweight and obese population is slightly changing through the life time, but as these changes are not very distinctive the assumption that it is equal to 1.33 (average value from Table 2) is taken into account.

It is also very well known that active life style has very good influence also to body mass and in contrary people who are obese are inclined to inactivity, but there is practically no quantitative data available regarding the statistical correlation on the population level among these two variables. The interesting exception represents the paper of Brock (Brock et al, 2009), where the association between insufficiently physically active and the prevalence of obesity is described for the USA in the form of linear regression model. Testing this description in comparison to information from Table 2 and presented activity response showed that it is expected the prevalence of obesity to be slightly lower in EU countries. Further nonlinearity can be presumed which can mainly be the reason of the fact that activity is essentially decreasing especially after the age of 45 (see Fig. 7).

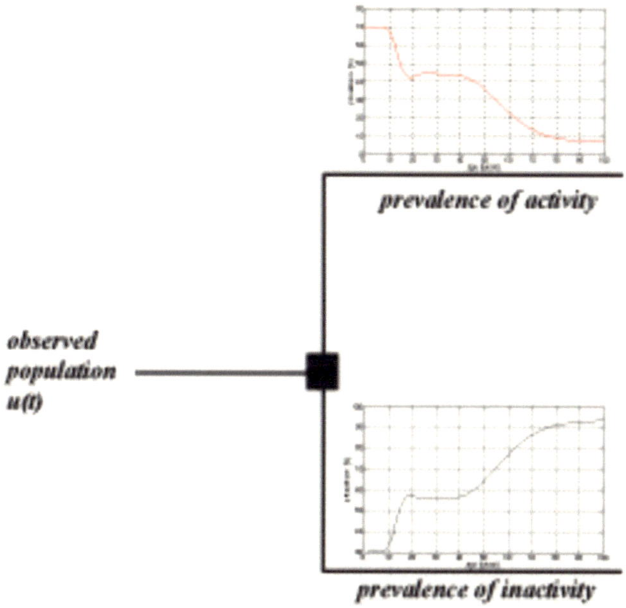

Fig. 8. Prevalence of activity and inactivity in observed population illustrated through decision tree

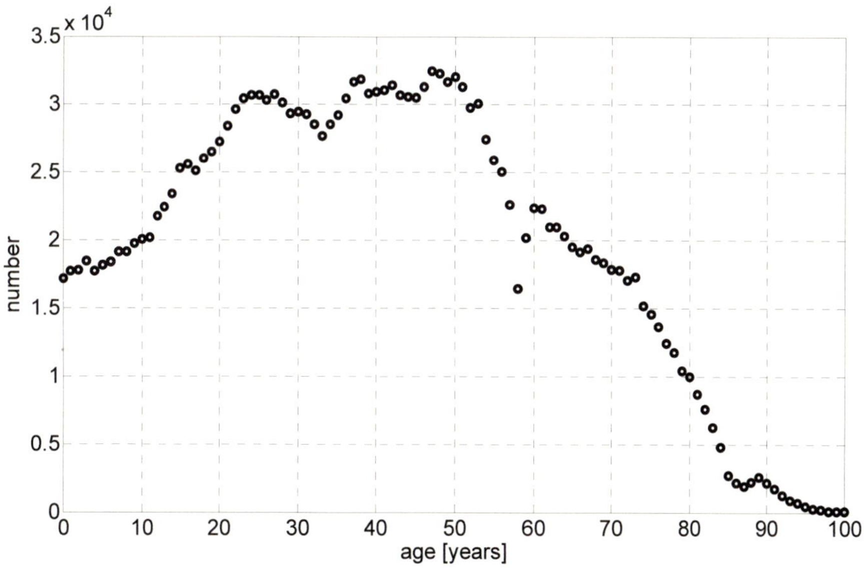

Fig. 9. Number of people in Slovenia

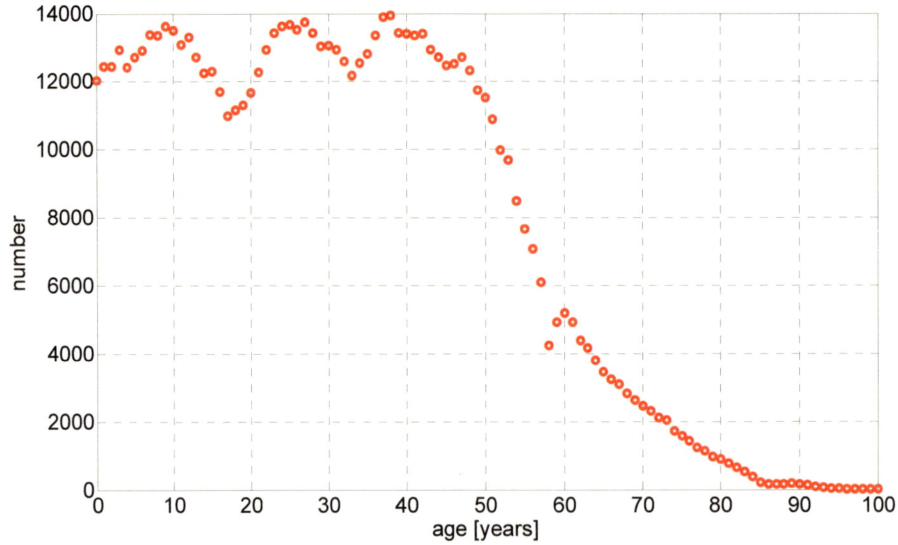

Fig. 10. Number of active people in Slovenia

Taking into account all mentioned data the mathematical model (11th order with time delays) of overweight and obese population was identified and responses are presented in Fig. 11. It is also possible to differ among overweight and obese taking into account mentioned ratio.

When prevalence functions are defined also the number of these people can be calculated (Fig. 12). Regarding the presented model in Slovenia live over 1 million people who have BMI equal to or greater than 25 or with other words almost 55% of population have higher body mass as recommended. Among these people around 300 000 are active while others are not.

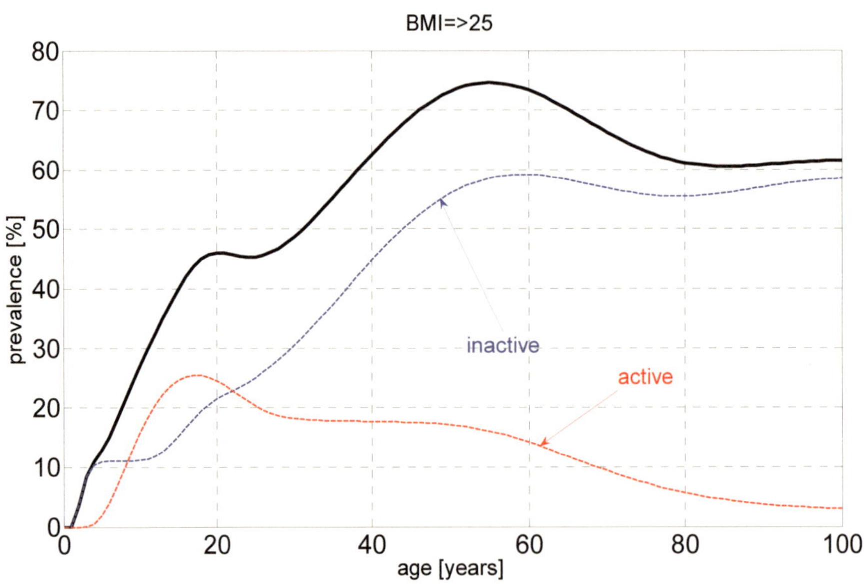

Fig. 11. Prevalence of population with BMI=>25

Both, inactivity and obesity are very important regarding the development of D2 (Valensi et al., 2005). It was discovered that most adults (85.4 - 86% in average) with diagnosed diabetes were overweight or obese (MMWR, 2004), 52% were obese, and 8.1% had morbid obesity (Daousi, 2006). Before this chronic disease is fully developed patients have a pre-diabetes which in general significantly differ from D2 regarding the fact that when strict life change is adopted taking into account corresponding diet and activity, sometimes complemented by drug treatment, patients can return to normal state. Sometimes this transition is (for example due to long lasting pre-diabetes) not possible, but in such situations D2 development is in most cases significantly postponed. Pre-diabetes is not a true disease but can be interpreted as a serious risk factor for developing D2 and cardiovascular diseases. Over 30% of people with pre-diabetes develop D2 within 5 years (Valensi, 2005). The average conversion rate was estimated at 5.8% per year with wide variations which depend on differences in age, BMI, ethnicity, etc.. It is very important to accent that several well-designed randomized controlled trials (Valensi, 2005) have been reported that categorically confirm the benefits of interventions in pre-diabetes. Standardized diet with reduced food intake, increased physical activity and sometimes also additional drug treatment can reduce the incidence of D2 for almost 60% (in mentioned studies from 25% to 58%). But, it is important to point out that intensive lifestyle modification was nearly twice as effective in preventing D2. It is therefore evident that active management of pre-diabetes can be very effective in preventing the progression of diabetes.
For modelling purposes the information given in Tables 3 (Narayanappa et al., 2011; Li, et al., 2009; NDS, 2011; Valensi et al., 2005) and 4 (Behl et al., 2004) was taken into account. Again the average data between men and women are presented.

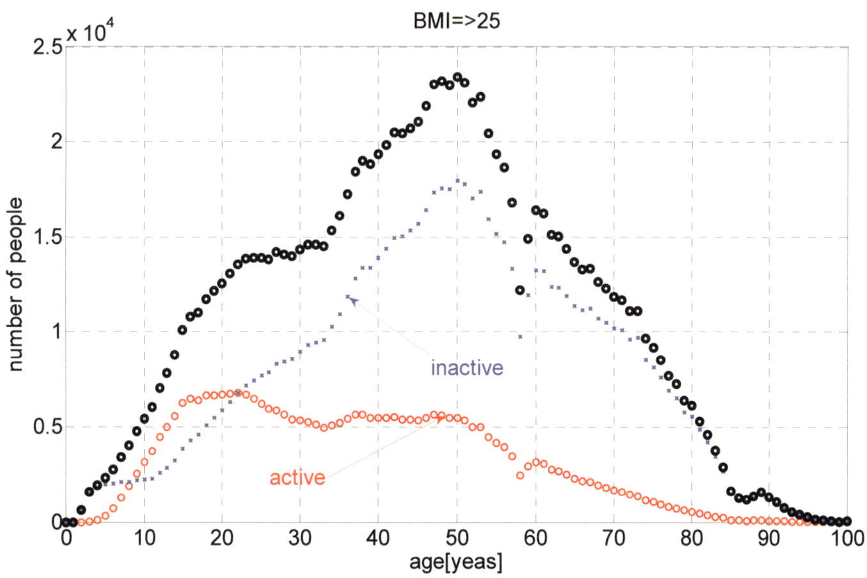

Fig. 12. Number of people in Slovenia with BMI=>25 (active and inactive)

age [years]	5-11	12-19	20+	40-75	65+
average prevalence [%]	3.7	16.1	35	40	50

Table 3. Prevalence of pre-diabetes

age [years]	25-34	35-44	45-54	55-64	65+
average prevalence [%]	3.5	4.2	8.9	15.5	19

Table 4. Prevalence of diabetes type 2

In Fig. 13 model responses are given regarding pre-diabetes (16th order model with time delays) and D2 (5th order with time delays), what further enable the calculation of observed patients with respect to their age, what shows Fig. 14. It can be concluded that in Slovenia live around 611 000 patients with pre-diabetes, or with other words, approximately 30% of the population is in such state. In addition almost 144 000 are D2-patients, or over 7% have developed this serious chronic disease. Among this group of patients 85.7% are overweight or even obese.

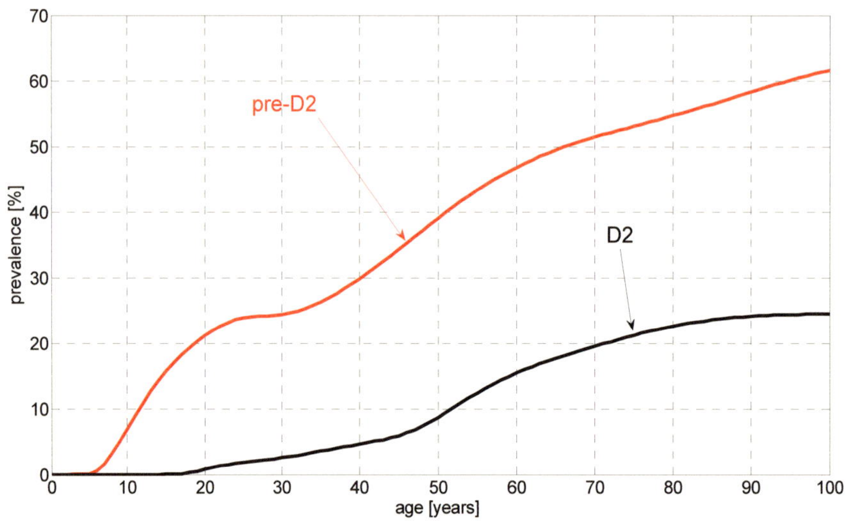

Fig. 13. Prevalence of pre-diabetes and D2

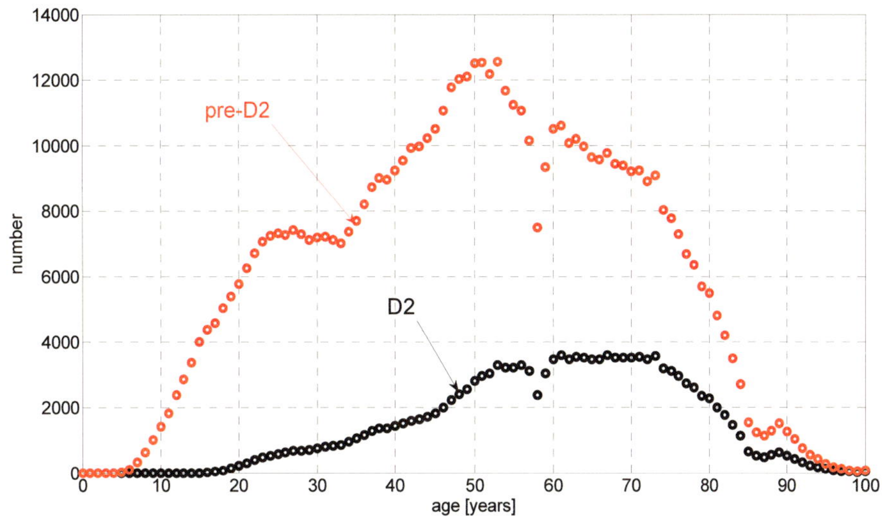

Fig. 14. Number of patients with pre-diabetes and D2 in Slovenia

In this design phase also some of expenses needed for observed patients can be indicated. For the population with higher mass it is possible to find out that a great majority of these people would like to loose their overweight. Some of them are experimenting with different diets, around 20% of adult population (from 18 to 60) also use drugs, and around 5% from the age window of 40 to 60 use the help of medical experts. In some special cases also surgical help is needed. In Slovenia in average around 100 such surgical operations per year can be expected. More and more frequent are also cosmetic surgical operations, but were not taken into account here as they are mainly performed in private institutions and data are not available.

It was estimated, that for one overweight or obese patient the year price for drugs is €447.96, what represents an economic burden of €66.88 million per year (for 20% of adult population between 18 to 60). As year treatment by medical expert represents economical burden of around €3000 for this group additional €63.4 million is used (for 5% from the age window of 40 to 60). Prices for surgical operations differ drastically. In Slovenia for such intervention €7200 is needed for one patient or €720 000 per year for the whole country. All together this represents €131 million per year of direct costs or in average around €130 each year for each from the group of obese or overweight persons.

An average year treatment price for one D2 patient was estimated to be €355 (Atanasijević-Kunc et al., 2008c) (general practitioner: 4 times / year, laboratory: 2 times / year, drugs), representing economical burden of over €51 million per year. It is important to observe that the maximum number of these patients can be expected inside the age window of 55 to 75. As population in Slovenia, similar to other EU countries, is getting older, in the future decades this burden can become even more serious.

To estimate such population changes mathematical model was developed taking into account average statistical parameters using data (fertility, mortality and migrations) from 2004 to 2007 as presented by Statistical Office of the Republic of Slovenia (SORS, 2011). Fertility was calculated regarding the number of people in the age window from 18 to 45. It was estimated that each year 2.2715% newborns are expected regarding the mentioned group of people. The realized prediction starts in 2003 and illustrates the expectations till the year 2052. The situation is illustrated in Fig. 15. An important observation from this figure is that the number of people after the age of 60 is expected to increase while the younger population, including also the majority of working people, is diminished. Combination of modelling results from Fig. 15 and the prevalence of D2 model is shown in Fig. 16.

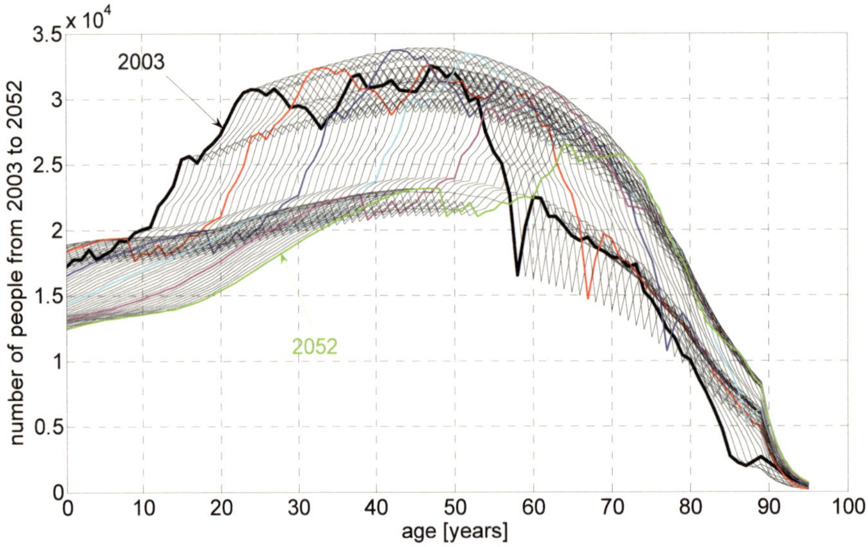

Fig. 15. Number of people in Slovenia from 2003 to 2052

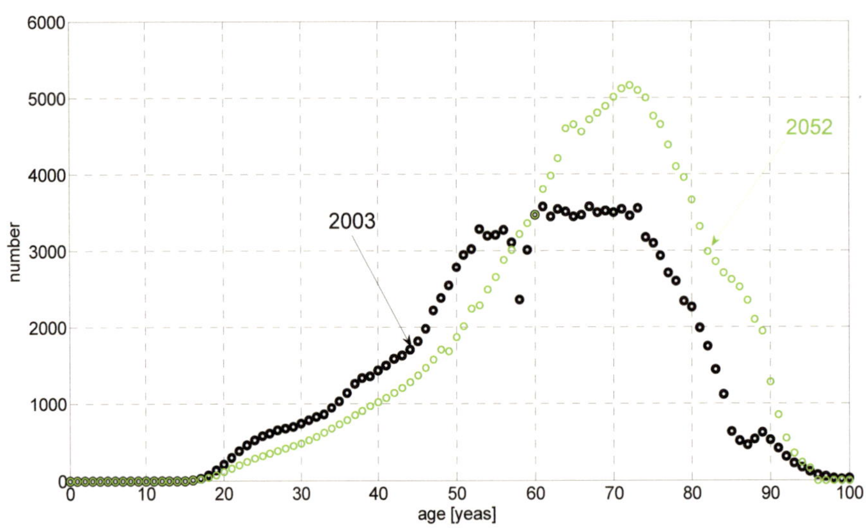

Fig. 16. Number of D2 patients from 2003 to 2052

The number of D2 patients in younger population is expected to decrease as the number of younger population is also decreasing, but after the age of 60 the number of D2 patients is essentially higher. The ratio between the number of D2 patients and the number of active people (people between 20 and 60) in 2003 equals 0.1208, while in 2052 it is expected to rise to 0.2036. This means that for active population only regarding D2 patients the economic burden is expected to increase for 68.5% if the prevalence of this disease remains unchanged.

Here it is important to point out also the following additional facts:

- As revealed in (NDS, 2011) the average medical expenditures for the people with diagnosed D2 are 2.3 times higher than that for the people without D2.
- The prevalence of several other chronic diseases and different complications are higher among older population (Atanasijević-Kunc et al., 2008a, 2008b, 2008c).

Therefore it would be of great importance to indicate and evaluate some solutions which would decrease this enormous social and economical burden.

The increase of activity is, regarding medical recommendation, the first step which can represent an improvement in desired direction, and the second is of course body mass reduction. To estimate the interdependence of mentioned variables in a quantitative manner two-compartment mathematical model was used (Chow & Hall, 2008), enabling to differ among fat-free body mass (*ffm*) and fat mass (*fm*). Equation for daily energy balance is:

$$eb(t) = ei(t) - ee(t) \tag{1}$$

where *ei(t)* represents daily energy intake and *ee(t)* daily energy expenditure in *kcal*. Energy intake depends on food and its caloric value:

$$ei(t) = k_1 ci(t) + k_2 fi(t) + k_3 pi(t) \tag{2}$$

ci(t) indicating carbohydrate intake, *fi(t)* fat intake and *pi(t)* protein intake while constants k_i are: k_1=4*kcal/gram*, k_2=9*kcal/gram*, k_3=4 *kcal/gram*. It is recommended that protein intake represents 20-30%, fat intake 15-20% and carbohydrate intake 55-60% of daily food intake.

Daily energy expenditure is calculated as follows:

$$ee(t) = tef(t) + pa(t) + rmr(t) \tag{3}$$

where *tef(t)* is thermic effect of feeding which usually ranges from 7 to 15% of the total energy intake (11% in our case), *pa(t)* represents energy spent on physical activity and *rmr(t)* is the so called resting metabolic rate. It refers to the energy needed to maintain basic physiological processes. It represents a substantial percentage (45-70%) of energy expenditure for the typical individual (HER, 2001). It mainly depends on *ffm(t)* and was approximated with:

$$rmr(t) = 500 + 22\,ffm(t) \tag{4}$$

The daily energy balance *eb(t)* is partitioned into one of two compartments for fat mass and for fat-free mass:

$$\frac{dfm(t)}{dt} = \frac{(1 - r(t))eb(t)}{\rho_{fm}} \tag{5}$$

$$\frac{dffm(t)}{dt} = \frac{r(t)eb(t)}{\rho_{ffm}} \tag{6}$$

where *r(t)* ratio is the parameter that assigns a percentage of the imbalance denoted by *eb(t)* to the compartments fat mass and fat-free mass, respectively (Dugdale & Payne, 1977):

$$r(t) = \frac{K}{K + fm(t)}; \quad K = 10.4\frac{\rho_{ffm}}{\rho_{fm}} \tag{7}$$

$$\rho_{ffm} = 1800\ kcal / kg$$
$$\rho_{fm} = 9400\ kcal / kg$$

It is important to mention that also more precise (and complex) mathematical models describing the influence of eating and physical activity to body mass exist. But in our case the goal was mainly to present the interdependence of different models and information which can be shared to obtain better insight into population behaviour what is also the reason why in this modelling step only an average person (between men and women) was taken into account. From the average height (1.72m regarding 11 European countries) and average BMI=32 also the average mass of this person is estimated to be 94.7kg. Regarding medical recommendations such person should loose around 30kg to satisfy BMI=22 in the middle of desired BMI interval. The initial fat mass was estimated from the regression equations (Jackson et al., 2002): *fm(0)=34.7 kg*.

Model response is given in Fig. 17 for observation time of 10 years. During the first year (365 days) energy intake is equal to energy expenditure (2460kcal) (for control purposes) and therefore the body mass remains unchanged. After the first year physical activity is increased from 370kcal per day (representing minimal physical activity) for 210 kcal per day. This energy expenditure can be realized by a half an hour walk, but without the increase of energy intake. Such minimal increase of activity, which is in general suitable also for obese persons, would change in three years BMI to 25.

In our case however, at the beginning of the third year of observation also the energy intake is decreased for 300 kcal per day, but only for one year. In this way desired range of BMI is reached during the second year as presented in Fig. 17. If the person remains active for half an hour per day he-she is reaching desired mass at the end of the third year.

What direct changes could such a regime of activity and diet represent for observed population and why the problems are expected in practice?

Let's take into account the following assumptions. 80% of obese and inactive people between the age of 20 to 50 are motivated to undertake the presented regime of increased activity and diet. With this they are immediately transferred into the group of active population, where they remain. After two years of activity they are also transferred out from obese population and they remain in the group of people with healthy body mass. Each year also 80% of 20 years old obese and inactive are motivated to join the motivated group.

The consequences of life - lasting increased activity together with corresponding diet are shown in Figs. 18 to 20. The increased number of active population (Fig. 18) would together with proposed diet slowly changing the number of overweight and obese people (Fig. 19).

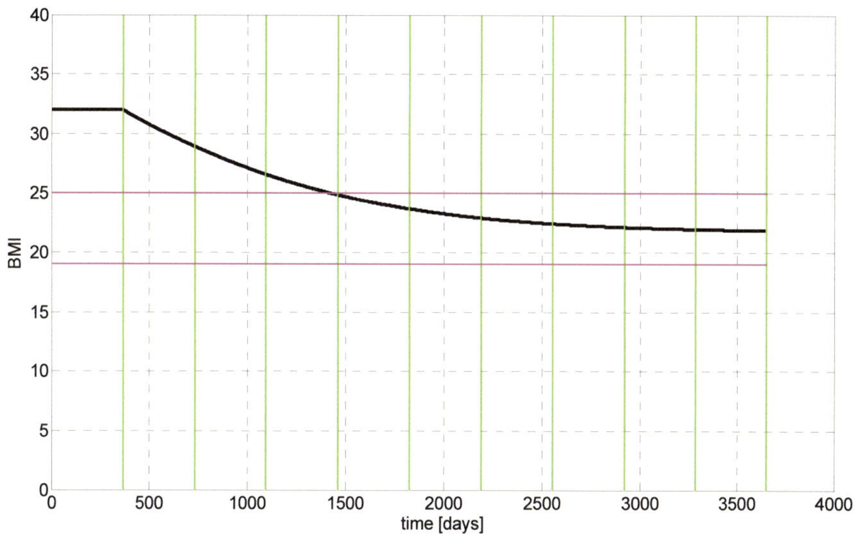

Fig. 17. BMI changing in an average person

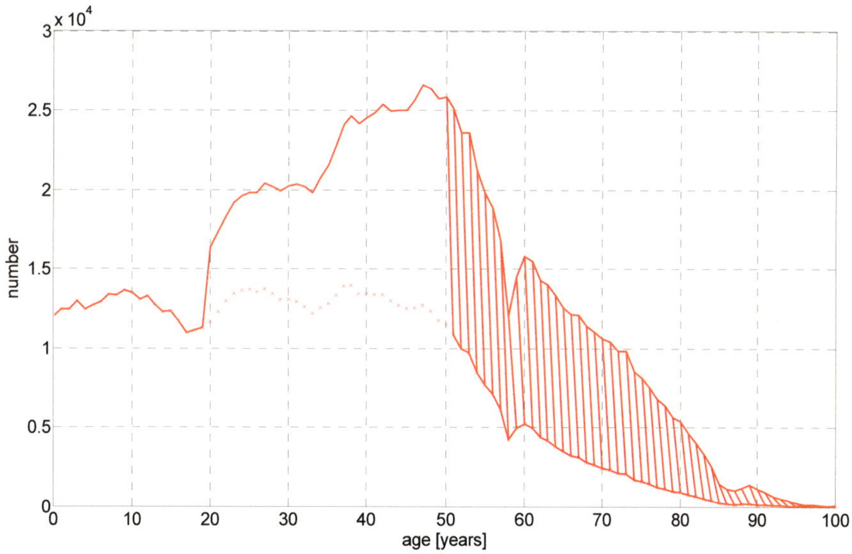

Fig. 18. Activity is increasing

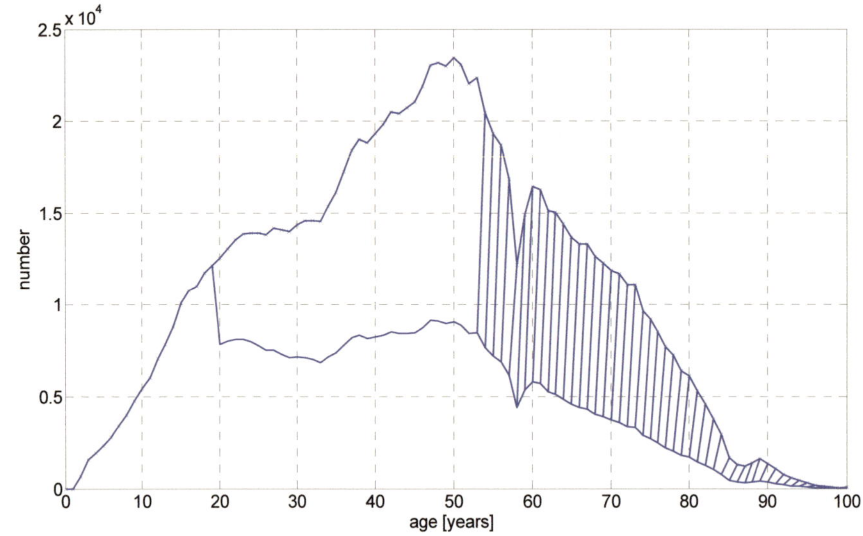

Fig. 19. Number of overweight and obese patients is decreasing

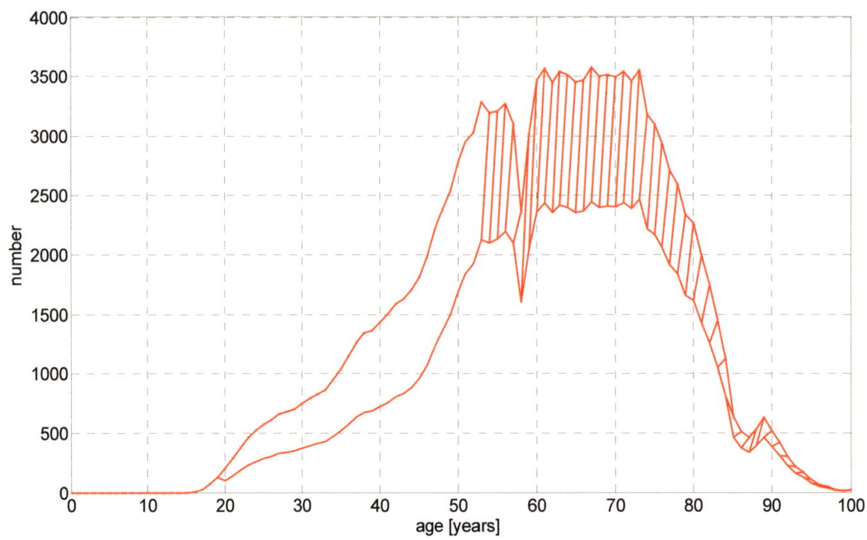

Fig. 20. Number of D2 patients is decreasing

The consequence would be that among this group of patients from pre-diabetes only 50% would develop D2, while other would return to the population with healthy body mass and without D2 (Fig 20).
In this way the number of obese and overweight people would be decreased for over 53% and the number of D2 patients for 35%. In the same proportion also the corresponding expenses would be reduced.
The proposed strategy has one important deficiency, namely the lack of patients' motivation and discipline as the success is completely dependent on these two important factors. Therefore our further goal is to extend the presented model with motivation aspects and expenses needed for its stimulation.

4. Conclusion

Four-level mathematical description structure is proposed which can be efficiently used for the estimation of the number of observed patients, the distribution regarding their age and for the estimation of their economical burden. It can comprise different mathematical descriptions important for observed processes. In our case it consists of dynamical decision tree describing the prevalence of population activity and inacivity, overweight and obesity, pre-diabetes and diabetes type 2. In combination with dynamical population model predicting the number of people, two-compartment dynamical model for estimation of body mass changes and evaluated treatment expenses also the number of observed patients and treatment burden were calculated for Slovenia. As similar results can be expected in the countries with comparable social and economical situation (the great majoity of EU countries), the following can be concluded for the population of one million people:

- over 60% are inacive,
- only 45% have body mass in normal range,
- overweight and obese patients spend around €65.5 million per year for body mass reduction,
- 30% of people has pre-diabetes,
- over 7% have developed diabetes type 2,
- direct tratment expenses for D2 patients are around €25.5 million,
- essential savings could be expected with minimal life-style changes,
- in this way the number of obese and overweight people could be decreased for over 53% and the number of D2 patients for over 35%.

It is obvious that motivation is the most important obstacle in achieving the efficient improvement in reduction of D2 patients and corresponding economical burden. Therefore our future interest will be directed in developing corresponding mathematical model to complement the presented structure and to indicate the potentially important further activities.

5. Acknowledgment

The authors sincerely thank prof. dr. Rihard Karba, University of Ljubljana, Faculty of Electrical Engineering, for the fruitful discussions and his suggestions which have significantly influenced the work.

6. References

ADA - American Diabetes Association (2007). Standards of medical care in diabetes—2007, *Diabetes Care*, 2007, Jan;30, Suppl 1:S4-S41, ISSN 0149-5992.

Arnold, R. J. G. (Editor) (2010). *Pharmacoeconomics, From Theory to Practice*, CRC Press, Taylor & Francis Group, Drug Discovery Series/13, ISBN 978-1-4200-8422, Boca Raton.

Atanasijević-Kunc, M.; Drinovec, J. & Mrhar, A. (2008a). Usage of Modelling and Simulation in Medicine and Pharmacy. *Journal of Slovene Medical Society*, Vol. 77, No. 1, (2008), pp. 57-71, ISSN 1318-0347.

Atanasijević-Kunc, M.; Drinovec, J.; Ručigaj, S. & Mrhar, A. (2008b). Modelling of the risk factors and chronic diseases that influence the development of serious health complications. *Journal of Slovene Medical Society*, Vol. 77, No. 8, (2008), pp. 487-498, ISSN 1318-0347.

Atanasijević-Kunc, M.; Drinovec, J.; Ručigaj, S. & Mrhar, A. (2008c). Modeling the influence of risk factors and chronic diseases on the development of strokes and peripheral arterial-vascular disease. *Simulation modelling practice and theory*, Vol. 16, No. 8, (2008), pp. 998 -1013, ISSN 1569-190X, doi: DOI:10.1016/j.simpat. 2008.03.008.

Atanasijević-Kunc, M.; Drinovec, J.; Ručigaj, S. & Mrhar, A. (2011). Simulation analysis of coronary heart disease, congestive heart failure and end-stage renal disease economic burden. *Mathematics and Computers in simuation*, pp. 1-14, ISSN 0378 - 4754,<http://dx.doi.org/10.1016/j.matcom.2010.10.024>, doi: 10.1016/j.matcom.2010.10.024.

Behl, G. F. E., Copeland, J. A., Wiggins, J. (2004). *The District of Columbia Diabetes Surveillance Report*, DC Department of Health, Washington, DC, September 2004, <http://dchealth.dc.gov/doh/lib/doh/services/special_programs/diabetes/pdf/ final data_and_stat_diabetes.pdf. #search=%22columbia%20diabetes%20 prevalence%22>.

Bellazzi R., Nucci G. & Cobelli C. (2001). The Subcutaneous Route to Insulin Dependent Diabetes Therapy: Closed-Loop and Partially Closed-Loop Control Strategies for insulin Delivery and Measuring Glucose Concentration. IEEE Engineering in Medicine and Biology Magazine, 2001, 20(1), pp.54-64, ISSN: 0739-5175.

Belič, A. (2009). Modelling in systems biology, neurology and pharmacy. *Mathematical and Computer Modelling of Dynamical Systems*, Vol. 15, No. 6, (2009), pp. 479 – 491, ISSN 1387-3954, <http://dx.doi.org/10.1080/13873950903375304>, doi:10.1080/13873950903375304.

Berghöfer, A., Pischon, T., Reinhold, T., Apovian, C. M., Sharma, A. M. & Willich, S. N. (2008). Obesity prevalence from a European perspective: a systematic review, *BMC Public Health*, 2008, 8:200, doi:10.1186/1471-2458-8-200, ISSN 1471-2458.

Boutayeb, A.; Twizell, E. H.; Achouayb, K. & Chetouani, A. (2004). A mathematical model for the burden of diabetes and its complications. *BioMedical Engineering OnLine*, Vol. 3, No. 20, (2004), doi:10.1186/1475-925X-3-20.

Boutayeb, A. & Chetouani, A. (2006). A critical review of mathematical models and data used in diabetology, *BioMedical Engineering OnLine*, Vol. 5, No. 43, (2006), ISSN: 1475-925X, doi:10.1186/1475-925X-5-43.

Boutayeb, A., Chetouani, A., Achouyab, K. & Twizell, E. H. (2006). A non-linear population model of diabetes mellitus. Journal of Applied Mathematics and computing, Vol. 21, pp. 127-139, ISSN 15985865.

British Heart Foundation Statistics Website (2008). Age differences and physical activity, <http://www.heartstats.org/atozpage.asp?id=4955>.

British Heart Foundation Statistics Website (2010). Trends in the prevalence of overweight and obesity, <http://www.heartstats.org/datapage.asp?id=1011>.

Briggs, A. & Sculpher, M. (1998). An Introduction to Markov Modeling for Economic Evaluation. *PharmacoEconomics*, 13(4), 1998 , pp. 397-409, ISSN 1170-7690.

Brock, D. W., Thomas, O., Cowan, C. D., Allison, D. B., Gaesser, G. A. & Hunter, G. R. (2009). Association Between Insufficiently Physically Active and the Prevalence of Obesity in the United States, *Journal of physical activity & health*, 2009, January, Vol. 6, No. 1, pp.1–5, ISSN 1543-3080.

Cassandras, C.G., Lafortune S. (1999). *Introduction to Discrete Evant Systems*. Kluwer Academic Publishers, Boston, ISBN 0-7923-8609-4.

Cellier, F. E.(1991). *Continuous System Modeling*. Springer-Verlag, New York, ISBN 0-387-97502-0.

Cellier, F. E. & Kofman, E. (2006). *Continuous System Simulation*, Springer Science + Business Media, New York, ISBN 0-387-26102-8.

Chow, C. C. & Hall, K. D. (2008). The dynamics of human body weight change, *PLoS Computational Biology*, Vol. 4, No. 3, pp. 1–13, ISSN 1553-734X.

Daousi, C., Casson, I. F., Gill, G. V., MacFarlane, I. A., Wilding, J. P. H.& Pinkney, J. H. (2006). Prevalence of obesity in type 2 diabetes in secondary care: association with cardiovascular risk factors, *Postgraduate Medical Journal*, 2006; Vol. 82, pp. 280-284 doi:10.1136/pmj.2005.039032, ISSN 00325473.

Defay, R., Delcourt, C., Ranvier, M., Lacroux, A. & Papoz, L. (2001). Relationships between physical activity, obesity and diabetes mellitus in a French elderly population: the POLA study, *International Journal of Obesity*, 2001, Vol. 25, No. 4, pp. 512-518, ISSN 0307-0565.

DPPRG - Diabetes Prevention Program Research Group, (2002). Reduction in the Incidence of Type 2 Diabetes with Lifestyle Intervention or Metformin, *The New England Journal of Medicine*, 2002, Vol. 346, pp. 393-403, ISSN 1533-4406.

Dugdale, A. & Payne, P. (1977). Pattern of lean and fat deposition in adults, *Nature*, Vol. 266, pp. 349–351, ISSN 0028-0836.

Eddy, D. M. & Schlessinger, L. (2003a). Archimedes, A trial-validated model of diabetes. *Diabetes Care*, Vol. 26, No. 11, (2003), pp. 3093–3101, Online ISSN 1935-5548

Eddy, D. M. & Schlessinger, L. (2003b). Validation of the Archimedes Diabetes Model. *Diabetes Care*, Vol. 26, No. 11, (2003), pp. 3102–3110, Online ISSN 1935-5548.

HER (2001). Human energy requirements, Report of a Joint FAO/WHO/UNU Expert Consultation, Rome, 17-24 October 2001, ISBN 92-5-105212-3, ISSN 1813-3932, <http://www.fao.org/docrep/007/y5686e/y5686e00.htm>.

Homer, J., Jones, A., Seville, D., Essien, J., Milstein, B. & Murphy, D. (2004). The CDC's Diabetes Systems Modeling Project: Developing a New Tool for Chronic Disease Prevention and Control. 22nd International Conference of the System Dynamics Society, July 25-29, 2004 (Oxford, England), <http://www.sustainabilityinstitute.org/pubs/Diabetes_System(ISDC04).pdf>.

Hoppensteadt, F. C. & Peskin, C. S. (2002). *Modeling and Simulation in Medicine and the Life Sciences*, Springer-Verlag, New York, ISBN 0-387-95072-9.

D'Inverno, M. & Luck, M. (2010). *Understanding Agent Systems*. Springer-Verlag, Berlin, ISBN 978-3-642-07382-3.

Jackson, A. S., Stanforth, P. R., Gagnon, J., Rankinen, T., Leon, A. S., Rao, D. C., Skinner, J. S., Bouchard, C. & Wilmore, J. H. (2002). The effect of sex, age and race on estimating percentage body fat from body mass index: The heritage family study, *International Journal of Obesity*, Vol. 26, pp. 789–796, doi:10.1038/sj.ijo.0802006, ISSN 0307-0565.

Kriska, A. M., Saremi, A., Hanson, R. L., Bennett, P. H., Kobes, S., Williams, D. E. & Knowler, W. C. (2003). Physical Activity, Obesity, and the Incidence of Type 2 Diabetes in a High-Risk Population, *American Journal of Epidemiology*, 2003, Vol. 158, No. 7, DOI: 10.1093/aje/kwg191, ISSN 0002-9262.

Kristöfel, P., Breitenecker, F., Gyimesi, M. & Popper, N. (2007). A System Dynamics Model for the Diabetes Prevalence in Austria, Proc. EUROSIM 2007, 9-13 Sept. 2007, Ljubljana, Slovenia, ISBN 978-3-901608-32-2.

Lam, Z. H., Hwang, K.S., Lee, J. Y., Chase, J. G. & Walker, G. C. (2002). Active insulin infusion using optimal and derivative weighted control. *Medical engineering physics*, 2002, Vol. 24, pp. 663-672, ISSN 1350-4533.

Levenson, J. W., Skerrett, P. J., Gaziano, J. M. (2002). Reducing the Global Burden of Cardiovascular Disease: The Role of Risk Factors. *Preventive Cardiology*, Fall 2002, Vol. 5, pp. 188-199, ISSN 1520-037X.

Li C., Ford, E. S., Zhao, G. & Mokdad, A. H. (2009). Prevalence of Pre-Diabetes and Its Association With Clustering of Cardiometabolic Risk Factors and Hyperinsulinemia Among U.S. Adolescents, Diabetes Care, Vol. 32, No. 2, 2009, pp. 342-347, ISSN: 1935-5548.

Makroglou, A.; Li, J. & Kuang, Y. (2006). Mathematical models and software tools for the glucose-insulin regulatory system and diabetes: an overview. *Applied Numerical Mathematics*, Vol. 56, Iss. 3-4, (2006), pp. 559-573, Selected Papers, The Third International Conference on the Numerical Solutions of Volterra and Delay Equations, ISSN 0168-9274.

Matko, D.; Karba, R. & Zupančič, B. (1992). Simulation and Modelling of Continuous Systems, A Case Study Approach, Prentice Hall, New York, ISBN 0-13-808064-X

Matlab, (2005). *Reference Guide*, The MathWorks Inc.

MMWR (2004). Prevalence of Overweight and Obesity Among Adults with Diagnosed Diabetes - United States, 1988--1994 and 1999—2002, (2004). *Morbidity and Mortality Weekly Report (MMWR)*, 53(45); pp. 1066-1068, 2004, Centers for Disease Control and Prevention (CDC), ISSN 0149-2195, <http://www.cdc.gov/mmwr/preview/mmwrhtml/mm5345a2.htm>.

Mokdad, A. H., Ford, E. S., Bowman, B. A., Dietz, W. H., Vinicor, F., Bales, V. S. & Marks, J. S. (2003). Prevalence of Obesity, Diabetes, and Obesity-Related Health Risk Factors, 2001, *JAMA, The Journal of the American Medical Association*, 2003; Vol. 289, No. 1, pp. 76-79, doi: 10.1001/jama.289.1.76, ISSN 00987484.

Narayanappa, D., Rajani, H. S., Mahendrappa, K. B. & Prabhakar, A. K. (2011). Prevalence of Prediabetes in School-Going Children, Indian Pediatrics, Vol. 48, 2011, pp. 295-299, ISSN 0019-6061.

NDS (2011). National Diabetes Statistics, 2011, U.S. Department of Health and Human Services, National Institutes of Health, NIH Publication No. 11-3892, February 2011, <http://diabetes.niddk.nih.gov/DM/PUBS/statistics/DM_Statistics.pdf>.

Shianga, K.D. & Kandeelc, F. (2010). A computational model of the human glucose-insulin regulatory system. Journal of Biomedical Research, Vol. 24, Iss. 5, (2010), pp. 347-364, ISSN 1552-4965.

Shih, H.C., Chou, P., Liu, C. M. & Tung, T. H. (2007). Estimation of progression of multi-state chronic disease using the Markov model and prevalence pool concept. BMC Medical Informatics and Decision Making, 2007, 7:34, doi:10.1186/1472-6947-7-34, ISSN 1472-6947.

Simulink (2005). *User's Guide*, The MathWorks Inc.

SORS (2011). Statistical Office of the Republic of Slovenia, <http://www.stat.si/eng/index.asp>.

Stahl, J. E. (2008). Modelling Methods for Pharmacoeconomics and Health Technology Assessment, An Overview and Guide, *Pharmacoeconomics*, 2008, Vol. 26, No. 2, pp. 131-148, ISSN 1170-7690.

Tarride, J. E., Hopkins, R., Blackhouse, G., Bowen, J. M., Bischof, M., Von Keyserlingk, C., O'Reilly, D., Xie, F. & Goeree, R. (2010). A Review of Methods Used in Long-Term Cost-Effectiveness Models of Diabetes Mellitus Treatment, *Pharmacoeconomics*, 2010, Vol. 28, No. 4, pp. 255-277, ISSN 1170-7690.

Tuomilehto, J., Lindström, J. E. J. G., Valle, T. T., Hämäläinen, H., Ilanne-Parikka, P., Keinänen-Kiukaanniemi, S., Laakso, M., Louheranta, A., Rastas, M., Salminen, V., Uusitupa, M. (2001). Prevention of type 2 diabetes mellitus by changes in lifestyle among subjects with impaired glucose tolerance, *The New England Journal of Medicine*, 2001, Vol. 344, No. 18, pp. 1343-1350, ISSN 1533-4406.

Valensi, P., Schwarz, P., Hall, M., Felton, A. M., Maldonato, A. & Mathieu, C. (2005). Pre-diabetes essential action: a European perspective, *Diabetes & Metabolism*, Vol 31, No. 6, 2005, pp. 606-620, ISSN 1262-3636, doi : DM-12-2005-31-6-1262-3636-101019-200516342.

WHO - World Health Organization (2000), Technical report series 894: Obesity: Preventing and managing the global epidemic. Geneva: World Health Organization. ISBN 92-4-120894-5, <http://whqlibdoc.who.int/trs/WHO_TRS_894_(part1).pdf>.

WHO - World health organization (2011a). Diabetes Programme, Prevalence data, <http://www.who.int/diabetes/facts/world_figures/en/index.html>.

WHO - World health organization (2011b), Obesity and overweight, Fact sheet N°311, March 2011, <http://www.who.int/mediacentre/factsheets/fs311/en/>.

2

Alzheimer's Disease and Type 2 Diabetes: Different Pathologies and Same Features

Marta Di Carlo[1], Pasquale Picone[1], Rita Carrotta[2], Daniela Giacomazza[2] and P.L. San Biagio[2]
[1]*Istituto di Biomedicina e Immunologia Molecolare (IBIM) – CNR*
[2]*Istituto di Biofisica (Palermo unit) – CNR*
Italy

1. Introduction

Protein aggregation is a very fascinating matter due to its implication in many human neurodegenerative diseases and its relevance in food and pharmaceutical industries. In some cases, the aggregation of protein is a natural phenomenon occurring in living organisms. For example, in the reaction leading from the globular (G) monomeric actin to its polymeric fibrillar (F) structure (Morris et al., 2009):

$$n\,(\text{G-Actin}) \rightarrow (\text{F-Actin})_n$$

or the case of polymerization of tropocollagen to obtain collagen fibrils, a process leading, in the case of type I Collagen, to the formation of long fibrils having a wave pattern (Yadavalli et al., 2010).

In general, a non-physiological aggregation, that is an aggregation process not naturally occurring, starts from "activated" molecules having secondary and/or tertiary structures different from those corresponding to the "native state" (Manno et al., 2006, 2010; Morris et al., 2009). Increasing evidence suggests that the non-physiological aggregation of proteins such beta-amyloid, alpha-synuclein, huntingtin and ataxin, superoxide-dismutase 1 (SOD1), Tau and Amylin, is responsible for the onset of many neurodegenerative pathologies such as Alzheimer's, Parkinson's and Huntington's diseases, Amyotrophic Lateral Sclerosis, Frontotemporal Lobar Degeneration (Figure 1) and Type 2 Diabetes (or diabetes mellitus), respectively (Chiti & Dobson, 2006).

The question of what triggers the transformation of a biologically active protein into a "pathogenic agent" with high self-assembly propensity is still unanswered. Some of the proposed explainations include:

i. the propensity of some proteins to assume a pathological conformation which increases with aging (Uversky, 2007; Saraiva, 2001);
ii. the persistently high cellular or plasma concentrations (Singleton et al., 2003; Farrer et al., 2004);
iii. an amino acid mutation or a genetic expansion of DNA sequences encoding proteins, as in the case of Huntington disease (Cummings & Zoghbi, 2000);
iv. an abnormal post-traslational modification of the protein responsible for the disease (Goedert et al., 1993);

v. the proteolitic cleavage of the precursor protein, as in the case of Abeta-peptide;
vi. the influence of environmental factors.

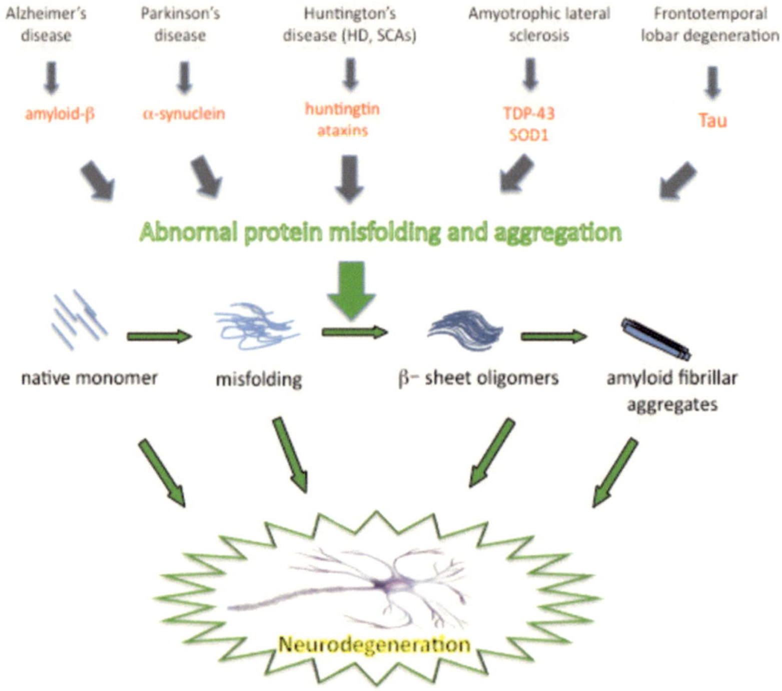

Fig. 1. *Protein misfolding and aggregation as the common molecular pathogenesis of neurodegenerative diseases.* Some genetic mutations responsible of neurodegenerative diseases render the causative proteins prone to misfold and to form beta-sheet-rich oligomers and amyloid fibrillar aggregates, resulting in their accumulation in the affected neurons and eventually leading to degeneration in the brain. This mechanism is retained common to a broad variety of neurodegenerative diseases, such as Alzheimer's, Parkinson's and Huntington disease, Amyothophic Lateral Sclerosis and Frontotemporal Lobar degeneration.

Type 2 diabetes (T2D) is classified as a metabolism disorder and it is often associated with microvascular and macrovascular complications, including retinopathy, nephropathy, neuropathy and cardiovascular disease. A diabetes affected person has an elevated quantity of glucose in the blood (hyperglycemia) that is caused by the inability of the body either to produce any insulin or enough insulin, or by the inability of the cells to respond properly to the insulin producted in the pancreas. This excess blood glucose eventually passes out of the body in the urine. So, even though the blood has plenty of glucose, the cells are incapable of getting it for their essential energy and growth requirements. There are three main types of diabetes: Type 1 diabetes (T1D) (referred to as *insulin-dependent* diabetes and *juvenile* diabetes), results from the body's failure to produce insulin, and presently requires the person to inject insulin. Type 2 diabetes (referred to as *non-insulin-dependent* diabetes mellitus, and *adult-onset* diabetes.) is associated with a reduced ability of insulin to stimulate glucose utilization (insulin resistance) and sometimes it is combined with an absolute insulin deficiency. The third type, gestational diabetes, is when pregnant women, who have never had diabetes before, have a high blood glucose level during pregnancy and it may precede development of T2D. Ninety percent of diabetes patients have T2D, which usually has its onset in adulthood. Diabetes is increasing and the World Health Organization estimates that there will be a doubling of cases by 2025, largely as a result of lack of physical activity and poor dietary habits, both of which are risk factors for the disease. Obesity, hypertension, hyper-cholesterolemia and hyperlipidemia are all associated with T2D (MedScape).

Alzheimer's disease (AD) is the most common form of dementia in the elderly. It is characterized by neuronal cell loss and increasing accumulation of neurofibrillary tangles (NTF) in neurons and amyloid fibers in neuritic plaques and in the walls of blood vessels (Wisniewski et al., 1997). Amyloid beta-peptides of varying length (39–43 residues) are produced by cleavage of a transmembrane protein, the amyloid beta-protein precursor (APP) (Wilquet & De Strooper, 2004). The 42 residue beta-peptide (Abeta-42) is the predominant form found in plaques and under physiological condition the ratio between Abeta42 and Abeta40 is about 1:10 (Iwatsubo et al., 1994). Abeta42 has a much greater neurotoxity than Abeta40 and its aggregation kinetics is faster than other beta-petides (Davis & Van Nostrand, 1996). The proteinaceous material is organized in structured linear aggregates (amyloid fibrils). A recent and now convincing belief is that small diffusible oligomers of Abeta-42, called ADDLs, are the determining pathogenic species causing synaptic dysfunction and eventually neuronal degeneration (Lambert et al., 1998; Picone et al., 2009)

AD accounts for 50–70% of all dementia cases and is characterized by cognitive deficits. This incurable, degenerative, and terminal disease was first described by the German psychiatrist and neuropathologist Alois Alzheimer in 1906. Several factors have been considered relevant for the AD pathogenesis and among these the most important is age. During life small variations occurring in cellular metabolism and structure can modify the functional state of susceptible neurons, leading to dramatic or even lethal changes. Thus, while the the monomeric Abeta is not neurotoxic, for not yet known reasons it starts to form supramolecular aggregates accumulating in the AD brain.

Familial AD is a rare form of dementia and is caused by autosomal dominant mutations in one or more of the genes encoding the amyloid precursor protein (APP), presenilin 1 or presenilin 2 (the latter two proteins form the catalytic core of γ-secretase) (Gotz et al., 2004). By contrast, late-onset AD might be caused by environmental and/or life style factors (Rocchi et al., 2003). Interestingly, late-onset AD is characterized not only by the neuropathological markers mentioned above, but also by vascular lesions, and hyperglycemia, hyperinsulinemia, insulin resistance, glucose intolerance, adiposity, atherosclerosis and hypertension (Haan, 2006).

Diabetes and AD are considered age-related diseases and are both increasing. In the USA, diabetes and AD affect ≈ 23.6 and ≈ 5.3 million people, respectively, and these numbers are projected to rise considerably. The Centers for Disease Control and Prevention predict that more than 29 million people in the US will be affected by diabetes by 2050, while the Alzheimer's association forecasts that by this date, 11–16 million Americans will have AD (Han & Li, 2010). Numerous studies report that patients with diabetes have an increased risk of developing AD compared with healthy individuals (Arvanitakis et al., 2004; Neumann et al., 2008; Roriz-Filho et al. 2009). In fact, some studies revealed that 80% of patients with AD exhibited either impairments in glucose tolerance or frank diabetes (Schrijvers et al., 2010). In particular, similarities between T2D and AD include: aging-related processes, degeneration, high cholesterol levels, peripheral and CNS insulin resistance, dysfunctional IR and IR-mediated signaling pathways, decreased glucose transport and metabolism, despite the higher non-metabolized glucose levels in cerebral blood (Hoyer, 1998; Salkovic-Petrisic & Hoyer, 2007; Schulingkamp et al., 2000). The inbalance between low and high glucose levels in T2D patients may be responsible for brain vascular damage and neurodegeneration thus facilitating the AD onset.

2. Alzheimer's disease and type 2 diabetes: Two amyloidogenic pathologies

AD and T2D are two pathologies characterized by the presence of large insoluble aggregates having an amyloidogenic fibrillar conformation, amylin in T2D pancreatic islets and Abeta and the microtubule protein Tau in the brain of AD patients. In particular, amylin aggregation is associated with pancreatic b-cell loss, whereas Abeta and Tau aggregation is associated with neuronal cell loss and synaptic dysfunction (Lupi & Del Prato, 2008; Schroeder & Koo, 2005; Resende et al., 2008a). The formation of amyloid aggregate occurs both in the intra- and extra-cellular environments; further the proteinaceous aggregates are strictly bound with membranes and calcified. Despite their common secondary structure conformation, it is well accepted that a correlation does not exit between amino acid sequence and tendency to amyloid structure formation; thus it is assumed that amyloid formation is a generic properties of all polypeptides (Chiti & Dobson, 2006).
In particular, amyloid fibers share the following features (Xu, 2007):

- all have a rope-like appearance;
- all show a dominant beta-sheet structure;
- their formation can be enhanced either by the stirring or the presence of seeds;
- all aggregate starts from spherical oligomers that in turn self-assemble linearly;
- all can incorporate a special kind of dye molecules such as Congo Red or Thioflavin T.

On a molecular lengthscale, Abeta can form aggregates of different shape originated in vitro under different conditions. These structures include amyloid fibrils (Ban et al., 2004), small oligomers (Walsh et al., 1999), spherical amyloid oligomers (Westlind-Danielsson & Arnerup, 2001) and annular pore-forming structures (Lashuel et al., 2002), amyloid protofibrils (Harper et al., 1997), beaded chain protofibrils (Huang et al., 2000) and spherocylindrical micelles (Lomakin et al., 1996; Yong et al., 2002).
X-ray fiber diffraction showed that amyloid fibrils contain beta-sheet structure lying orthogonally to the major fibril axis (Serpell, 2000). In the early 2000s, Tycko's group (Antzutkin et al., 2000; Balbach et al., 2002) obtained, for the first time, evidence of an extended parallel beta-sheet organization for the Abeta40 fibrils using solid-state NMR. They showed that the methyl carbons of Ala-21 and Ala-30 must be placed in groups of at least four with internuclear distances of less than 5.5 Å. Although beta-sheets are the main constituent of the amyloid fibrils they are not the only structure present in the fibrils. Liquid state NMR, FTIR and CD measurements in Abeta40 have demonstrated the existence of a turn formed by the amino acids at position 26-29. Little information is known about the Abeta42 fibril structure and many mutant peptides have been synthetized to obtain an explanation about its secondary structure. The results have showed that the residues at positions 15–21 and 24–32 are involved in the beta-sheet formation and that the turn at positions 22 and 23 plays a crucial role in the aggregation of Abeta42.

The islet amyloid polypetide (IAPP), identified for the first time in 1987 (Westermark et al.) and also known as amylin, is secreted by the beta cells of the pancreatic islets of Langerhans, which also secrete the insulin. The occurrence of IAPP in the membranes of beta-cells and the presence of alterations in the membranes of the same cells (Lorenzo et al., 1994; Janson et al., 1999) suggest that this interaction is responsible for the cytotoxic effect of these formations. The primary sequence of the peptide is well conserved in organisms and, in particular human and mouse IAPPs differ by only six amino acids but the latter does not form fibrils neither in vitro nor in vivo. The development of IAPP deposits is deeply associated with T2D because more than 90% of T2D patients presents this type of amyloid formations as evidenced by autopsy and, further, the amount of aggregates appears to be correlated with the pathology seriousness.

Human IAPP (hIAPP) consists of 37 amino acids with a S-S bridge between the Cys 2 and Cys 7. As in Abeta, IAPP is non-toxic in its monomeric form but it exhibits high toxicity levels when it aggregates into beta-rich amyloid structures. As in other amyloid peptides, the mechanism of fibrillation occurs through the formation of nuclei with a lag phase whose duration is concentration-dependent and proceeds by addition of monomers or oligomers to both fibril terminals. The secondary structure of hIAPP mainly consists of unstructured regions, with small alpha-helical and beta-sheet components (Goldsbury et al., 2000). Recently has been suggested that hIAPP oligomers in presence of membranes could exhibit an alpha-helical structure (Knight et al., 2006).

The three dimensional structure of hIAPP has been extensively studied with different techniques and the results show that, similarly to other amyloid proteins, the amylin mature amyloid fibrils show a relevant amount of beta-structure (McLean, 1992; Goldsbury, 2000). Studies on the mechanism of hIAPP fibrillation indicate that during the process, hIAPP undergoes a conformational change from an unstructured peptide to beta-sheets and alpha-helical structures (Goldsbury, 2000).

The IAPP decapeptide sequence between residues 20-29 seems to play an important role in the fibrillization process (Westermark et al., 1990) even if it does not appear to be the only region involved in fibril formation. In fact, recent studies have evidenced the importance of the residues in position 13-18 in the interaction leading to the formation of fibrils (Gilead & Gazit, 2008). Also the aromatic-aromatic interactions between residues 15, 23 and 37 seem to be important in amyloid formation althought not essential for fiber formation as evidenced using IAPP with a triple mutation (Marek et al., 2007).

3. The effect of oxidative stress

The brain has a high energy demand and, although it represents only 2% of body weight, it accounts for 20% of total body oxygen consumption. This energy requirement is largely driven by neuronal request of energy to maintain the ion gradients across the plasma membrane, which are critical for the generation of action potentials. This intense energy requirement is continuous; even brief periods of oxygen or glucose deprivation result in neuronal death. Diabetes mellitus leads to functional and structural changes in the brain, which appear to be most pronounced in the elderly. Furthermore, increased age is associated with insulin resistance. Increasing data support the idea that mitochondrial function declines with aging and in age-related diseases such as diabetes and AD.

Normal glucose metabolism is required for the performance of cognitive functions, and impairments in glucose metabolism might contribute to cognitive dysfunction. Imaging studies have revealed that patients with AD and individuals at risk of developing this disease typically have reductions in glucose metabolism in temporal and parietal brain regions and hippocampus (Garrido et al., 2002). Moreover, compared to healthy individuals, patients with AD often have increased plasma insulin levels and/or a decreased cerebrospinal fluid (CsF)-to-plasma insulin ratio. These findings indicates that glucose metabolism and insulin signaling are important in normal brain function. The negative effect of impaired glucose metabolism on cognitive functioning can be caused by an increase in oxidative stress that is associated with mitochondrial dysfunction.

Mitochondria are essential subcellular organelles for generating the energy that fuels normal cellular functioning. At the same time, the mitochondria have a strategic task because, depending on environmental factors, they can decide whether to continue the healthy life of the cell or to terminate it by apoptosis activation. Mitochondria are essential for neuronal function because the limited glycolytic capacity of these cells makes them highly dependent on aerobic oxidative phosphorylation for their energetic needs. However, oxidative phosphorylation is a major source of endogenous free radicals. A variety of reactive oxygen species (ROS) and reactive nitrogen species (RNS) are produced in vivo through both enzymatic and non-enzymatic routes. ROS include hydrogen peroxide, hydroxyl radical, superoxide ion and singlet oxygen, products of normal cellular respiration. The hydroxyl radical is a highly reactive species and has a relatively short life time. It is abundantly produced in the mitochondria during respiration cycles and reacts with the proteins, lipids, and nucleic acids during their production. Peroxynitrous acid is one of the major RNS found intracellularly and it is involved in the rapid nitration of aromatic residues of proteins, such as tyrosine, to give 3-nitrotyrosine, which may alter the protein structure. Further it is also a marker of oxidative stress (Smith et al., 1997). Under normal conditions, antioxidant defenses can counteract oxidative stress damage. In the absence of an appropriate compensatory response from the endogenous antioxidant network, the system becomes redox imbalanced, leading to the activation of a stress-sensitive intracellular signaling pathway and, in extreme conditions, to apoptosis. Increased oxidative damage and impaired antioxidant defenses are prominent both in the onset of AD and diabetes (Smith et al., 1996; Evans et al. 2002). Abnormal glucose metabolism can also increase the production of free radicals such as reactive oxygen species (ROS) and reactive nitrogen species (RNS). This overproduction of free radicals can exhaust the antioxidant capacity of the cell and lead to a condition known as oxidative stress, which is a hallmark of both T1D and T2D and a contributing factor to diabetic neuropathy (Russell et al., 2008; Vincent et al., 2004). Oxidative stress is not only associated with diabetes and its complications, but has been linked to insulin resistance, the subnormal response to a given amount of insulin (West, 2000).

ROS-induced and RNS-induced protein modifications and/or lipid peroxidations result in cell damage that can lead to cell death, and they are increased in patients with diabetes or AD compared with healthy controls (Pratico et al., 2004). Brain and cerebrospinal fluid (CSF) levels of lipid peroxidation biomarkers, including malondialdehyde and 4-hydroxynonenal (two highly toxic products generated in part by lipid oxidation and ROS), are both higher in individuals with AD and diabetes mellitus than in healthy people (Reddy et al., 2009; Slatter et al., 2000). Furthermore, levels of oxidized proteins are increased in the frontal and parietal lobes and in the hippocampus of patients with mild cognitive impairment compared with healthy controls, indicating that oxidative damage might occur early in the development of AD (Butterfield et al., 2007). ROS, as mentioned earlier, are also involved in the damage of

DNA. Minor modifications of the nucleic acid bases are repaired through base excision repair involving DNA glycosylase and AP endonuclease, which are located in nuclei and mitochondria. The progression of AD is associated with the diminished expression of these DNA repair enzymes (Nakabeppu et al., 2004). The accumulation of the oxidatively damaged nucleic acids and proteins likely exceeds the limit of cellular repair and detoxification mechanisms and leads to the onset or progression of diabetic and neurological pathologies. In general, accumulation of oxidatively damaged proteins, lipids, and nucleic acids correlates with the onset of age-related diseases, especially in diabetes and AD (Stadtman, 2001), indicative of a common pathological mechanism.

Oxidative stress and lipid peroxidation seem to be able to induce Abeta accumulation: studies in a mouse model of AD have demonstrated that brain lipid peroxidation increases before that Abeta levels increase (Pratico et al., 2001) and that the onset of Abeta deposition is associated with an increase in the level of RNS (Apelt et al., 2004). Further evidence supporting this hypothesis has been obtained from studies of a mouse model of AD in which mutations in the genes encoding APP and presenilin 1 cause an increase in Abeta42 production. In these animals, lipid and protein peroxidation is evident at the disease onset (Matsuoka et al., 2001). In a triple-transgenic animal model of AD, in which mice develop Abeta plaques, tangles and cognitive defects, a decrease in antioxidant capacity and an increase in lipid peroxidation were noted before the development of AD pathology (Resende et al., 2008). Oxidative stress seems to affect APP either directly, by increasing APP levels, or indirectly, by modulating APP processing, and both mechanisms could increase levels of Abeta. Studies in transgenic mice and postmortem brain tissue from patients with AD suggest also that an increase in Abeta production leads to a rise in the production of ROS and that oxidative stress occurs early in the development of the disease.

4. The mitochondrial dysfunction

Several studies are consistent with the view that diabetes-related mitochondrial dysfunction is exacerbated by aging and/or by the presence of neurotoxic agents, such as Abeta. This suggests that diabetes and aging are risk factors for the neurodegeneration induced by this peptide. Mitochondrial dysfunction could be one of the common underlying mechanisms explaining the association between diabetes and AD. Mitochondrial dysfunction and the resulting energy deficit trigger the onset of neuronal degeneration and death. Mitochondria serve also as high capacity Ca^{2+} sink, which allows them to follow the changes in cytosolic Ca^{2+} loads and helps in maintaining cellular Ca^{2+} homeostasis, required for normal neuronal function (Rizzuto et al., 2000). Conversely, excessive Ca^{2+} uptake inside mitochondria has been shown to increase ROS production, inhibit ATP synthesis, release cytochrome C, and induce mitochondrial permeability transition (Brustovetsky et al., 2002). The mitochondrial permeability transition (MPT) is defined as the sudden increase of inner mitochondrial membrane permeability to solutes of molecular mass lower than 1500 Da (Bernardi et al., 1994). Strong evidence now exists that the MPT is due to the opening of a nonselective megachannel (estimated to be 2–3 nm in diameter). Because the chemiosmotic theory is based on the impermeability of the inner mitocondrion membrane to solutes that are not specifically transported, MPT would collapse the mitochondrial membrane potential ($\Delta\Psi m$) and uncouple the electron transport system from the production of ATP. Additionally, MPT results in mitochondrial swelling and can lead to the release of proapoptotic proteins. Importantly, Ca^{2+}, P_i, oxidative stress, and low inner membrane potential promote the onset of MPT, whereas cyclosporin A, Mg^{2+}, ADP, and the existence of a high membrane potential oppose the onset (Bernardi et al., 1994).

Increasing data support the idea that mitochondrial function declines with aging and in age-related diseases, such as diabetes and AD (Calabrese et al., 2001). Some data show the existence of an age-related impairment of the respiratory chain and an uncoupling of oxidative phosphorylation in brain mitochondria isolated from Goto-Kakizaki (GK) rats, as model of T2D (Moreira et al., 2003). Furthermore, aging exacerbates the decrease in the energetic levels promoted by diabetes. The maintenance of oxidative phosphorylation capacity is extremely important in the brain since a large amount of the energy required for the normal functioning of neurons is provided by mitochondria. Moreover, the CNS requires a large amount of ATP for the transmission of impulses along the neural pathway, thus indicating that mitochondrial function impairment can result in neurodegeneration and loss in neuronal metabolic control (Calabrese et al., 2001).

5. Advanced glycation end products (AGE)

Abnormal glucose metabolism and oxidative stress contribute to the formation of advanced glycation end products (AGE). This process occurs through the Maillard reaction or "non-enzymatic browning", a complex series of reactions between reducing carbohydrates with lysine side chains and N-terminal amino groups of proteins. This process initially leads to rather labile Schiff bases which as a rule rearrange to the more stable Amadori products. The Amadori compounds are slowly degraded, in complex reaction pathways via dicarbonyl intermediates, to a plethora of compounds (Ledl & Schleicher, 1990) designated summarily as "advanced glycation end products" (AGEs); this overall reaction sequence proceeds both in vitro and in vivo. In long-lived tissue proteins, these chemical modifications accumulate with age and may contribute to pathophysiologies associated with aging and long-term complications of diabetes and atherosclerosis (Lederer & Klalber, 2000).

Practically, AGEs comprise a heterogeneous group of molecules formed by irreversible, non-enzymatic reactions between sugars and the free amino groups of proteins, lipids and nucleic acids. Auto-oxidation of glucose leads to the formation of oxygen radicals, which are intermediates in the AGE pathway and the predominant source of endogenous AGEs. AGEs may exist as protein cross-links or as modification of the side chains of a single protein, and significantly alter protein conformations leading to protein inactivation. Numerous AGEs have been isolated and characterized by spectroscopic analysis after cleavage from the protein backbones. AGEs involving protein cross-links include: pentosidine, a dimer of arginine and lysine; methylglyoxal-lysine dimer (MOLD), a dimer of two lysine residues; and methylglyoxal-derived imidazolium cross-link (MODIC) and glyoxal-derived imidazolium cross-link (GODIC), dimers of arginine and lysine residues. Examples of AGEs resulting from the single protein modification are pyrraline and Nε -(carboxymethyl)lysine (CML), the lysine-residue modified products, and argpyrimidine, an arginine-residue modified protein. Although many other AGEs, including the hydroimidazolone adduct MG-H1, have been characterized in diabetes, some of them have common occurrence in AD (Rabbani et al., 2008).

The formation and accumulation of AGEs occur during normal aging; however, these processes are exacerbated in patients with diabetes and the binding of AGE to its receptor (receptor for AGEs or RAGE) induces a series of biological processes that cause further diabetic complications (Singh et al., 2001). AGE immunoreactivity is present in both Abeta plaques and NFTs in patients with AD. Furthermore, hippocampal neurons from patients with this neurodegenerative disease contain Abeta-positive, AGE-positive and RAGE positive granules. (Sasaki et al., 2001). Whether the modifications of Abeta and tau by AGEs are a primary or secondary event in AD is a controversial topic. Nevertheless, AGEs are widely accepted to be active participants in the progression of AD, since AGE-induced glycation of Abeta and tau protein has been shown to cause the Abeta aggregation and the formation of NFTs, respectively (Ledesma et al., 1994). Moreover, diabetic mice with cognitive impairments exhibit increased RAGE expression in neurons and glia compared with wild-type control mice (Toth et al. 2006), and in one clinical study, AGE immunostaining was increased in postmortem brain slices from patients with AD and diabetes compared with non-diabetic patients with AD (Girones et al., 2004).

The question of whether AGEs are the cause or consequence of the pathology is not clear, although there is likely a primary role of oxidative stress in both pathologies. However, it should be pointed out that glycoxidation and oxidative stress are mutually dependent and reinforce each other. Thus, while the sources of oxidative stress may widely differ in diabetes and AD, and while a number of AGEs accumulate in both conditions, other AGEs found in diabetes have yet to be characterized in AD.

6. Antioxidant therapy in Alzheimer's disease and diabetes

Given the importance of mitochondria as the primary source of oxidative stress in AD and diabetes, the use of antioxidants may also be useful. However, the broad occurrence of both diseases, the non-regenerative nature of the CNS and the fact that AD diagnosis often does not occur until late in the disease progression, suggest that the ideal antioxidant should be used as a prophylactic treatment for the aged population. Oxidative stress is one of the earliest events in the neurological and pathological changes of AD, while the effects of oxidative stress are manifested in the slow accumulation of AGEs in diabetes. Thus, antioxidant therapy in combination with AGE inhibitor therapy may be effective approaches for AD and diabetes-related complications. Oxidative stress leads to irreversible protein aggregation and consequent neuronal degeneration in AD (Liu et al., 2007). Advanced lipoxidation products, such as HNE, bind to phosphorylated tau protein to form paired helical filaments, accelerating the formation of neurofibrillary tangles. Oxidative stress also results in the covalent crosslinking of tau filaments to form large aggregates that are resistant to proteolytic cleavage. Larbig and coworkers reported a series of inhibitors for tau protein aggregation (Larbig et al., 2007). Remarkably, thiazolium-based compounds, which are also AGE inhibitors and potentially useful for diabetic therapy, are effective inhibitors of tau aggregation.

Extensive studies of pharmacological interventions based on biological antioxidants have been carried out both for AD and diabetes (Lee et al., 2010; Maritim et al., 2002). Common antioxidants include the vitamins A, C, and E, glutathione, and the enzymes superoxide dismutase, catalase, glutathione peroxidase, and glutathione reductase. Other antioxidants include lipoic acid, mixed carotenoids, coenzyme Q10, several bioflavonoids, antioxidant minerals (copper, zinc, manganese, and selenium), and the cofactors (folic acid; vitamins B1, B2, B6 and B12). They work in synergy with each other and against different types of free radicals. Vitamin E suppresses the propagation of lipid peroxidation; vitamin C, with vitamin E, inhibits hydroperoxide formation; metal complexing agents, such as penicillamine, bind transition metals involved in some reactions in lipid peroxidation.

Vitamins A, C, and E are interesting antioxidant molecules because are diet-derived and directly detoxify free radicals. They also interact in recycling processes to generate reduced forms of the vitamins. Tocopherol is reconstituted when ascorbic acid recycles the tocopherol radical; dihydroascorbic acid, which is generated, is recycled by glutathione. Under some conditions, these vitamins also foster toxicity by producing pro-oxidants. Vitamin E, a component of the total peroxyl radical-trapping antioxidant system, reacts directly with peroxyl and superoxide radicals and singlet oxygen and protects membranes from lipid peroxidation (Weber et al., 1997). A deficiency of vitamin E is concurrent with increased peroxides and aldehydes in many tissues. There have been conflicting reports about vitamin E levels in diabetic animals and human subjects. Plasma and/or tissue levels of vitamin E are reported to be unaltered, increased, or even decreased by diabetes (Asayama et al., 1994).
Some AGE inhibitors and AGE crosslink breakers have been utilized as potential therapies. Some attention to AGE inhibitors was focused on aminoguanidine, which blocks electrophilically activated 1,3-dicarbonyl compounds, the precursors of AGEs (Thomas et al. 2005; Webster et al., 2005). This compound was not approved by the US Food and Drug Administration due to adverse side effects in diabetic patients during Phase III clinical trials, and the search to find alternatives continues. Pyridoxamine (vitamin B6, pyridorin) and thiamin pyrophosphate have been proposed as potential alternatives to aminoguanidine (Ahmed et al., 2007; Androver at al., 2008). Furthermore, these compounds are also good metal ion chelators and attenuate oxidative stress. N-acetylcysteine and lipoic acid act as inhibitors through attenuation of oxidative stress. While the AGE-inhibitory effect of these compounds is not clearly understood, a similar mechanism may operate in the case of AGEs. Carnosine, homocarnosine, and related compounds are potentially suitable as AGE inhibitors although further studies are needed to prove their efficacy in diabetes and AD (Reddy et al., 2005). Carnosine protects superoxide dismutase, catalase, and α-crystallin from non-enzymatic glycation and protein crosslinking (Hipkiss, 2007). OPB-9195 inhibits AGE formation, especially pentosidine and NΣ-(carboxymethyl)lysine (CML), apparently through carbonyl trapping and metal ion chelation (Wada et al., 2001). Thiazolium-based compounds such as alagebrium chloride (ALT-711) and N-phenyacyl-1,3-thiazolium bromide (PTB) are effective AGE crosslink breakers, and are potentially useful drugs for diabetes and AD (Susic, 2007). It should, however, be pointed out that the mechanisms of the action of the latter compounds are not clearly understood. In addition to their action as crosslink breakers of AGEs derived from 1,2-dicarbonyl compounds, they may also act as antioxidants through chelation of transition metal ions. The development of these drugs as therapeutics thus depends on the detailed understanding of their mechanisms of action. An alternative strategy involves removal of AGEs through the soluble receptors for AGEs (sRAGEs). Poor glycemic control in diabetes results in decreased concentrations of sRAGES, and upon insulin treatment, significant improvements in the levels of sRAGEs were observed, with concomitant decrease in AGEs (Devangelio et al., 2007). Treatment of diabetic patients with rosiglitazone, a 2,4-thiazolidine dione derivative, results in increase of plasma sRAGEs, comparable to controls (Tan et al., 2007). Significant amounts of plasma sRAGEs are also produced when angiotensin converting enzyme inhibitors (ACEi; e.g., perindopril) were used for the treatment of diabetes (Tan et al., 2006). However, the protective effect of sRAGEs has been questioned recently as their level are much higher in experimental animal models than those found in vivo, suggesting they may be only markers of inflammation (Humpert et al., 2007). Following the trend in using natural antioxidants, a recent paper has examined the effects of banana (Musa sp. var. elakki bale) flower and

pseudostem on hyperglycemia and AGEs in streptozotocin-induced diabetic rats. The results indicate that fructosamine and AGEs formed during diabetes were inhibited in treated groups when compared with the diabetic group (Bhaskar et al., 2011).
However, the results of clinical trials of antioxidant therapy are not clear because of duration of treatment as well as recruitment of patients at different stages of the diseases. In spite of inconsistency in the conclusions of clinical trials on the beneficial effects of antioxidants on these pathologies, epidemiological studies indicate that antioxidants may reduce the risk of their insurgence. It is suggested that a combination of antioxidants might be of greater potential benefit, especially if these agents work in different cellular compartments or have complementary activity (e.g. Vitamins E, C, and ubiquinone). If oxidative stress plays as important a role in AD and diabetes pathologies as the literature suggests, regular intake of antioxidants may be beneficial much before any sign or symptoms of the disease are visible.

7. Insulin resistance, Tau hyperphosphorylation and the amyloid cascade

In addition to being a modulator of food intake and energy homoeostasis, insulin is also an important neurothrophic factor. It modulates brain activity, particularly for such high glucose demanding functions such as memory. As mentioned above, T2D is associated with cognitive impairment. This form of diabetes is characterized by insulin resistance, hyperinsulinemia and impaired insulin signaling. Insulin resistance is the common link of the components of the much invoked metabolic syndrome (a cluster of high adiposity, abnormal glucose level, dyslipidemia, hypertension and high inflammation) and it is known to cause common diseases such as stroke, heart disease, and cancer. Given the aging of the population and the epidemic of elevated insulin resistance, evidenced by the rise in elevated adiposity, prediabetes, and diabetes, it is alarming that insulin resistance could contribute to AD. Many epidemiologic studies have found an association of elevated adiposity, insulin resistance, and T2D with cognitive impairment and dementia (Baker et al., 2011). However, there are several important questions to be addressed for investigators studying the relation of insulin resistance and AD. For example is not clear if the association between insulin resistance and AD is causal. However, one of the links found is that defects in brain insulin signaling have been reported in AD and it has been proposed that insulin resistance could be an early marker of AD (Baker et al., 2011) (Figure 2).

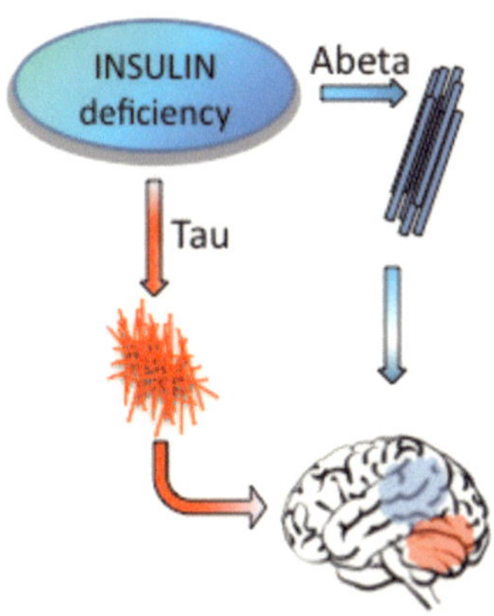

Fig. 2. Insulin deficency can lead to Abeta plaques formation and Tau hyperphos-phorylation

Insulin crosses the blood-brain barrier, and might even be produced locally in the brain, exerting its effects on cells by binding to a specific cell surface receptor. Insulin receptors are expressed throughout the CNS, expecially in the hippocampus and cortex, even if their function in the brain is not fully understood. Binding of insulin to its receptor activates the intrinsic tyrosine kinase activity of the cytoplasmic domain of the insulin receptor. This leads to autophosphorylation of tyrosine residues, which initiates several intracellular signaling cascades. In the brain, insulin influences the release and reuptake of neurotransmitters, and also appears to improve learning and memory (Zhao et al., 2004). The initial components of the insulin receptor signaling cascade in the brain are largely similar to those of the periphery. The downstream targets of the cascade are quite different, however, probably involving, among others, neuronal glutamate receptors (Zhao et al., 2004). Neurodegeneration and cognitive impairment in T2D and AD could be caused, in part, by damage to insulin receptor signaling (de la Monte & Wands, 2005). In fact, decreases in the sensitivity of such receptors are known to affect the expression and metabolism of Abeta and tau and impaired insulin receptor activity and hyperinsulinemia are observed in patients with AD and in animal models of this disease (Frolic et al., 1998). In addition, dysfunction of insulin receptor signaling is associated with impairments in Abeta oligomer clearance (Zhao, 2009) and increases the rate of NFT development (Lesort & Johnson, 2000). In fact, insulin transiently increases tau phosphorylation in primary cortical neurons, and hyperinsulinemia results in tau hyperphosphorylation in rat brains. Furthermore, insulin receptor substrate 2 knockout mice demonstrate typical pathological signs of T2D and have an increased number of NFTs in hippocampal neurons compared with control wild-type mice (Schubert, 2003). Thus, impaired insulin signaling could increase tau phosphorylation and cleavage. Insulin receptor signaling leads to the activation of two major signaling pathways, the mitogen-activated protein kinase (MAPK) pathway and the Akt signaling pathway. MAPK signaling is a required component of cell differentiation, cell proliferation and cell death, whereas Akt signaling is involved in the regulation of cell growth, cell proliferation, protein synthesis (via the mammalian target of rapamycin signaling pathway) and cell survival (through the inhibition of several proapoptotic agents).

Akt signaling induces the inhibition of glycogen synthase kinase-3β (GSK-3β) phosphorylates and, hence, inactivates glycogen synthase, a key enzyme in glycogenesis (Balaraman et al., 2006). Thus, under normal conditions, insulin signaling via the insulin receptor leads to GSK-3β inactivation, whereas insulin resistance leads to GSK-3β dephosphorylation and activation (Balaraman et al., 2006). The regulation of GSK-3β in the hippocampus and cortex changes in response to changes in glucose and insulin concentrations and in T2D an increase in GSK-3β activity might lead to insulin resistance by reducing glucose clearance (Lee & Kim, 2007). Increased GSK-3β activation might also lead to an elevation in Abeta production (resulting from a GSK-3β-mediated increase in presenilin 1 activity) and an increase in tau phosphorylation associated with NFT formation (Balaraman et al., 2006; Phiel et al., 2003). In contrast, inhibition of GSK-3β attenuates APP processing and inhibits hyperphosphorylated tau-associated neurodegeneration in cell-culture and animal models of AD (Phiel et al., 2003).

Another important link between insulin resistance and the amyloid cascade may be related to the insulin degrading enzyme (IDE). This enzyme is a metalloprotease responsible for insulin degradation and is also the main enzyme responsible for Abeta degradation (Farris et al., 2003). IDE is secreted to the extracellular space by microglial cells in the brain, where it degrades Abeta peptide, thus reducing the rate of aggregation and the plaque formation (Qiu et al., 1998). IDE levels have been reported to be decreased in the brains of AD patients (Cook et al., 2003). It has also been hypothesized that hyperinsulinemia in people with pre-diabetes and T2D effectively sequesters IDE, reducing Abeta peptide degradation. This would increase levels of Abeta, and promote many of the pathological features associated with Alzheimer's disease. Supporting this model, the affinity for the binding of insulin to IDE is much greater than that for the Abeta (Qiuet al., 1997). In patients with Alzheimer's disease, IDE expression in the hippocampus is substantially reduced, with regards to controls, in particular among patients with the APOEvar epsilon4 genotype. This latter observation could explain the potential interaction between diabetes and the APOEvar epsilon4 genotype in multiplying the risk of dementia (Cook et al., 2003). Curiously, although the presence of the APOEvar epsilon4 is associated with an increased incidence of Alzheimer's disease, it seems that insulin resistance is only a significant risk factor for AD in those patients without APOEvar epsilon4 (Craft et al., 1998). Subjects with AD without the APOEvar epsilon4 also had improved memory scores when they had hyperinsulinemia, which was not the case for people with at least one APOEvar epsilon4 allele (Craft et al., 1999).

However, unexpectedly, recent clinicopathological studies have shown no evidence that the pathological hallmarks of AD, including amyloid plaque, were increased in the brains of diabetic patients. This suggests that T2D could affect the pathogenesis of AD through mechanisms other than modulation of Abeta metabolism even if the underlying mechanisms for this association remain largely unknown (Takeda et al., 2011).

8. FOXO: A common biomarker for AD and T2D

There is ongoing interest in defining mechanisms that govern insulin resistance and AD. The O subfamily of Forkhead/winged helix transcription factors (FOXO) plays important roles in regulating key physiological functions, including cell proliferation, cell differentiation, and survival together to cell cycle arrest and apoptosis. (Accili et al., 2004; Huang et al., 2007: van der Horst & Tindall, 2007). Thus, FOXO transcription factors are key players in cell death/life pathways. In addition, FOXO works in a complex way to regulate insulin signaling and glucose and lipid metabolism (Accili et al., 20004; Barthel et al., 2005). An additional layer of complexity exists in the transciptional activity of FOXO that is regulated by insulin through the phosphatidyl inositol 3 kinase (PI3K)/Akt signaling pathway. Both insulin and insulin-like growth factor-1 (IGF-1), through activation of their receptors, induce PI3K/Akt-dependent phosphorylation of FOXO, which facilitates its interaction with 14-3-3 protein, leading to nuclear exclusion and eventual ubiquitylation-dependent proteasomal degradation (Matzusaki et al., 2006). In particular, in presence of insulin, activated Akt translocates to the nucleus where directly phosphorylates FOXO at distinct sites stimulating interaction with 14-3-3 protein (Greer and Brunet, 2005). This chaperone protein promotes the nuclear export and inhibits the nuclear import of FOXO proteins, driving the cells towards cell survival (van der Heide et al., 2004). In contrast, FOXO proteins, under conditions of oxidative stress, are phosphorylated by other protein kinases, including Mst1 and JNK, able to disrupt its interaction with 14-3-3, promoting FOXO nuclear translocation and thereby inducing cell death in neurons, thus opposing Akt's action (Sunayama et al., 2005). Thus, it is well established that Akt plays a key role in repressing FOXO transcriptional activity. Immediately upstream from FOXO, the activity of

Akt itself is governed by several protein kinases and phosphatases. Akt is activated by phosphorylation at Thr-308 within its catalytic domain by 3-phosphoinositide-dependent protein kinase-1 (PDK1) and by phosphorylation at Ser-473 within a C-terminal hydrophobic motif by mammalian target of rapamycin (mTOR) (Stokoe et al., 1997; Sarbassov et al., 2005). Some studies show that phospho-Thr-308 and phospho-Ser-273 are dephosphorylated by protein phosphatase 1 (PP1), protein phosphatase 2A (PP2A), and pleckstrin homology (PH) domain leucine rich repeat protein phosphatase (PHLPP), a member of the protein phosphatase 2C family (Gao et al., 2005). Akt regulates a variety of key physiological functions, and there is strong evidence suggesting that defective Akt signaling contributes to development of insulin resistance (Zdychova & Komers, 2005).

However, although it is clear that FOXO governs multiple events in the insulin signaling cascade, mediating both positive and negative effects, the underlying molecular mechanisms are unknown. Some evidence has been reported that FOXO3 activation is also able to increase basal levels of Akt phosphorylation and kinase activity thus it is capable to activating its own inhibitor, providing a feedback regulation (Ni et al., 2007) . Moreover, FOXO transcription factors are involved in both the insulin action and the cellular response to oxidative stress, thereby providing a potential integrative link between AD and insulin resistence (Manolopoulos et al., 2010). Both insulin resistence and oxidative stress due to Abeta stimulus, may promote the transcriptional activity of FOXO proteins, resulting in hyperglycaemia and a further increased production of ROS.

The consecutive activation of c-Jun N-terminal kinases and inhibition of Wingless (Wnt) signalling may result in the formation of Abeta plaques and tau protein phosphorylation. Wnt inhibition may also result in a sustained activation of FOXO proteins with induction of apoptosis and neuronal loss, thereby completing a vicious circle from oxidative stress, insulin resistence and hyperglycaemia back to the formation of ROS and consecutive neurodegeneration. Thus, it has been proposed that FOXO proteins may provide a potential molecular target for the treatment of both insulin resistence and AD (Manolopoulos et al., 2010). Recently it has been demostrated that insulin plays a protective role by inhibiting mithocondrial dysfunction and apoptosis activation triggered by Abeta oligomers (Di Carlo et al., 2010) (Figure 3).

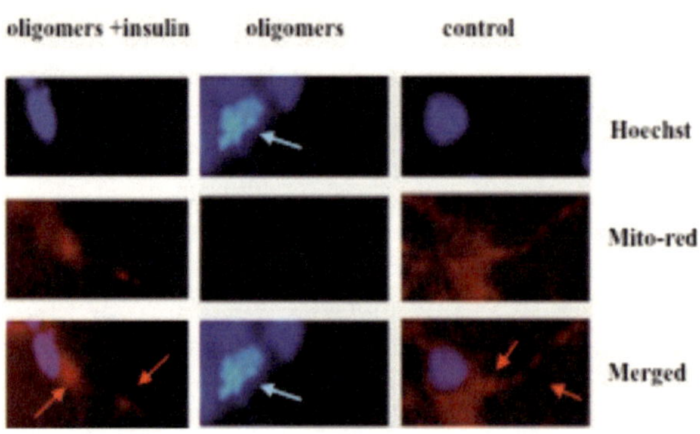

Fig. 3. *Insulin recovers mitochondrial respiratory activity reduced by rAb42 oligomers.* LAN5 untreated (control), treated with rAb42 oligomers oligomers), and rAb42 oligomers and insulin (oligomers+insulin) were incubated with Mito Red and Hoechst 33258. The images of each sample were merged. Mitochondrial activity is indicated by red arrows, fragmentation of nuclei is indcate by blu arrows.

Moreover, unpublished results indicate that insulin counteracts oxidative stress induced by amyloid beta by activation of Akt survival pathway. Akt traslocates from the cytoplasm to nucleus where phophorylates FOXO3a that, in turn, moves from the nucleus to the cytoplasm inhibiting, in this way the transcription of the FOXO-dependent genes. Since after Abeta-induced oxidative stress are usually activated pro-apoptotic genes, their trascriptional inhibition helps the survival program (Picone et al., 2011). Moreover, it has been suggested that since insulin signalling in the brain is known to decline with age, the outcome of the balance of different molecules, as Akt and FOXO, represents a risk factor for AD that is well suited for therapeutic intervention. By restoring the balance of molecules to favour neuron survival, new drugs, designed to specifically enhance CNS insulin signalling, would provide a new and potentially significant class of AD therapeutics.

9. Conclusions

The present chapter highlights the overlap and the many points of intersection existing between T2D and AD. Insulin resistence in the CNS results in the dysregulation of multiple extracellular and intracellular signaling cascades and molecular mechanisms, which in turn could lead to decrease in neuronal and synaptic functions up to neurodegeneration. An understanding of how each molecular pathway intersects and affects the others is essential for the development of future drug intervention strategies for these pathologies.

10. Acknowledgments

The present work was supported by a Grant from the Italian Ministry of Universty and Scientific Research for Programs of Relevant National Interest (PRIN 2008 - prot. 20083Y34Y7) *"Development of a molecular strategy for the prevention of protein aggregation and fibrillogenesis: a biophysical approach"*

11. References

Accili, D., Arden, K.C. (2004) FOXOs at the crossroads of cellular metabolism, differentiation, and transformation. *Cell*, Vol. 117, pp. 421–426

Adrover, M., Vilanova, B., Frau, J., Munoz, F. & Donoso, J. (2008) The pyridoxamine action on Amadori compounds: A reexamination of its scavenging capacity and chelating effect. Bioorg. Med. Chem., Vol. 16, pp. 5557–5569.

Ahmed, N., Thornalley, P.J. (2007) Advanced glycation endproducts: what is their relevance to diabetic complications? *Diabetes Obes. Metab.*, Vol. 9, pp. 233–245.

Antzutkin, O.N., Balbach, J.J., Leapman, R.D., Rizzo, N.W., Reed, J. & Tycko, R. (2000) Multiple quantum solid-state NMR indicates a parallel, not antiparallel, organization of b-sheets in Alzheimer's b-amyloid fibrils. *Proc. Natl. Acad. Sci. USA*, Vol. 97, pp. 13045–13050.

Apelt, J., Bigl, M., Wunderlich, P. & Schliebs, R. (2004) Aging-related increase in oxidative stress correlates with developmental pattern of betasecretase activity and beta-amyloid plaque formation in transgenic Tg2576 mice with Alzheimer-like pathology. *Int. J. Dev. Neurosci.*, Vol. 22, pp. 475–484

Arvanitakis, Z., Wilson, R.S., Bienias, J.L., D. A. Evans, D.A. & Bennett, D.A. (2004) Diabetes mellitus and risk of Alzheimer disease and decline in cognitive function. *Archives of Neurology*, Vol. 61, pp. 661–666.

Asayama, K., Nakane, T., Uchida, N., Hayashibe, H., Dobashi, K. & Nakazawa, S. (1994) Serum antioxidant status in streptozotocin-induced diabetic rat. *Horm. Metab. Res.*,Vol. 26, pp. 313–315.

Baker, L.D., Cross, D.J., Minoshima, S., Belongia, D., Watson, G.S. & Craft, S. (2011) Insulin resistance and Alzheimer-like reductions in regional cerebral glucose metabolism for cognitively normal adults with prediabetes or early type 2 diabetes. *Arch. Neurol.*, Vol. 68, pp. 51-57.

Balaraman, Y., Limaye, A. R., Levey, A. I. & Srinivasan, S. (2006) Glycogen synthase kinase 3β and Alzheimer's disease: pathophysiological and therapeutic significance. *Cell. Mol. Life Sci.*, Vol. 63, pp. 1226–1235

Balbach, J. J., Petkova, A. T., Oyler, N. A., Antzutkin, O. N., Gordon, D. J., Meredith, S. C., & Tycko, R. (2002) Supramolecular structure in full-length Alzheimer's b-amyloid fibrils: evidence for a parallel b-sheet organizatioin from solid-state nuclear magnetic resonance. *Biophys. J.*, Vol. 83, pp. 1205–1216

Ban, T., Hoshino, M., Takahashi, S., Hamada, D., Hasegawa, K., Naiki H. & Goto Y. (2004) Direct observation of Ab amyloid fibril growth and inhibition. *J. Mol. Biol.*, Vol. 344, pp. 757–767

Barthel A, Schmoll D, Unterman TG (2005) FOXO proteins in insulin action and metabolism. *Trends Endocrinol. Metab.*, Vol. 16, pp. 183–189

Bernardi, P., Broekemeier, K.M., Pfeiffer, D.R. (1994) Recent progress on regulation of the mitochondrial permeability transition pore; a cyclosporin-sensitive pore in the inner mitochondrial membrane. J. Bioenerg. Biomembr., Vol. 26, pp. 509–17.

Bhaskar, J.J., Shobha, M.S., Sambaiah, K. & Salimath, P.V. (2011) Beneficial effects of banana (Musa sp. var. elakki bale) flower and pseudostem on hyperglycemia and advanced glycation end-products (AGEs) in streptozotocin-induced diabetic rats. J. Physiol. Biochem. April 8, ahead of print

Brustovetsky, N., Brustovetsky, T., Jemmerson, R. & Dubinsky, J.M. (2002) Calcium-induced cytochrome c release from CNS mitochondria is associated with the permeability transition and rupture of the outer membrane. *J. Neurochem.*, Vol. 80, pp. 207–18

Butterfield, D. A., Reed, T.T., Perluigi, M., De Marco, C., Coccia, R., Keller, J.N., Markesbery, W.R. & Sultana, R. (2007) Elevated levels of 3-nitrotyrosine in brain from subjects with amnestic mild cognitive impairment: implications for the role of nitration in the progression of Alzheimer's disease. *Brain Res.*, Vol. 1148, pp. 243–248.

Calabrese, V., Scapagnini, G., Giuffrida Stella A.M., Bates, T.E. & Clark, J.B. (2001) Mitochondrial involvement in brain function and dysfunction: relevance to aging, neurodegenerative disorders and longevity. *Neurochem Res.* Vol. 26, pp. 739–764.

Chiti, F. and Dobson C.M. (2006) Protein misfolding, functional amyloid and human disease. *Ann. Rev. Biochem.*, Vol. 75, pp. 333-366

Cook, D.G., Leverenz, J.B., McMillan, P.J., Kulstad, J.J., Ericksen, S., Roth, R.A., Schellenberg, G.D., Jin, L.W., Kovacina, K.S. & Craft, S. (2003) Reduced hippocampal insulindegrading enzyme in late-onset Alzheimer's disease is associated with the apolipoprotein E-epsilon4 allele. *Am. J. Pathol.*, Vol. 162, pp. 313–319.

Craft S., Asthana, S., Schellenberg, G., Cherrier, M., Baker, L.D., Newcomer, J., Plymate, S., Latendresse, S., Petrova, A., Raskind, M., Peskind, E., Lofgreen C. & Grimwood K. (1999) Insulin metabolism in Alzheimer's disease differs according to apolipoprotein E genotype and gender. *Neuroendocrinology*, Vol. 70, pp. 146–152.

Craft S., Peskind, E., Schwartz, M.W., Schellenberg, G.D., Raskind, M. & Porte, D. Jr. (1998) Cerebrospinal fluid and plasma insulin levels in Alzheimer's disease: relationship to severity of dementia and apolipoprotein E genotype. *Neurology*, Vol. 50, pp. 164–168.

Cummings, C.J. and Zoghbi, H.Y. (2000) Trinucleotide repeats: mechanisms and pathophysiology. *Annu. Rev. Genomics Hum. Genet.*, Vol. 1, pp. 281-328

Davis, J. & Van Nostrand, W. E. (1996) Enhanced pathologic properties of Dutch-type mutant amyloid beta-protein. *Proc. Natl. Acad. Sci. USA*, Vol. 93, pp. 2996–3000

de la Monte, S. M. and Wands, J. R. J. (2005) Review of insulin and insulin-like growth factor expression, signaling, and malfunction in the central nervous system: relevance to Alzheimer's disease. *Alzheimers Dis.*, Vol. 7, pp. 45–61.

Devangelio, E., Santilli, F., Formoso, G., Ferroni, P., Bucciarelli, L., Michetti, N., Clissa, C., Ciabattoni, G., Consoli, A. & Davi, G. (2007) Soluble RAGE in type 2 diabetes: association with oxidative stress. *Free Radic. Biol. Med.*, Vol. 43, pp. 511–518.

Di Carlo, M., Picone, P., Carrotta, R., Giacomazza, D. & San Biagio, P.L. (2010) Insulin promotes survival of amyloid-beta oligomers neuroblastoma damaged cells via caspase 9 inhibition and Hsp70 upregulation., *J. Biomed. Biotechnol.*, art. #147835

Evans, J.L., Goldfine, I.D., Maddux, B.A. & Grodsky, G.M. (2002) Oxidative stress and stress-activated signaling pathway: a unifying hypothesis od Type 2 diabetes. *Endocrine Reviews*, Vol. 25, pp. 599-622.

Farrer, M., Kachergus, J., Forno, L., Lincoln, S., Wang, D.S., Hulihan, M., Maraganore, D., Gwinn-Hardy, K.,Wszolek Z, Dickson D & Langston J.W. (2004) Comparison of kindreds with parkinsonism and alpha-synuclein genomic multiplications. *Ann. Neurol.*, Vol. 55, pp. 174–179.

Farris, W., Mansourian, S., Chang, Y., Lindsley, L., Eckman, E.A., Frosch, M.P., Eckman, C.B., Tanzi, R.E., Selkoe, D.J. & Guenette, S. (2003) Insulin-degrading enzyme regulates the levels of insulin, amyloid beta-protein, and the beta-amyloid precursor protein intracellular domain in vivo. *Proc. Natl. Acad. Sci.*, Vol. 100, pp. 4162–4167.

Frölich, L., D. Blum-Degen, D., Bernstein, H.-G. , Engelsberger, S., Humrich, J., Laufer, S., Muschner, D., Thalheimer, A., Turk, A., Hoyer, S., Zöchling, R., Boissl, K.W., K. Jellinger, K. & Riederer, P. (1998) Brain insulin and insulin receptors in aging and sporadic Alzheimer's disease. *J. Neural Trasm.*, Vol. 105, pp. 423-438

Gao, T., Furnari, F. and Newton, A. C. (2005). PHLPP: a phosphatase that directly dephosphorylates Akt, promotes apoptosis, and suppresses tumor growth. *Mol. Cell*, Vol. 18, pp. 13–24.

Garrido, G. E., Furule, S.S., Buchpiguel, C.A., Bottino, C.M.C., Almeida, O.P., Cid, C.G., Camargo, C.H.P., Castro, C.C., Glabus, M.F. & Busatto, G.F. (2002) Relation between medial temporal atrophy and functional brain activity during memory processing in Alzheimer's disease: a combined MRI and SPECT study. *J. Neurol. Neurosurg. Psychiatry*, Vol. 73, pp. 508–516.

Gilead, S. and Gazit E. (2008) The role of the 14-20 domain of the islet amyloid polypeptide in amyloid formation, in *Experimental Diabetes Research* Westermark, G.T., Westermark, P. and Kahn S.A. eds. Indawi Pub. Corp. Article ID 256954, Retrived from <http://www.hindawi.com/journals/edr/2008/>

Girones, X., Guimerà, A., Cruz-Sanchez, C.-Z., Ortega, A., Sasaki, N., Makita, Z., Lafuente, J.V., Kalaria, R. & Cruz-Sanchez, F.F. (2004) Nε-carboxymethyllysine in brain aging, diabetes mellitus, and Alzheimer's disease. *Free Radic. Biol. Med.*, Vol. 36, pp. 1241–1247

Goedert, M., Jakes, R., Crowther, R.A., Six, J., Lubke, U., Vandermeeren, M., Cras, P., Trojanowsky, J.Q. & Lee, V.M.-Y. (1993) The abnormal phosphorylation of tau protein at Ser-202 in Alzheimer disease recapitulates phosphorylation during development *Proc. Natl. Acad. Sci. USA*, Vol. 90, pp. 5066-5070

Goldsbury, C., Goldie, K., Pellaud, J., Seelig, J., Frey, P., Muller, S.A., Kistler, J., Cooper, G.J. & Aebi, U. (2000) Amyloid fibril formation from full-length and fragments of amylin. *J. Struct. Biol.*, Vol. 130, pp. 352-362

Gotz, J., Schild, A., Hoerndli, F. & Pennanen, L. (2004) Amyloid-induced neurofibrillary tangle formation in Alzheimer's disease: insight from transgenic mouse and tissue-culture models. *Int. J. Dev. Neurosci.*, Vol. 22, pp. 453–465

Greer, E.L. and Brunet, A. (2005) FOXO transcription factors at the interface between longevity and tumor suppression. *Oncogene*, Vol. 24, pp. 7410-7425

Haan, M. N. (2006) Therapy Insight: type 2 diabetes mellitus and the risk of late-onset Alzheimer's disease. *Nat. Clin. Pract. Neurol.*, Vol. 2, pp. 159–166.

Han, W. and Li, C. (2010) Linking type 2 diabetes and Alzheimer's disease. *Proc. Natl. Acad. Sci. USA.*, Vol. 107, pp. 6557-6558

Harper, J.D., Wong, S.S., Lieber, C.M. & Lansbury, P.T.J. (1997)Observation of metastable Ab-amyloid protofibrils by atomic force microscopy. *Chem. Biol.*, Vol. 4, pp. 119-125

Hipkiss, A.R. (2007) Could carnosine or related structures suppress Alzheimer's disease? J. Alzheimers Dis., Vol. 11, pp. 229–240

Hoyer, S. (1998) Risk factors for Alzheimer's disease during aging. Impacts of glucose/energy metabolism. *J. Neural. Transm. Suppl.* 54, pp. 187-194

Huang, H. and Tindall, D.J. (2007) Dynamic FOXO transcription factors. *J.Cell Sci.*, Vol. 120, 2479-2487.

Huang, T.H.J., Yang, D.S., Plaskos, N.P., Go, S., Yip, C.M., Fraser, P.E. & Chakrabartty, A. (2000) Structural studies of soluble oligomers of the Alzheimer b-amyloid peptide. *J. Mol. Biol.* Vol. 297, pp. 73–87

Iwatsubo, T., Odaka, A., Suzuki, N., Mizusawa, H., Nukina, N. & Ihara, Y. (1994) Visualization of Abeta42(43) and Abeta40 in senile plaques with end-specific Abeta monoclonals: evidence that an initially deposited species is Abeta42(43). *Neuron*, Vol. 13, pp. 45–53

Janson, J., Ashley, R.H., Harrison, D., McIntyre, S. & Butler, P.C. (1999) The mechanism of islet amyloid polypeptide toxicity is membrane disruption by intermediate-sized toxic amyloid particles. *Diabetes*, Vol. 48, pp. 491-498.

Hnight, J.D., Hebda, J.A. and Minraker, A.D. (2006) Conserved and cooperative assembly of membrane-bound alpha-helical states of islet amyloid polypeptide. *Biochemistry*, Vol. 45, pp. 9496-9508

Lambert, M.P., Barlow, A.K., Chromy, B.A., Edwards, C., Freed, R., Liosatos, M., Morgan, T.E., Rozovsky, I., Trommer, B., Viola, K.L.,Wals, P., Zhang, C., Finch, C.E. & Krafft, G.A. (1998) Diffusible, nonfibrillar ligands derived from Ab1–42 are potent central nervous system neurotoxins. *Proc. Natl. Acad. Sc.i USA*, Vol. 95, pp. 6448–6453

Larbig, G., Pickhardt, M., Lloyd, D.G., Schmidt, B. & Mandelkow, E. (2007) Screening for inhibitors of tau protein aggregation into Alzheimer paired helical filaments: a ligand based approach results in successful scaffold hopping. Curr. Alzheimer Res. Vol. 4, pp. 315–323.

Lashuel, H.A., Hartley, D., Petre, B.M., Walz, T. & Lansbury, P.T.J. (2002) Amyloid pores from pathogenic mutations. *Nature*, Vol. 418, pp. 291-291

Lederer, M.O. and Klalber, R.G. (1999) Cross-linking of proteins by maillard processes: characterization and detection of lysine–arginine cross-links derived from glyoxal and methylglyoxal *Bioorganic & Medicinal Chemistry*, Vol. 7, pp. 2499-2507

Ledl, F. and Schleicher, E. (1990) New Aspects of the Maillard Reaction in Foods and in the Human Body. *Angew. Chem.,Int. Ed. Engl.*, Vol. 29., pp. 565-594

Lee, H.P., Zhu, X., Casadesus, G., Castellani, R.J., Nunomura, A., Smith, M.A., Lee, H.G. & Perry, G. (2010) Antioxidant approaches for the treatment of Alzheimer's disease. *Expert. Rev. Neurother.*, Vol. 10, pp. 1201-1208

Lee, J. and Kim, M. S. (2007) The role of GSK3 in glucose homeostasis and the development of insulin resistance. *Diabetes Res. Clin. Pract.*, Vol. 77 , pp. S49–S57.

Lesort, M. and Johnson, G. V. (2000) Insulin-like growth factor-1 and insulin mediate transient site selective increases in tau phosphorylation in primary cortical neurons. *Neuroscience*, Vol. 99, pp. 305–316

Liu, Q., Xie, F., Rolston, R., Moreira, P.I., Nunomura, A., Zhu, X., Smith, M.A. & Perry, G. (2007) Prevention and treatment of Alzheimer disease and aging: antioxidants. *Mini Rev. Med. Chem.*, Vol. 7, pp. 171–180.

Lomakin, A., Chung, D.S., Benedek ,G.B., Kirschner, D.A. & Teplow, D.B. (1996) On the nucleation and growth of amyloid b-protein fibrils: Detection of nuclei and quantitation of rate constants. *Proc. Natl. Acad. Sci. USA*, Vol. 93, pp. 1125–1129

Lorenzo, A., Razzaboni, B., Weir, G.C. & Yankner, B.A. (1994) Pancreatic islet toxicity of amylin ssociated with type-2 diabetes mellitus. *Nature*, Vol. 368, pp. 756-760

Lupi, R. and Del Prato, S. (2008) Beta-cell apoptosis in type 2 diabetes: quantitative and functional consequence. *Diabetes Metab.*, Vol. 34, pp. S56-S64

Manno, M., Craparo, E.F., Martorana, V., Bulone, D. & San Biagio, P.L. (2006) Kinetics of insulin aggregation: disentaglement of amyloid from large-size cluster formation. *Biophys. J.*, Vol. 90, pp. 4585-4591

Manno, M., Giacomazza, D., Newman, J., Martorana, V. & San Biagio, P.L. (2010) Amyloid gels: precocious appearance of elastic properties during the formation af an insulin fibrillar network. *Langmuir*, Vol. 26, pp. 1424-1426

Manolopoulos, K.N., Klotz, L.-O., Korsten, P., Bornstein, S.R. & Barthel, A. (2010) Linking Alzheimer's disease to insulin resistance: the FOXO response to oxidative stress. *Mol. Psychiatry*, Vol. 15, pp. 1046-1052

Marek, P., Abedini A., Song, B., Kanungo, M., Johson M.E., Gupta R., Zaman W., Wong, S.S. & Raleigh, D.P. (2007) Aromatic interactions are not required for amyloid fibril formation by islet amyloid polypeptide but do influence the rate of fibril formation and fibril morphology. *Biochemistry*, Vol. 46, pp. 3255-3261

Maritim, A.C., Sanders, R.A. and Watkins, J.B. (2003) Oxidative stress, antioxidants and diabetes: a review. *J. Biochem. Mol. Toxicol.*, Vol. 17, pp. 24-38

Matsuoka, Y., Picciano, M., La Francois, J. & Duff, K. (2001) Fibrillar β-amyloid evokes oxidative damage in a transgenic mouse model of Alzheimer's disease. *Neuroscience*, Vol. 104, pp. 609–613.

Matsuzaki, H., Daitoku, H., Hatta, M., Tanaka, K. & Fukamizu, A. (2003) Insulin-induced phosphorylation of FKHR (FOXO1) targets to proteasomal degradation. *Proc. Natl. Acad. Sci. USA*, Vol. 100, pp. 11285–11290.

McLean, L.R. and Balasubramanian, A. (1992) Promotion of b-structure by interaction f diabetes associated polypeptide (amylin) with phosphatidylcholine. *Biochimica et Biophysica Acta*, Vol. 1122, pp. 317-320

Moreira, P.I., Santos, M.S., Moreno, A.M., Seiça, R. & Oliveira, C.R. (2003) Increased vulnerability of brain mitochondria in diabetic (Goto-Kakizaki) rats with aging and amyloid-beta exposure. *Diabetes*, Vol. 52, pp. 1449–56.

Morris, A.M., Watzky, M.A. and Finke, R.G. (2009) Protein aggregation kinetics, mechanism, and curve-fitting: A review of the literature. *Biochimica et Biophysica Acta*, Vol. 1794, pp. 375-397

Nakabeppu, Y., Tsuchimoto, D., Ichinoe, A., Ohno, M., Ide, Y., Hirano, S., Yoshimura, D., Tominaga, Y., Furuichi, M. & Sakumi, K. (2004) Biological significance of the defense mechanisms against oxidative damage in nucleic acids caused by reactive oxygen species: from mitochondria to nuclei. *Ann. N.Y. Acad. Sci.*, Vol. 1011, pp. 101–111.

Nazario, B. (June, 02 2009) Type 2 Diabetes Overview, In *MedScape*, Available from: <http://diabetes.webmd.com/guide/type-2-diabetes>

Neumann K.F., Rojo L., Navarrete L.P., Farias G., Reyes P. & Maccioni R.B. (2008) Insulin resistance and Alzheimer's disease: molecular links & clinical implications. *Current Alzheimer Research*, Vol. 5, pp. 438–447

Ni, Y.G., Wang N., Cao, D.J., Sachan, N., Morris, D.J., Gerard, R.D., Kuro-o, M., Rothermel, B.A., Hill, J.A. (2007) FOXO transcription factors activate Akt and attenuate insulin signaling in heart by inhibiting protein phosphatases. *Proc. Natl. Acad. Sci. U.S.A.*, Vol. 104, pp. 20517-20522

Phiel, C. J., Wilson, C. A., Lee, V. M. & Klein, P. S. (2003) GSK-3α regulates production of Alzheimer's disease amyloid-β peptides. Nature, Vol. 423, pp. 435–439.

Picone, P., Carrotta, R., Montana, G., Nobile, M.R., San Biagio, P.L. & Di Carlo, M. (2009) Abeta oligomers and fibrillar aggregates induce different apoptotic pathways in LAN5 neuroblastoma cell cultures. *Biophys. J.*, Vol. 96, pp. 4200-4211

Picone, P., Giacomazza, D., Vetri, V., Carrotta, R., Militello, V., San Biagio, P.L. & Di Carlo, M. Aging Cell, Accepted doi: 10.1111/j.1474-9726.2011.00724.x.

Pratico, D. and Sung, S. (2004) Lipid peroxidation and oxidative imbalance: early functional events in Alzheimer's disease. *J. Alzheimers Dis.*, Vol. 6, pp. 171–175

Pratico, D., Uryu, K., Leight, S., Trojanoswki, J. Q. & Lee, V. M. (2001) Increased lipid peroxidation precedes amyloid plaque formation in an animal model of Alzheimer amyloidosis. *J. Neurosci.*, Vol. 21, pp. 4183–4187.

Qiu, W.Q., Walsh, D.M., Ye, Z., Vekrellis, K., Zhang, J., Podlisny, M.B., Rosner, M.R., Safavi, A., Hersh, L.B. & Selkoe, D.J. (1998) Insulin-degrading enzyme regulates extracellular levels of amyloid beta-protein by degradation. *J. Biol. Chem.*, Vol. 273, pp. 32730-32738

Qiu, W.Q., Ye, Z., Kholodenko, D., Seubert, P. & Selkoe, D.J. (1997) Degradation of amyloid beta-protein by a metalloprotease secreted by microglia and other neural and non-neural cells. *J. Biol. Chem.*, Vol. 272, pp. 6641-6646.

Rabbani, N. and Thornalley, P.J. (2008) The dicarbonyl proteome: proteins susceptible to dicarbonyl glycation at functional sites in health, aging, and disease. *Ann. N.Y. Acad. Sci.*, Vol. 1126, pp. 124-127.

Reddy, V.P., Garrett, M.R., Perry, G. & Smith, M.A. (2005) Carnosine: a versatile antioxidant and antiglycating agent. Sci. Aging. Knowledge Environ., Vol. 2005, pp. pe12

Reddy, V.P., Zhu, X., Perry, G. & Smith, M. A. (2009) Oxidative stress in diabetes and Alzheimer's disease. *J. Alzheimers Dis.*, Vol. 16, pp. 763-774.

Resende R., Ferreiro R., Pereira C. & Resende de Oliveira, C. (2008a) Neurotoxic effect of oligomeric and fibrillar species of amyloid-beta peptide 1-42: involvement of endoplasmic reticulum calcium release in oligomer-induced cell death. *Neuroscience*, Vol. 155, pp. 725-737

Resende R., Moreira; P.I., Proença T., Deshpande, A., Busciglio, J., Pereira C. & Resende Oliveira, C. (2008b) Brain oxidative stress in a triple-transgenic mouse model of Alzheimer disease. *Free Radic. Biol. Med.*, Vol. 44, pp. 2051-2057

Rizzuto, R., Bernardi, P. and Pozzan, T. (2000) Mitochondria as all-round players of the calcium game. *J. Physiol.*, Vol. 529, pp. 37-47.

Rocchi A., Pellegrini S., Siciliano G. & Murri L. (2003) Causative and susceptibility genes for Alzheimer's disease: a review. *Brain Res. Bull.*, Vol. 61, pp. 1-24

Roriz-Filho J.S., Sà-Roriz T.M., Rosset I., Camozzato, A.L., Santos, A.C., Chaves, M.L., Moriguti, J.C. & Roriz-Cruz, M. (2009) (Pre)diabetes, brain aging, and cognition. *Biochimica et Biophysica Acta*, Vol. 1792, pp. 432-443

Russell, J.W., Berent-Spillson A., Vincent, A.M., Freimann, C.L., Sullivan, K.A. & Feldman, E.L. (2008) Oxidative injury and neuropathy in diabetes and impaired glucose tolerance. *Neurobiol. Dis.*, Vol. 30, pp. 420-429.

Salkovic-Petrisic M. and Hoyer S. (2007) Central insulin resistance as a trigger for sporadic Alzheimer-like pathology: an experimental approach. *J. Neural. Transm.* Suppl. 72, pp. 217-233.

Saraiva, M.J. (2001) Transthyretin amyloidosis: a tale of weak interactions. *FEBS Lett.*, Vol. 498, pp. 201-203.

Sarbassov, D.D., Guertin, D.A., Ali, S.M., Sabatini, D.M. (2005) Phosphorylation and regulation of Akt/PKB by the rictor-mTOR complex. *Science*, Vol. 307, pp. 1098-1101.

Schrijvers E.M.C., Witteman J.C.M., Sijbrands E.J.G., Hofman A., Koudstaal P.J. & Breteler M.M.B. (2010) Insulin metabolism and the risk of Alzheimer disease. *Neurology*, Vol. 75, pp. 1982-1987

Schroeder, B. E. and Koo, E. H. (2005) To think or not to think: synaptic activity and Abeta release. *Neuron.* , Vol. 48, pp. 873-875.

Schubert, M., Brazil, D.P., Burks, D.J., Kushner, J.A., Ye, J., Flint, C.L., Farhang-Fallah, J., Dikkes, P., Warot, X.M., Rio, C., Corfas, G. & White, M.F. (2003) Insulin receptor substrate-2 deficiency impairs brain growth and promotes tau phosphorylation. *J. Neurosci.*, Vol. 23, pp. 7084-7092.

Schulingkamp R.J., Pagano T.C., Hung D. & Raffa R.B. (2000) Insulin receptors and insulin action in the brain: review and clinical implications. *Neurosci Biobehav. Rev.*, Vol. 24, pp. 855-872.

Serpell, L.C. (2000) Alzheimer's amyloid fibrils: structure and assembly. *Biochim. Biophys. Acta*, Vol. 1502, pp. 16–30.

Singleton, A.B., Farrer, M., Johnson, J., Singleton, A., Hague, S., Kachergus, J., Hulihan, M., Peuralinna, T., Dutra, A., Nussbaum, R., Lincoln, S., Crawley, A., Hanson, M., Maraganore, D., Adler, C., Cookson, M.R., Muenter, M., Baptista, M., Miller, D., Blancato, J., Hardy, J. & Gwinn-Hardy, K. (2003) Alpha-Synuclein locus triplication causes Parkinson's disease. *Science*, Vol. 302, pp. 841-841

Slatter, D.A., Bolton, C.H. and Bailey, A.J. (2000) The importance of lipid derived malondialdehyde in diabetes mellitus. *Diabetologia*, Vol. 43, pp. 550–557

Smith, M.A., Perry, G., Richey, P.L., Sayre, L.M., Anderson, V.E., Beal, M.F. & Kowall, N. (1996) Oxidative damage in Alzheimer's. *Nature*, Vol. 382, pp. 120-121.

Smith, M.A., Richey Harris, P.L., Sayre, L.M., Beckman, J.S. & Perry, G. (1997) Widespread peroxynitrite-mediated damage in Alzheimer's disease. J. Neurosci., Vol. 17, pp. 2653–2657

Stadtman, E.R. (2001) Protein oxidation in aging and age-related diseases. *Ann. N.Y. Acad. Sci.*, Vol. 928, pp. 22-38

Stokoe, D., Stephens, L.R., Copeland, T., Gaffney, P.R.J., Reese, C.B., Painter, G.F., Holmes, A.B., McCormick, F. & Hawkins, P.T. (1997) Dual Role of Phosphatidylinositol-3,4,5-trisphosphate in the Activation of Protein Kinase B. *Science*, Vol. 277, pp. 567–570.

Sunayama, J., Tsuruta, F., Masuyama, N. & Gotoh, Y. (2005) JNK antagonizes Akt-mediated survival signals by phosphorylating 14-3-3. *Journal of Cell Biology*, Vol. 170, pp. 295-304.

Susic, D. (2007) Cross-link breakers as a new therapeutic approach to cardiovascular disease. *Biochem. Soc. Trans.*, Vol. 35, pp. 853–856.

Takeda, S., Sato, N., Rakugi H. & Morishita R. (2011) Molecular mechanisms linking diabetes mellitus and Alzheimer disease: beta-amyloid peptide, insulin signaling, and neuronal function. Mol. BioSyst., DOI: 10.1039/C0MB00302F

Tan, K.C., Chow, W.S., Tso, A.W., Xu, A., Tse, H.F., Hoo, R.L., Betteridge, D.J. & Lam, K.S. (2007) Thiazolidinedione increases serum soluble receptor for advanced glycation end-products in type 2 diabetes. *Diabetologia*, Vol. 50, pp. 1819–1825.

Tan, K.C., Shiu, S.W., Chow, W.S., Leng, L., Bucala, R. & Betteridge, D.J. (2006) Association between serum levels of soluble receptor for advanced glycation end products and circulating advanced glycation end products in type 2 diabetes. *Diabetologia*, Vol. 49, pp. 2756–2762

Thomas, M.C., Baynes, J.W., Thorpe, S.R. & Cooper, M.E. (2005) The role of AGEs and AGE inhibitors in diabetic cardiovascular disease. Curr. Drug Targets, Vol. 6, pp. 453–474.

Toth, C., Schmidt, A.M., Tuor, U.I., Francis, G., Foniok, T., Brussee, V., Kaur, J., Yan, S.F., Martinez, J.A., Barber, P.A., Buchan, A. & Zochodne, D.W. (2006) Diabetes, leukoencephalopathy and rage. *Neurobiol. Dis.*, Vol. 23, pp. 445–461.

van der Heide, L.P., Hoekman, M.F. and Smidt, M.P. (2004) The ins and outs of FOXO shuttling: mechanisms of FOXO translocation and transcriptional regulation. *Biochemical Journal*, Vol. 380, pp. 297–309.

van der Horst, A. and Burgering, B.M. (2007) Stressing the role of FOXO proteins in lifespan and disease. *Nat. Rev. Mol. Cell. Biol.*, Vol. 8, pp. 440–450.

Vincent, A. M., Russell, J. W., Low, P. & Feldman, E. L. (2004) Oxidative stress in the pathogenesis of diabetic neuropathy. *Endocr. Rev.*, Vol. 25, pp. 612–628.

Uversky, V.N. (2007) Neuropathology, biochemistry, and biophysics of alpha-synuclein aggregation. *J. Neurochem.*, Vol. 103, pp. 17–37.

Wada, R., Nishizawa, Y., Yagihashi, N., Takeuchi, M., Ishikawa, Y., Yasumura, K., Nakano, M. & Yagihashi, S. (2001) Effects of OPB-9195, anti-glycation agent, on experimental diabetic neuropathy. Eur. J. Clin. Invest., Vol. 31, pp. 513–520.

Walsh, D.M., Hartley, D.M., Fezoui, Y., Condron M.M., Lomakin, A., Benedek, G.B., Selkoe, D.J. & Teplow, D.B. (1999) Amyloid beta-protein fibrollogenesis. Structure and biological activity of protofibrillar intermediates. *J. Biol. Chem.*, Vol. 274, pp. 25945-25952

Weber, P., Bendich, A. and Machlin, L.J. (1997) Vitamin E and human health: rationale for determining recommended intake levels. Nutrition, Vol. 13, pp. 450–460.

Webster, J., Urban, C., Berbaum, K., Loske, C., Alpar, A., Gartner, U., de Arriba, S.G., Arendt, T. & Munch, G. (2005) The carbonyl scavengers aminoguanidine and tenilsetam protect against the neurotoxic effects of methylglyoxal. Neurotox. Res., Vol. 7, pp. 95–101.

West, I.C. (2000) Radicals and oxidative stress in diabetes. Diabet. Med., Vol. 17, pp. 171–180

Westermark, P., Engstrom, U., Johnson, K. H., Westermark, G. T. & Betsholtz, C. (1990) Islet amyloid polypeptide - Pinpointing amino-acid-residues linked to amyloid fibril formation. *Proc. Natl. Acad. Sci. U.S.A.*, Vol. 87, pp. 5036–5040.

Westermark, P., Wernstedt, C., Wilander, E., Hayden, D.W., O'Brian, T.D. & Johnson, K.H. (1987) Amyloid fibrils in human insulinoma and islets of Langherans of the diabetic cat are derived from a neuropeptide-like protein also present in normal islet cells. *Proc. Natl. Acad. Sci. USA*, Vol. 84, pp. 3881-3885

Westlind-Danielsson, A. and Arnerup, G. (2001) Spontaneous in vitro formation of supramolecular b-amyloid structures, "b-amy balls", by b-amyloid 1-40 peptide. *Biochemistry*, Vol. 40, pp. 14736-14743

Wisniewski T., Ghiso J. and Frangione B. (1997) Biology of Aβ amyloid in Alzheimer's disease. *Neurobiology of Disease*, Vol. 4, pp. 313–328

Wilquet V. and De Strooper B. (2004) Amyloid-beta precursor protein processing in neurodegeneration. *Neurobiology*, Vol. 14, pp. 582–588

Yadavalli, V.K., Svintradze, D.V., Pidaparti, R.M. (2010) Nanoscale measurements of the assembly of collagen to fibrils. *Int. J. Biol. Macromol.*, Vol. 46, pp. 458-464

Yong, W., Lomakin, A., Kirkitadze, M.D., Teplow, D.B., Chen, S.-H. & Benedek, G.B. (2002) Structure determination of micelle-like intermediates in amyloid b-protein fibril assembly using small angle neutron scattering. *Proc. Natl. Acad. Sci. USA*, Vol. 99, pp. 150–154

Xu, S. (2007) Aggregation drives "misfolding" in protein amyloid fiber formation. *Amyloid*, Vol. 14, pp. 119-131

Zdychova, J. and Komers, R. (2005) Emerging role of Akt kinase/protein kinase B signaling in pathophysiology of diabetes and its complications. *Physiol. Res.*, Vol. 54, pp. 1–16.

Zhao, W.Q., Chen, H., Quon, M.J. & Alkon, D.L. (2004) Insulin and the models of learning and memory. *Eur. J. Pharmacol.*, Vol. 490, pp. 71–81.

Zhao, W.Q., Lacor, P.N., Chen, H., Lambert, M.P., Quon, M.J., Krafft, G.A. & Klein, W.L. (2008) Insulin receptor dysfunction impairs cellular clearance of neurotoxic oligomeric ab. J. Biol. Chem., Vol. 284, pp. 18742–18753

3

Insulin Resistance and Alzheimer's Disease

Sung Min Son, Hong Joon Shin and Inhee Mook-Jung
Department of Biochemistry & Biomedical Sciences,
Seoul National University College of Medicine, Seoul
Korea

1. Introduction

Alzheimer disease (AD) is known as a form of type III diabetes due to its similar cellular responses and pathogenesis. Insulin alters normal brain function and peripheral glucose metabolism, and conditions that are related to insulin dysregulation, such as obesity, diabetes mellitus, and cardiovascular disease, have potentially harmful effects on brain function. Many reports have demonstrated that insulin resistance increases age-related memory impairments and is a risk factor for AD. The molecular and cellular link between insulin resistance and AD, however, is unknown. We discuss the potential mechanisms of these metabolic disorders in the pathogenesis of AD. Glucose homeostasis is critical for energy maintenance, neurogenesis, neuronal survival, and synaptic plasticity, which are required for learning and memory. During insulin resistance, one develops reduced sensitivity to insulin, resulting in hyperinsulinemia, and this impairment in insulin signaling mediates the pathogenesis of AD, which manifests as brain inflammation, oxidative stress, alterations in amyloid beta (Aβ) levels, and cell death. Human and experimental animal studies have noted that drugs that modulate insulin resistance decrease the accumulation of Aβ in the brain and the cognitive impairments that are associated with AD. Therapeutic strategies that target the link between insulin resistance and AD might benefit the development of future AD drugs.

2. Insulin signaling

2.1 Introduction

Insulin is a peptide hormone that comprises 51 amino acids and is synthesized in and secreted from pancreatic β-cells in the islet of Langerhans (Huang et al., 2010). Its rapid release is generally triggered by increased levels of glucose in the blood, despite other mechanisms that release insulin; normal blood glucose levels range from 4.4 to 6.1 mmol/L (82 to 110 mg/dL).

Of its many functions, the most significant effects of insulin are its promotion of cellular growth and differentiation, activation or repression of transcription, and regulation of protein kinases and phosphatases (Saltiel and Pessin, 2002). Defects in insulin signaling can affect many diseases, such as type 2 diabetes mellitus (T2DM), metabolic syndrome, and Alzheimer disease (AD). Although most studies have examined the function of insulin and the dysregulation of insulin secretion or insulin receptor signaling in peripheral tissue, it has recently been reported to cause serious mental illness (Huang et al., 2010).

2.2 General effects of insulin signaling

Insulin increases glycogen and lipid synthesis in liver and muscle cells and simultaneously inhibits glycogenolysis and gluconeogenesis in the liver during feeding (Saltiel and Kahn, 2001). These actions are mediated by its binding to membrane-bound insulin receptors (IRs), members of the tyrosine kinase receptor family (Saltiel and Pessin, 2002). The binding of insulin to the alpha subunit of IR induces a conformational change, resulting in the autophosphorylation of tyrosine residues in the beta subunit of the receptor (Van Obberghen et al., 2001). This ligation leads to the subsequent tyrosine phosphorylation of insulin receptor substrates 1-4 (IRS1-4), Shc, Gab-1, Cbl, and APS (Saltiel and Pessin, 2002), and activates downstream cytoplasmic effectors, such as the lipid kinase phosphatidylinositol 3-kinase (PI 3-kinase) and mitogen-activated protein kinase (MAPK) (Cole et al., 2007; Plum et al., 2005).

During insulin-mediated glucose uptake, the phosphorylated residues of insulin receptor and IRS1, 2, and 3 are recognized by the Src homology 2 (SH2) domain (Bevan, 2001) of the p85 regulatory subunit of PI 3-kinase. The catalytic subunit of PI 3-kinase, p110, phosphorylates phosphatidylinositol (4,5) bisphosphate (PtdIns(4,5)P2), leading to the formation of Ptd(3,4,5)P3 (Lizcano and Alessi, 2002). Ptd(3,4,5)P3 then binds to the plasma membrane and associates with phosphoinositol-dependent kinase-1 (PDK-1) and induces the phosphorylation and activation of protein kinase B (PKB)/Akt, a serine-threonine kinase. Activated Akt enters the cytoplasm, where it evokes the phosphorylation and inactivation of glycogen synthase kinase 3 (GSK3), which promotes glycogen synthesis.

By activating PI3-kinase and AKT (Lizcano and Alessi, 2002), insulin affects the translocation of glucose transporter 4 (GLUT4) from intracellular stores to the plasma membrane: When insulin concentrations are low, GLUT4 exists in cytoplasmic vesicles. After insulin binds to its receptors, GLUT4-containing vesicles fuse with the plasma membrane, and the newly inserted GLUT4 takes up glucose efficiently. In parallel, there is a PI 3-kinase independent pathway that recruits GLUT4 to the plasma membrane, led by the phosphorylation of the proto-oncogene Cbl, which is associated with the adaptor protein c-Cbl-associated protein (CAP) (Saltiel and Kahn, 2001).

Insulin promotes the uptake and synthesis of fatty acids in the liver and prevents lipolysis by inhibiting the intracellular lipase that hydrolyzes triglycerides to release fatty acids. Although insulin promotes the synthesis of glycogen in the liver, further synthesis is suppressed when the liver is saturated with glycogen. Any additional glucose that is taken up is then shunted into pathways that lead to fatty acid synthesis (Saltiel and Kahn, 2001).

One study has indicated that lipid synthesis requires increased expression of the transcription factor steroid regulatory element-binding protein (SREBP)-1c (Shimomura et al., 1999), which is synthesized as a membrane protein in the endoplasmic reticulum (ER) (Sato, 2010). Insulin is believed to induce SREBP-1c proteolytic activity and, consequently, insulin-mediated lipogenesis (Sato, 2010). Further, insulin inhibits lipid metabolism by decreasing cellular concentrations of cAMP through activation of a cAMP-specific phosphodiesterase in adipocytes (Kitamura et al., 1999).

Insulin stimulates amino acid uptake into cells, inhibits protein degradation, and promotes protein synthesis (Saltiel and Kahn, 2001) by stimulating components of the translational machinery, including eukaryotic initiation factors (eIFs) and eukaryotic elongation factors (eEFs) (Proud, 2006). This entails the activation of PKB, leading to the phosphorylation and inactivation of GSK3, which in turn promotes phosphorylation and inhibition of a guanine nucleotide exchange factor, eIF2B, to regulate the initiation of translation (Proud, 2006).

Moreover, PKB phosphorylates the tuberous sclerosis complex 1 (TSC1)-TSC2 complex, relieving its inhibition of the mammalian target of rapamycin (mTOR) (Proud, 2006), which promotes protein synthesis through p70 ribosomal S6 kinase (p70S6k) and inhibition of eIF-4E binding protein (4E-BP1), and thereby governs ribosomal protein translation (Proud, 2006).

2.3 Insulin in the brain

The brain is the primary consumer of glucose, requiring two-thirds of total circulating glucose daily (Peters, 2011); thus, the regulation of glucose homeostasis by insulin in the central nervous system (CNS) is paramount for normal brain function. Insulin, by a saturable transport process that is mediated by insulin receptor, can cross the blood-brain barrier (BBB), which governs the transduction between the CNS and peripheral tissues (Neumann et al., 2008). Although insulin is synthesized locally in the brain (Banks et al., 1997; Devaskar et al., 1994; Rulifson et al., 2002), its function is unknown.

IRs in the CNS are widely expressed throughout the brain in neurons and glial cells, at particularly high concentrations in the cerebral cortex, hippocampus, hypothalamus, and olfactory bulb (Neumann et al., 2008). They have disparate functions, molecular weights, and structures from IRs in peripheral organs (Heidenreich et al., 1983), but it is unknown whether the counter effects of insulin in the CNS compared with those in peripheral tissues are attributed to such differences. Insulin increases glucose and inhibits feeding in the CNS, but decreases glucose and stimulates feeding in peripheral tissue (Florant et al., 1991). A recent report observed that impaired brain insulin activity might affect unrestrained lipolysis that initiates and exacerbates type 2 diabetes mellitus in humans (Scherer et al., 2011).

2.4 Role of insulin in cognitive function

In humans, brain insulin enhances learning, memory, and, in particular, verbal memory (Benedict et al., 2004). Insulin signaling in the limbic system and hypothalamus is especially important for cognitive function (Zhao et al., 1999), independent of changes in peripheral glucose (Craft et al., 1999; Kern et al., 1999). These functions have been supported by evidence that insulin modulates the concentrations of neurotransmitters, which influence cognition, such as Ach (acetylcholine) (Kopf and Baratti, 1999). Insulin also alters synaptic plasticity by regulating the endocytosis of 3-hydroxy-5-methylisoxazole-4-propionic acid (AMPA) receptor, which causes long-term depression (LTD) of excitatory synaptic transmission in the hippocampus and cerebellum (Huang et al., 2003; Man et al., 2000; Wang and Linden, 2000), and by enhancing N-methyl-D-aspartate (NMDA) receptor-mediated synaptic transmission at hippocampal CA1 synapses (van der Heide et al., 2005).

2.5 Insulin-like growth factor (IGF)

Insulin-like growth factors are polypeptides that are similar in sequence to proinsulin (Clemmons, 2007). Insulin-like growth factor 1, which stimulates cell growth and proliferation, especially in nerve cells, binds to IGF receptor and IRs (Jones et al., 2009). IGF-1 functions similarly to insulin receptor. IGF-1, a tyrosine kinase, initiates signaling cascades through IRS and enhances insulin activity (Clemmons, 2007).

Deficiency of or irresponsiveness to IGF-1 causes not only growth failure but also dyslipidemia (Twickler et al., 2003), insulin resistance (Conti et al., 2002; Twickler et al.,

2003), and obesity (Rasmussen et al., 1995). According to recent longitudinal studies, these phenotypes are closely related to a high risk of neurodegenerative disorders, such as dementia and AD (Luchsinger et al., 2004; Ott et al., 1996; Ronnemaa et al., 2008). Similarly, mice in which IGF-1 has been deleted develop increased Aβ levels in the brain, suggesting that IGF-1 promotes the clearance of Aβ (Carro et al., 2002). Moreover, IGF-1 mediates transient site-selective increases in tau phosphorylation—hyperphosphorylated tau is a pathological hallmark of AD—in primary cortical neurons via GSK-3 pathways (Lesort and Johnson, 2000).

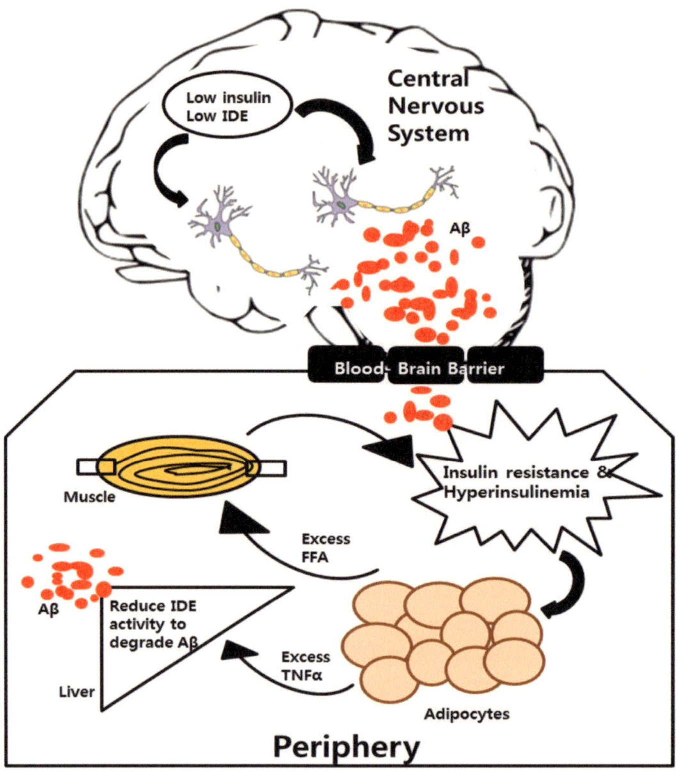

Fig. 1. Schematic diagram of the effects of peripheral insulin resistance on insulin, insulin-degrading enzyme (IDE) and Aβ levels. Peripheral insulin resistance and hyperinsulinemia triggers an excess release of FFA from adipocytes to liver and muscles. A three-fold increase of FFAs reduce insulin-dependent skeletal muscle glucose uptake by 50% (Roden et al., 1996), thereby hampering further insulin signal transduction (Hotamisligil et al., 1996; Schinner et al., 2005). In addition, Increased peripheral FFA levels invoke elevations in TNFα in the periphery and in the CNS, which may result in increased accumulation of Aβ. Chronic elevations in plasma Aβ may result in increased transport of Aβ into the brain. In contrast, peripheral hyperinsulinemia decrease insulin transport into the CNS. Low insulin level in CNS, and low level of IDE may contribute to the formation of senile plaques via disability to degrade Aβ peptides (Jones et al., 2009), further promoting intraneuronal Aβ accumulation, which is the hallmark of AD. <modified from Craft's paper (Craft, 2007)>

2.6 Insulin-degrading enzyme (IDE)

Insulin-degrading enzyme is the chief enzyme that degrades excess insulin and other substrates, including Aβ, a peptide that is implicated in the pathogenesis of AD (Wang et al., 2010). IDE knockout mice experienced decreased Aβ degradation, hyperinsulinemia, and hyperglycemia (Farris et al., 2003). As insulin levels rise, IDE expression increases to prevent the chronic activation of insulin (Zhao et al., 2004). Reduced IDE activity might contribute to the formation of senile plaques through the inability to degrade Aβ peptides (Jones et al., 2009).

3. Insulin resistance

3.1 Definition of insulin resistance

Insulin resistance is a physiological condition in which one loses or reduces his sensitivity to insulin—that is, it becomes less effective at lowering glucose levels in the blood. There are several representative phenotypes of insulin resistance that are used to diagnose diabetes, such as hyperinsulinemia (elevated levels of insulin that are required to maintain normal glucose levels in the bloodstream) and hyperglycemia (elevated glucose levels in the bloodstream that result from the failure of insulin to mediate glucose uptake or insufficient production of insulin by β-cells). Thus, insulin resistance reduces glycogen storage in muscle and fat cells and decreases hepatic glucose uptake.

High cortisol and uric acid levels and low vitamin D levels (Chiu et al., 2004; Vuorinen-Markkola and Yki-Jarvinen, 1994) are believed to be dietary conditions that precipitate insulin resistance. In addition, insulin resistance is closely related to obesity, hypertension, polycystic ovarian syndrome, dyslipidemia, and atherosclerosis (Saltiel and Pessin, 2002).

3.2 Peripheral effects of insulin resistance

Advanced glycation end products (AGEs) production is a pathological phenotype that results from hyperglycemia (Jager et al., 2007). Activation of the jun-N-terminal kinase (JNK) pathway by the binding of AGEs to their receptor (RAGE) leads to serine phosphorylation of IRS proteins and disrupts the imbalance in glucose levels further (Han et al., 2011). In addition to excess AGE production, prolonged hyperglycemia activates the transcription factor nuclear factor kappa B (NF-kB), which regulates proinflammatory and antiapoptotic pathways by modulating the transcription of cytokine and antioxidant genes (Baeuerle and Baltimore, 1996); it also controls the expression of genes that mediate immune responses and proliferation.

Peripheral insulin resistance mediates the progression to hyperglycemia and affects other functions of insulin. In particular, it affects reduced uptake of circulating lipids and increased hydrolysis of stored triglycerides. Such dysfunctional lipid homeostasis has been identified as a significant trigger of insulin resistance (Jones et al., 2009)

Because insulin resistance is linked to metabolic syndrome, which is generally characterized as overweightedness and obesity, and is often observed in persons with hyperglycemia and visceral adiposity, visceral fat is believed to accelerate insulin insensitivity, since visceral fat is less sensitive to the antilipolytic activity of insulin than subcutaneous fat (Jones et al., 2009), thereby triggering excessive release of free fatty acids (FFAs) (Schulingkamp et al., 2000) into the bloodstream. FFAs increase 3-fold above basal levels, reducing insulin-dependent skeletal muscle glucose uptake by 50% (Roden et al., 1996). This phenomenon, a direct cause of insulin resistance, induces inhibits serine phosphorylation of IRS and decreases its chances of binding to insulin receptor, further hampering insulin signaling (Hotamisligil et al., 1996; Schinner et al., 2005).

3.3 Central insulin resistance

As discussed, an abnormality in peripheral insulin is a risk factor for memory loss and neurodegeneration. In addition, chronic exposure of neurons to high insulin levels has a negative impact on memory, according to animal model studies. Chronic hyperinsulinemia impairs BBB function and IR activity and reduces insulin transport to the brain (Strachan et al., 1997). In contrast, some studies have noted that acute increases in brain insulin enhance memory (Craft et al., 1999; Park et al., 2000).

4. Link between insulin resistance and Alzheimer disease

Many studies have suggested that patients with diabetes have a higher risk of AD. Luchsinger et al. found that hyperinsulinemia increased risk for AD (Luchsinger et al., 2004). Also, it has been shown that high levels of insulin and insulin resistance are associated with a higher risk of AD in Rotterdam study, a population-based cohort study (Ott et al., 1999; Schrijvers et al., 2010). Although relationship between diabetes and AD remains controversial (Profenno et al., 2010), the abnormalities in insulin metabolism, which influence the onset of AD mechanistically, are believed to mediate AD through their influence on the synthesis and degradation of Aβ, tau hyperphosphorylation, oxidative stress and/or inflammation.

4.1 Impaired insulin/IGF-1 system in the AD brain

By positron emission tomography (PET) of early-stage AD and mild cognitive impairment (MCI), glucose uptake and metabolism decline significantly in the cortex (Jagust et al., 1991). According to another study, cerebral glucose utilization and blood flow fall by 45% and 18%, respectively, in the early stages of AD. In late-stage AD, cerebral blood flow is reduced by 65% (Hoyer and Nitsch, 1989). These data indicate that brain metabolism is altered in the AD brain, resembling T2DM. In addition, AD patients experience decreases in insulin in the CSF, reflecting dysregulation in insulin transport to the brain (Messier and White, 1987).

The AD brain also exhibits reduced expression of IR and IGF-1R, IRS, and trophic factors (Steen et al., 2005). IGF-1R expression decreases in AD brains in proportion to disease severity, and IGF-1 mRNA levels decline in late-stage AD (Frolich et al., 1998). IRS1/2 expression is decreased in the AD brain (Bosco et al., 2011; Squire, 1986). Because IRS1 and 2 regulate insulin and IGF-1 signaling, these findings suggest that insulin/IGF-1 signal transduction is altered in the AD brain.

There is much evidence of altered insulin signaling in AD. Inhibition of insulin/IGF-1 signaling in AD blocks the Wnt pathway (Doble and Woodgett, 2003), which mediates normal physiological processes in animals (Gogolla et al., 2009). Further, decreased PI3K signaling reduces GLUT4 translocation, inhibiting glucose uptake (Johnston et al., 2003). Since the brain depends on glucose as an energy source, altered glucose metabolism reduces the synthesis of acetyl-CoA and, ultimately, acetylcholine, an important neurotransmitter (Gibson et al., 1981). This decrease disrupts synaptic transmission and, consequently, impairs memory (Craft et al., 2003).

4.2 Insulin resistance and APP processing

Recent studies have indicated that abnormalities in insulin metabolism mediate the onset of AD through their influence on the synthesis and degradation of Aβ peptides (Table 1). Insulin significantly upregulates extracellular levels of Aβ40 and Aβ42 peptides through acceleration of amyloid precursor protein (APP)/Aβ trafficking from the Golgi/*trans*-Golgi network (TGN), a major site of Aβ generation, to the plasma membrane (Gasparini et al., 2001). Also, certain downstream signaling pathways of IR might also regulate the generation of Aβ peptides by modulating the expression or activity of β-secretase or γ-secretase (Phiel et al., 2003; Zhang et al., 2011), major components of APP processing (Edbauer et al., 2003; Vassar et al., 1999).

Under AD-like conditions, the expression levels of the neurotrophin receptors TrkA (tyrosine kinase receptor A) and p75NTR (p75 neurotrophin receptor) change markedly, increasing Aβ production by stabilizing β-secretase through the activation of sphingomyelinase (Puglielli et al., 2003). Chronic treatment of neuronal cells with IGF-1 (which induces insulin resistance) results in alteration in expression of TrkA and p75NTR, as in AD brains, increasing Aβ production (Costantini et al., 2006). Aβ is a ligand of p75NTR (Yaar et al., 1997), and Aβ stimulates p75NTR-mediated cell death in vitro and in vivo (Coulson, 2006; Sotthibundhu et al., 2008).

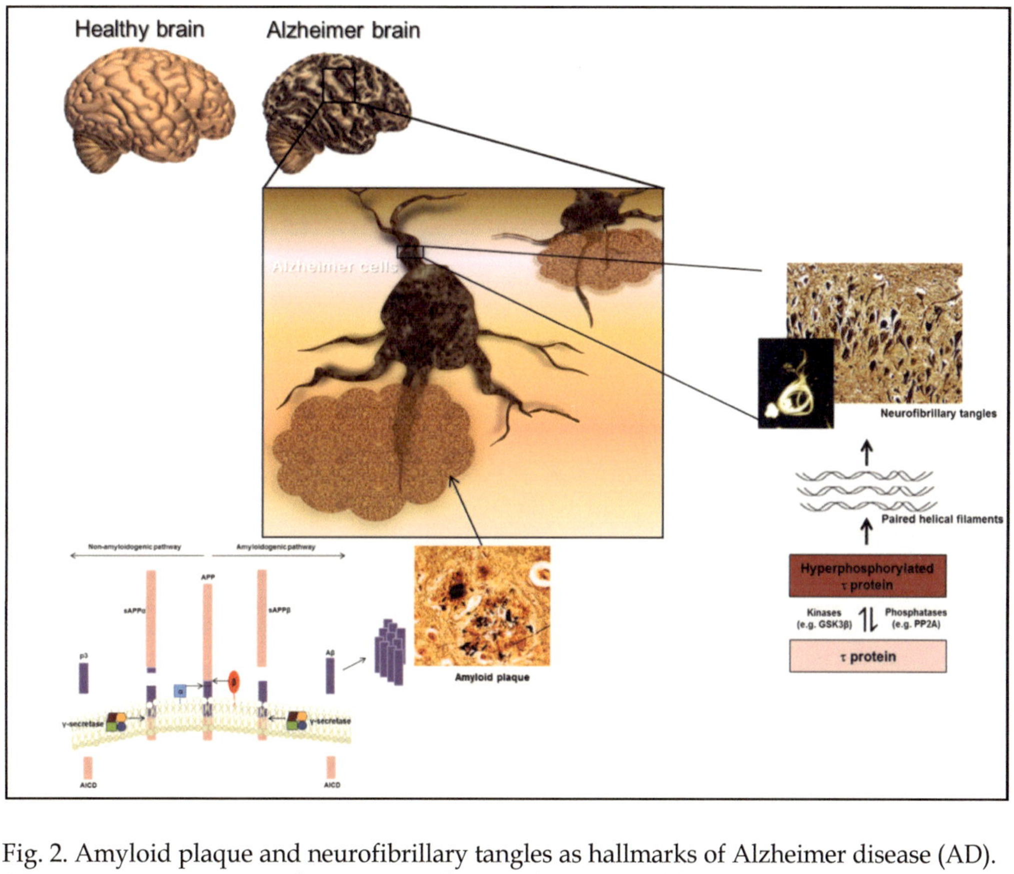

Fig. 2. Amyloid plaque and neurofibrillary tangles as hallmarks of Alzheimer disease (AD). AD is a progressive neurodegenerative disease characterized by senile plaques, neurofibrillary tangles and neuronal loss. Abnormal aggregates of amyloid-beta peptide (Aβ) are found in extracellular senile plaques and associated with neurodegeneration in AD. Neurofibrillary tangles are aggregates of the microtubule-associated protein (MAP) tau protein which is hyperphosphorylated by kinases and accumulated inside the neurons themselves.

In AD brains, Aβ accumulates on not only alterations in Aβ generation but also dysfunction of Aβ clearance. Several mechanisms of Aβ clearance have been examined: 1) Enzymatic degradation by microglia or endopeptidases, such as IDE (Qiu and Folstein, 2006), neprilysin (Iwata et al., 2000), endothelin-converting enzyme (ECE) (Eckman et al., 2003), angiotensin-converting enzyme (ACE) (Lehmann et al., 2005), matrix metalloproteinase-9 (MMP-9), and plasmin (Nalivaeva et al., 2008); 2) Influx into receptor-mediated transport across the BBB primarily via RAGE (Deane et al., 2003; Han et al., 2011); and 3) Receptor-mediated BBB transport by binding to low-density lipoprotein receptor-related protein-1 (LRP1) after ligation with apolipoprotein E (APOE) or α2-macroglobulin (α2M), to be delivered to peripheral sites of degradation (Shibata et al., 2000).

With regard to insulin resistance, insulin induces the accumulation of Aβ by limiting Aβ degradation through direct competition for IDE. IDE is a zinc metalloendopeptidase that preferentially cleaves proteins that tend to form β-pleated sheet-rich amyloid fibrils, such as Aβ peptides (Qiu and Folstein, 2006). IDE activity in the brain correlates negatively with Aβ levels (Farris et al., 2003), and IDE expression is decreased in the AD brain (Cook et al., 2003). Insulin regulates the levels of IDE, and insulin resistance reduces Aβ clearance by down-regulating IDE expression or competing with it for binding (Farris et al., 2003; Ho et al., 2004). A recent report has indicated that Aβ oligomers disrupt IR signaling, resulting from a rapid and substantial loss of neuronal IRs on dendrites by Aβ oligomer (Zhao et al., 2008). There is also evidence that Aβ reduces insulin binding to IRs and induces insulin resistance (Xie et al., 2002).

4.3 Insulin resistance and tau phosphorylation

AD is a multifactorial disease in which protein alterations, oxidative stress, inflammation, dysregulated immunity, impaired neuronal-glial communication, and increase of neurotoxic agents triggering neuronal death. AD is defined by Aβ pathology (Aβ plaques) and tau pathology [neurofibrillary tangles (NFTs)], but whether tau mediates AD pathology has been discussed for many years. Nevertheless, there is increasing evidence that when tau proteins assume pathological forms, they compromise neuronal function and affect cell death. These results suggest that tau is an important mediator of Aβ toxicity and AD pathology (Pritchard et al., 2011).

Microtubule (MT)-associated protein (MAP) tau is the major MT-associated phosphor-protein in normal neuronal cells (Cleveland et al., 1977). Normally, tau proteins assemble with tubulin to stabilize microtubules and vesicular transport. Neurofibrillary tangles are hyperphosphorylated and aggregated forms of tau proteins. When it is hyperphosphorylated, tau becomes insoluble and lacks affinity for microtubules, leading to neurodegeneration (Iqbal et al., 2005).

The kinases that regulate tau phosphorylation are grouped according to specificity: 1) proline-directed protein kinases, such as cyclin-dependent kinase 5 (CDK5), glycogen synthase kinase 3β (GSK3β), MAPK1, p38, JNK, and ERK2; and 2) nonproline-directed protein kinases, such as cAMP-dependent protein kinase A (PKA), PKC, CaMKII, CKII, and MAP/microtubule affinity-regulating kinase (MARK) (Baudier et al., 1987; Drewes et al., 1992; Goedert et al., 1997; Hanger et al., 1992; Morishima-Kawashima et al., 1995).

Tau hyperphosphorylation can also be induced by decreased dephosphorylation. Several protein phosphatases (PPs), including PP1, PP2A, PP2B, and PP5, catalyze tau dephosphorylation (Drewes et al., 1993; Liu et al., 2005). The appearance of tau hyperphosphorylation in the brain reflects an early stage of AD (Maccioni et al., 2010).

Insulin and IGF-1 are related to the phosphorylation state of tau (Table 1). Transient insulin treatment increases tau phosphorylation temporarily, correlating with the sequential activation and deactivation of GSK3β in SH-SY5Y cells (Lesort et al., 1999). Further, tau phosphorylation in primary cortical neurons is regulated by insulin and IGF-1 (Lesort and Johnson, 2000). In IRS-2 knockout mice, defects in IRS-2 signaling promotes neuronal death and induces the hyperphosphorylation of tau, suggesting that tau-mediated neurodegeneration is regulated by the IRS-2 branch of the insulin-IGF signaling pathway (Schubert et al., 2003).

Neuron-specific deletion of insulin receptor (neuronal/brain-specific insulin receptor knockout (NIRKO)) in mice leads to tau hyperphosphorylation (Schubert et al., 2004). However, the patterns of phosphorylation in NIRKO mice and IRS-2 knockout mice differ, suggesting that tau phosphorylation is regulated not only by insulin resistance, but also by other factors (e.g., hyperinsulinemia, hyperglycemia, inflammation) (Schubert et al., 2003; Schubert et al., 2004). There are other evidences on the relationship between insulin signaling and tau hyperphosphorylation. In IGF-1 knockout mice, tau is hyperphosphorylated at Ser202 and Ser396, implicating IGF-1 as protective against tau hyperphosphorylation (Cheng et al., 2005). Separately, the peripheral administration of insulin induced site-specific tau phosphorylation (at Ser202), which occurred rapidly after acute insulin administration but prolonged (Freude et al., 2005).

4.4 Insulin resistance and oxidative stress

The increase in oxidative stress and the resulting activation of many signaling pathways are associated with AD (Markesbery and Carney, 1999; Nunomura et al., 2001).

Oxidative stress is manifested by damage to proteins (Smith et al., 1991; Smith et al., 1996), lipids (Sayre et al., 1997), and nucleic acids (DNA, RNA) (Gabbita et al., 1998; Mecocci et al., 1994; Nunomura et al., 1999). In AD, neurons that show increased oxidative damage have significantly more mtDNA, indicating that mtDNA sustains high oxidative stress in AD (Hirai et al., 2001).

Mitochondria from the brains of AD patients experience structural damage and are the site of Aβ accumulation (Gouras et al., 2005; Hirai et al., 2001). Further, important mitochondrial enzymes become impaired in the brains of AD transgenic mice (Caspersen et al., 2005). Dysregulated mitochondria release oxidizing free radicals, with peroxidation of membrane lipids and the output of toxic aldehydes that cause considerable oxidative stress in AD (Smith et al., 1996).

Oxidative stress is a common feature in AD and insulin resistance. In Drosophila, oxidative stress increases signaling through c-Jun N-terminal kinase (JNK), which is a related pathway of AD and insulin resistance (Ozcan et al., 2004). Hydrogen peroxide-induced JNK activation induces γ-secretase activation, and increases Aβ generation (Shen et al., 2008). Insulin resistance leads to greater oxidative stress, DNA damage, mitochondrial dysfunction, and, ultimately, cell death (de la Monte, 2009). In AD patient brains, the expression of pro-oxidant enzymes that catalyze the generation of reactive nitrogen (RNS) and oxygen species (ROS), such as nitric oxide synthase (NOS) and NADPH oxidase (NOX), rises significantly, which accelerates insulin resistance in the brain (de la Monte and Wands, 2006).

4.5 Insulin resistance and inflammation

There are many reports that inflammation mediates the progress of AD. In brains of AD model mice and AD patients, Aβ plaque and NFTs activate astrocytes and microglia, resulting in the release of inflammatory molecules (cytokines and chemokines) and the production of complement, and ultimately causing neuroinflammation (Eikelenboom et al., 2002; Hoozemans et al., 2002; McGeer and McGeer, 2003; Tansey et al., 2007). In fact, in AD, neurons themselves induce the production of inflammatory molecules, such as interleukin (IL)-1, IL-6, TNF-α, and complement proteins (Li et al., 2000; Tchelingerian et al., 1996; Yu et al., 2002).Further, Aβ can attract and activate microglia, affecting the recruitment of microglia to Aβ plaques, and increase the secretion of proinflammatory molecules, such as IL-1, IL-6, and IL-8 (Rogers and Lue, 2001). Astrocytes are also activated by Aβ peptide to produce proinflammatory cytokines and chemokines in AD (Smits et al., 2002). Conversely, inflammatory cytokines, such as IL-6, regulate APP processing, resulting in elevation of Aβ42 levels (Papassotiropoulos et al., 2001).

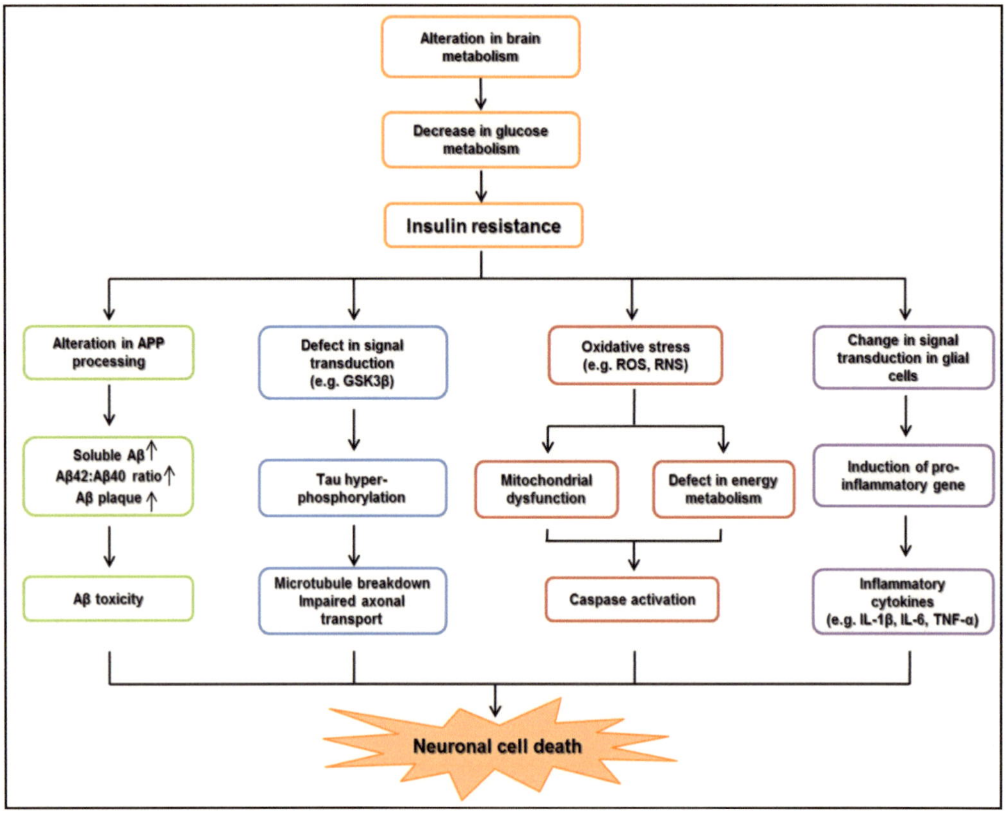

Fig. 3. Schematic representation of molecular pathways linking insulin resistance and Alzheimer disease. Peripheral insulin resistance leads to decrease insulin signaling in CNS, followed by alteration in brain metabolism. Increased Aβ toxicity, Tau hyperphosphorylation, oxidative stress and neuroinflammation are attributed to central insulin resistance, which leads to neurodegeneration.

Chronic administration of insulin induces inflammatory responses, although low doses of insulin is anti-inflammatory (Krogh-Madsen et al., 2004), suggesting that insulin contributes to inflammation. Several reports have noted that insulin modulates many inflammatory networks. Co-administration of insulin and lipopolysaccharide has a synergistic effect on the release of inflammatory cytokines, such as IL-1β and IL-6 (Soop et al., 2002). Insulin can regulate norepinephrine uptake in the locus coeruleus by modulating the expression of norepinephrine transporter protein (NET) (Figlewicz et al., 1993). Because norepinephrine is an endogenous anti-inflammatory neuromodulator that prevents IL-1β expression (Heneka et al., 2002), chronic administration of insulin might have abnormal inflammatory effects.

5. Clinical studies on insulin resistance and AD

Much evidence suggests that insulin resistance and peripheral hyperinsulinemia are risk factors for AD, implicating them as novel targets (Craft, 2005; Watson and Craft, 2003). For example, optimal doses of insulin and glucose in patients with AD improve declines in cognition (Watson et al., 2005). Using hyperinsulinemic-euglycemic clamps, intravenous insulin infusion in older subjects and in AD patients improves memory (Craft et al., 2003). Recently, intranasal administration of insulin was shown to improve cognitive function and modulate APP processing, resulting in increased Aβ40/Aβ42 ratio (Reger et al., 2008).

1. Aβ metabolism	
Insulin increases the extracellular level of Aβ by promoting its secretion.	(Gasparini et al., 2001)
Insulin increases the extracellular level of Aβ by inhibiting its degradation via insulin-degrading enzyme (IDE).	(Gasparini et al., 2001)
Chronic treatment with IGF-1 increases Aβ production by switching from TrkA to p75NTR.	(Costantini et al., 2006)
IGF-1 reduces BACE-1 expression in PC12 cells via activation of PI3K and ERK1/2 signaling pathways.	(Zhang et al., 2011)
IGF-1 enhanced APP phosphorylation at Thr668, contributing to the neuronal degeneration in AD.	(Araki et al., 2009; Chang et al., 2006)
Infusion of insulin under glucose clamp originated a rapid increase in CSF Aβ levels in older subject	(Watson and Craft, 2003)
Systemic administration of IGF-1 increases CSF Aβ levels.	(Carro et al., 2002)
IGF-1 increases neuronal excitability and release of Aβ is enhanced by neuronal activity.	(Gomez, 2008)
2. Tau hyperphosphorylation	
Insulin and IGF-1 treatment results in increase in tau phosphorylation in primary cortical neurons.	(Lesort and Johnson, 2000)
Peripheral administration of insulin induces site-specific tau phosphorylation (Ser202).	(Freude et al., 2005)
In IGF-1 knockout mice, tau is hyperphosphorylated at Ser202 and Ser396.	(Cheng et al., 2005)
In IRS-2 knockout mice, IRS-2 regulates tau-mediated neurodegeneration.	(Schubert et al., 2003)
Neuronal/brain-specific insulin receptor knockout (NIRKO) in mice leads to tau hyperphosphorylation.	(Schubert et al., 2004)

Table 1. The direct role for insulin or IGF-1 as a possible mediator of AD.

In addition to insulin, insulin-sensitizing compounds have been used as pharmacological treatments. Thiazolidinediones (TZDs) act as agonists of nuclear receptor PPAR-γ (peroxisome proliferator-activated receptor-gamma) and improve insulin sensitivity by reducing circulating insulin, FFA levels, and glucose uptake. TZDs are also anti-inflammatory drugs that decrease the levels of many inflammatory mediators (Jiang et al., 2008; Neumann et al., 2008; Rojo et al., 2008). Pioglitazone and rosiglitazone are some of the TZDs that are available for clinical use. The dual function of TZDs also affects hallmarks of AD pathogenesis, such as Aβ levels and tau hyperphosphorylation. PPAR-γ agonists, such as pioglitazone and indomethacin, can regulate Aβ42 levels and Aβ plaque loads (Heneka et al., 2005; Sastre et al., 2003).

Troglitazone decreases tau phosphorylation at Ser202 and Ser396/404 through a PPAR-γ-dependent/independent mechanism (d'Abramo et al., 2006). In a recent report, rosiglitazone reduced tau phosphorylation through JNK inhibition (Yoon et al., 2010).

TZDs improve memory in animal models and patients with AD. Rosiglitazone, a TZD, attenuates learning and memory deficits in Tg2576 mouse, an animal model of AD (Pedersen et al., 2006). Recently, pioglitazone was noted to preserve cognitive function in AD (Sato et al., 2009). This pilot study on 42 patients who were treated with 15-30 mg pioglitazone daily or placebo observed cognitive improvement in the pioglitazone groups. In another study, 511 AD patients were assigned to receive 2, 4, or 8 mg rosiglitazone (rosiglitazone group) or nothing (control group) (Risner et al., 2006); the rosiglitazone group improved cognition significantly, and this result was restricted to non-APOE ε4 carriers.

Insulin-sensitizing hormones, such as ghrelin, also affect AD pathogenesis. Ghrelin is a 28-amino-acid endogenous hormone that is a ligand of growth hormone secretagogue receptor 1a (GHSR-1a) (Kojima et al., 1999). Several studies have shown that ghrelin reduces tau hyperphosphorylation in high-glucose-induced neurons (Chen et al., 2010), and ghrelin enhances hippocampus-dependent memory in rodents (Carlini et al., 2010). Recently, Moon et al. observed that ghrelin ameliorates cognitive dysfunction in oligomeric Aβ42-injected mice (Moon et al., 2011). These and other reports demonstrate that brain insulin resistance leads to AD pathologies and thus suggest that insulin-sensitizing agents, such as the TZDs and ghrelin, are useful therapeutic agents.

6. Conclusion

Insulin resistance is characterized by chronic peripheral insulin elevations, central reduction of insulin levels and abnormality of insulin activity. Insulin modulates not only peripheral glucose metabolism but also normal brain function, and thereby conditions related to insulin dysregulation, such as obesity and diabetes mellitus, have deleterious effects on brain function. According to recent longitudinal studies, insulin resistance increases the risk of memory deficit and AD. Potential mechanisms linking insulin resistance to AD pathogenesis include the alteration in APP processing, defects in signal transduction related to both neuronal function (e.g. GSK3β) and cellular toxicity including oxidative stress and inflammation. Identification of underlying mechanisms for relevance of insulin resistance to AD is exigent goal to develop effective therapeutic strategies targeting AD. Many evidences have noted that agents modulating insulin resistance, including TZDs and insulin-sensitizing hormones, alleviate cognitive impairments associated with AD. Therapeutic strategies focused on preventing or regulating insulin resistance may thus benefit the development of drugs for AD.

7. Acknowledgement

This work was supported by Proteomics (FPR08B1-200), WCU-Neurocytomics, and KHID-ROAD grants.

8. References

Araki, W., Kume, H., Oda, A., Tamaoka, A. and Kametani, F. (2009). IGF-1 promotes beta-amyloid production by a secretase-independent mechanism. *Biochem Biophys Res Commun* 380, 111-4.

Baeuerle, P. A. and Baltimore, D. (1996). NF-kappa B: ten years after. *Cell* 87, 13-20.

Banks, W. A., Jaspan, J. B., Huang, W. and Kastin, A. J. (1997). Transport of insulin across the blood-brain barrier: saturability at euglycemic doses of insulin. *Peptides* 18, 1423-9.

Baudier, J., Lee, S. H. and Cole, R. D. (1987). Separation of the different microtubule-associated tau protein species from bovine brain and their mode II phosphorylation by Ca2+/phospholipid-dependent protein kinase C. *J Biol Chem* 262, 17584-90.

Benedict, C., Hallschmid, M., Hatke, A., Schultes, B., Fehm, H. L., Born, J. and Kern, W. (2004). Intranasal insulin improves memory in humans. *Psychoneuroendocrinology* 29, 1326-34.

Bevan, P. (2001). Insulin signalling. *J Cell Sci* 114, 1429-30.

Bosco, D., Fava, A., Plastino, M., Montalcini, T. and Pujia, A. (2011). Possible implications of Insulin Resistance and Glucose metabolism in Alzheimer's disease pathogenesis. *J Cell Mol Med.*

Carlini, V. P., Ghersi, M., Schioth, H. B. and de Barioglio, S. R. (2010). Ghrelin and memory: differential effects on acquisition and retrieval. *Peptides* 31, 1190-3.

Carro, E., Trejo, J. L., Gomez-Isla, T., LeRoith, D. and Torres-Aleman, I. (2002). Serum insulin-like growth factor I regulates brain amyloid-beta levels. *Nat Med* 8, 1390-7.

Caspersen, C., Wang, N., Yao, J., Sosunov, A., Chen, X., Lustbader, J. W., Xu, H. W., Stern, D., McKhann, G. and Yan, S. D. (2005). Mitochondrial Abeta: a potential focal point for neuronal metabolic dysfunction in Alzheimer's disease. *FASEB J* 19, 2040-1.

Chang, K. A., Kim, H. S., Ha, T. Y., Ha, J. W., Shin, K. Y., Jeong, Y. H., Lee, J. P., Park, C. H., Kim, S., Baik, T. K. et al. (2006). Phosphorylation of amyloid precursor protein (APP) at Thr668 regulates the nuclear translocation of the APP intracellular domain and induces neurodegeneration. *Mol Cell Biol* 26, 4327-38.

Chen, Y., Cao, C. P., Li, C. R., Wang, W., Zhang, D., Han, L. L., Zhang, X. Q., Kim, A., Kim, S. and Liu, G. L. (2010). Ghrelin modulates insulin sensitivity and tau phosphorylation in high glucose-induced hippocampal neurons. *Biol Pharm Bull* 33, 1165-9.

Cheng, C. M., Tseng, V., Wang, J., Wang, D., Matyakhina, L. and Bondy, C. A. (2005). Tau is hyperphosphorylated in the insulin-like growth factor-I null brain. *Endocrinology* 146, 5086-91.

Chiu, K. C., Chu, A., Go, V. L. and Saad, M. F. (2004). Hypovitaminosis D is associated with insulin resistance and beta cell dysfunction. *Am J Clin Nutr* 79, 820-5.

Clemmons, D. R. (2007). Modifying IGF1 activity: an approach to treat endocrine disorders, atherosclerosis and cancer. *Nat Rev Drug Discov* 6, 821-33.

Cleveland, D. W., Hwo, S. Y. and Kirschner, M. W. (1977). Physical and chemical properties of purified tau factor and the role of tau in microtubule assembly.*J Mol Biol*116, 227-47.

Cole, A. R., Astell, A., Green, C. and Sutherland, C. (2007). Molecular connexions between dementia and diabetes. *Neurosci Biobehav Rev* 31, 1046-63.

Conti, E., Andreotti, F., Sestito, A., Riccardi, P., Menini, E., Crea, F., Maseri, A. and Lanza, G. A. (2002). Reduced levels of insulin-like growth factor-1 in patients with angina pectoris, positive exercise stress test, and angiographically normal epicardial coronary arteries. *Am J Cardiol* 89, 973-5.

Cook, D. G., Leverenz, J. B., McMillan, P. J., Kulstad, J. J., Ericksen, S., Roth, R. A., Schellenberg, G. D., Jin, L. W., Kovacina, K. S. and Craft, S. (2003). Reduced hippocampal insulin-degrading enzyme in late-onset Alzheimer's disease is associated with the apolipoprotein E-epsilon4 allele. *Am J Pathol* 162, 313-9.

Costantini, C., Scrable, H. and Puglielli, L. (2006). An aging pathway controls the TrkA to p75NTR receptor switch and amyloid beta-peptide generation. *EMBO J* 25, 1997-2006.

Coulson, E. J. (2006). Does the p75 neurotrophin receptor mediate Abeta-induced toxicity in Alzheimer's disease? *J Neurochem* 98, 654-60.

Craft, S. (2005). Insulin resistance syndrome and Alzheimer's disease: age- and obesity-related effects on memory, amyloid, and inflammation. *Neurobiol Aging* 26 Suppl 1, 65-9.

Craft, S. (2007). Insulin resistance and Alzheimer's disease pathogenesis: potential mechanisms and implications for treatment. *Curr Alzheimer Res* 4, 147-52.

Craft, S., Asthana, S., Cook, D. G., Baker, L. D., Cherrier, M., Purganan, K., Wait, C., Petrova, A., Latendresse, S., Watson, G. S. et al. (2003). Insulin dose-response effects on memory and plasma amyloid precursor protein in Alzheimer's disease: interactions with apolipoprotein E genotype. *Psychoneuroendocrinology* 28, 809-22.

Craft, S., Asthana, S., Newcomer, J. W., Wilkinson, C. W., Matos, I. T., Baker, L. D., Cherrier, M., Lofgreen, C., Latendresse, S., Petrova, A. et al. (1999). Enhancement of memory in Alzheimer disease with insulin and somatostatin, but not glucose. *Arch Gen Psychiatry* 56, 1135-40.

d'Abramo, C., Ricciarelli, R., Pronzato, M. A. and Davies, P. (2006). Troglitazone, a peroxisome proliferator-activated receptor-gamma agonist, decreases tau phosphorylation in CHOtau4R cells. *J Neurochem* 98, 1068-77.

de la Monte, S. M. (2009). Insulin resistance and Alzheimer's disease. *BMB Rep* 42, 475-81.

de la Monte, S. M. and Wands, J. R. (2006). Molecular indices of oxidative stress and mitochondrial dysfunction occur early and often progress with severity of Alzheimer's disease. *J Alzheimers Dis* 9, 167-81.

Deane, R., Du Yan, S., Submamaryan, R. K., LaRue, B., Jovanovic, S., Hogg, E., Welch, D., Manness, L., Lin, C., Yu, J. et al. (2003). RAGE mediates amyloid-beta peptide transport across the blood-brain barrier and accumulation in brain. *Nat Med* 9, 907-13.

Devaskar, S. U., Giddings, S. J., Rajakumar, P. A., Carnaghi, L. R., Menon, R. K. and Zahm, D. S. (1994). Insulin gene expression and insulin synthesis in mammalian neuronal cells. *J Biol Chem* 269, 8445-54.

Doble, B. W. and Woodgett, J. R. (2003). GSK-3: tricks of the trade for a multi-tasking kinase. *J Cell Sci* 116, 1175-86.

Drewes, G., Lichtenberg-Kraag, B., Doring, F., Mandelkow, E. M., Biernat, J., Goris, J., Doree, M. and Mandelkow, E. (1992). Mitogen activated protein (MAP) kinase transforms tau protein into an Alzheimer-like state. *EMBO J* 11, 2131-8.

Drewes, G., Mandelkow, E. M., Baumann, K., Goris, J., Merlevede, W. and Mandelkow, E. (1993). Dephosphorylation of tau protein and Alzheimer paired helical filaments by calcineurin and phosphatase-2A. *FEBS Lett* 336, 425-32.

Eckman, E. A., Watson, M., Marlow, L., Sambamurti, K. and Eckman, C. B. (2003). Alzheimer's disease beta-amyloid peptide is increased in mice deficient in endothelin-converting enzyme. *J Biol Chem* 278, 2081-4.

Edbauer, D., Winkler, E., Regula, J. T., Pesold, B., Steiner, H. and Haass, C. (2003). Reconstitution of gamma-secretase activity. *Nat Cell Biol* 5, 486-8.

Eikelenboom, P., Bate, C., Van Gool, W. A., Hoozemans, J. J., Rozemuller, J. M., Veerhuis, R. and Williams, A. (2002). Neuroinflammation in Alzheimer's disease and prion disease. *Glia* 40, 232-9.

Farris, W., Mansourian, S., Chang, Y., Lindsley, L., Eckman, E. A., Frosch, M. P., Eckman, C. B., Tanzi, R. E., Selkoe, D. J. and Guenette, S. (2003). Insulin-degrading enzyme regulates the levels of insulin, amyloid beta-protein, and the beta-amyloid precursor protein intracellular domain in vivo. *Proc Natl Acad Sci U S A* 100, 4162-7.

Figlewicz, D. P., Szot, P., Israel, P. A., Payne, C. and Dorsa, D. M. (1993). Insulin reduces norepinephrine transporter mRNA in vivo in rat locus coeruleus. *Brain Res* 602, 161-4.

Florant, G. L., Singer, L., Scheurink, A. J., Park, C. R., Richardson, R. D. and Woods, S. C. (1991). Intraventricular insulin reduces food intake and body weight of marmots during the summer feeding period. *Physiol Behav* 49, 335-8.

Freude, S., Plum, L., Schnitker, J., Leeser, U., Udelhoven, M., Krone, W., Bruning, J. C. and Schubert, M. (2005). Peripheral hyperinsulinemia promotes tau phosphorylation in vivo. *Diabetes* 54, 3343-8.

Frolich, L., Blum-Degen, D., Bernstein, H. G., Engelsberger, S., Humrich, J., Laufer, S., Muschner, D., Thalheimer, A., Turk, A., Hoyer, S. et al. (1998). Brain insulin and insulin receptors in aging and sporadic Alzheimer's disease. *J Neural Transm* 105,423-38.

Gabbita, S. P., Lovell, M. A. and Markesbery, W. R. (1998). Increased nuclear DNA oxidation in the brain in Alzheimer's disease. *J Neurochem* 71, 2034-40.

Gasparini, L., Gouras, G. K., Wang, R., Gross, R. S., Beal, M. F., Greengard, P. and Xu, H. (2001). Stimulation of beta-amyloid precursor protein trafficking by insulin reduces intraneuronal beta-amyloid and requires mitogen-activated protein kinase signaling. *J Neurosci* 21, 2561-70.

Gibson, G. E., Peterson, C. and Jenden, D. J. (1981). Brain acetylcholine synthesis declines with senescence. *Science* 213, 674-6.

Goedert, M., Hasegawa, M., Jakes, R., Lawler, S., Cuenda, A. and Cohen, P. (1997). Phosphorylation of microtubule-associated protein tau by stress-activated protein kinases. *FEBS Lett* 409, 57-62.

Gogolla, N., Galimberti, I., Deguchi, Y. and Caroni, P. (2009). Wnt signaling mediates experience-related regulation of synapse numbers and mossy fiber connectivities in the adult hippocampus. *Neuron* 62, 510-25.

Gomez, J. M. (2008). Growth hormone and insulin-like growth factor-I as an endocrine axis in Alzheimer's disease. *Endocr Metab Immune Disord Drug Targets* 8, 143-51.

Gouras, G. K., Almeida, C. G. and Takahashi, R. H. (2005). Intraneuronal Abeta accumulation and origin of plaques in Alzheimer's disease. *Neurobiol Aging*26,1235-44.

Han, S. H., Kim, Y. H. and Mook-Jung, I. (2011). RAGE: The beneficial and deleterious effects by diverse mechanisms of actions. *Mol Cells* 31, 91-7.

Hanger, D. P., Hughes, K., Woodgett, J. R., Brion, J. P. and Anderton, B. H. (1992). Glycogen synthase kinase-3 induces Alzheimer's disease-like phosphorylation of tau: generation of paired helical filament epitopes and neuronal localisation of the kinase. *Neurosci Lett* 147, 58-62.

Heidenreich, K. A., Zahniser, N. R., Berhanu, P., Brandenburg, D. and Olefsky, J. M. (1983). Structural differences between insulin receptors in the brain and peripheral target tissues. *J Biol Chem* 258, 8527-30.

Heneka, M. T., Galea, E., Gavriluyk, V., Dumitrescu-Ozimek, L., Daeschner, J., O'Banion, M. K., Weinberg, G., Klockgether, T. and Feinstein, D. L. (2002). Noradrenergic depletion potentiates beta -amyloid-induced cortical inflammation: implications for Alzheimer's disease. *J Neurosci* 22, 2434-42.

Heneka, M. T., Sastre, M., Dumitrescu-Ozimek, L., Hanke, A., Dewachter, I., Kuiperi, C., O'Banion, K., Klockgether, T., Van Leuven, F. and Landreth, G. E. (2005). Acute treatment with the PPARgamma agonist pioglitazone and ibuprofen reduces glial inflammation and Abeta1-42 levels in APPV717I transgenic mice. *Brain* 128, 1442-53.

Hirai, K., Aliev, G., Nunomura, A., Fujioka, H., Russell, R. L., Atwood, C. S., Johnson, A. B., Kress, Y., Vinters, H. V., Tabaton, M. et al. (2001). Mitochondrial abnormalities in Alzheimer's disease. *J Neurosci* 21, 3017-23.

Ho, L., Qin, W., Pompl, P. N., Xiang, Z., Wang, J., Zhao, Z., Peng, Y., Cambareri, G., Rocher, A., Mobbs, C. V. et al. (2004). Diet-induced insulin resistance promotes amyloidosis in a transgenic mouse model of Alzheimer's disease. *FASEB J* 18, 902-4.

Hoozemans, J. J., Veerhuis, R., Rozemuller, A. J. and Eikelenboom, P. (2002). The pathological cascade of Alzheimer's disease: the role of inflammation and its therapeutic implications. *Drugs Today (Barc)* 38, 429-43.

Hotamisligil, G. S., Peraldi, P., Budavari, A., Ellis, R., White, M. F. and Spiegelman, B. M. (1996). IRS-1-mediated inhibition of insulin receptor tyrosine kinase activity in TNF-alpha- and obesity-induced insulin resistance. *Science* 271, 665-8.

Hoyer, S. and Nitsch, R. (1989). Cerebral excess release of neurotransmitter amino acids subsequent to reduced cerebral glucose metabolism in early-onset dementia of Alzheimer type. *J Neural Transm* 75, 227-32.

Huang, C. C., Lee, C. C. and Hsu, K. S. (2010). The role of insulin receptor signaling in synaptic plasticity and cognitive function. *Chang Gung Med J* 33, 115-25.

Huang, C. C., You, J. L., Lee, C. C. and Hsu, K. S. (2003). Insulin induces a novel form of postsynaptic mossy fiber long-term depression in the hippocampus. *Mol Cell Neurosci* 24, 831-41.

Iqbal, K., Alonso Adel, C., Chen, S., Chohan, M. O., El-Akkad, E., Gong, C. X., Khatoon, S., Li, B., Liu, F., Rahman, A. et al. (2005). Tau pathology in Alzheimer disease and other tauopathies. *Biochim Biophys Acta* 1739, 198-210.

Iwata, N., Tsubuki, S., Takaki, Y., Watanabe, K., Sekiguchi, M., Hosoki, E., Kawashima-Morishima, M., Lee, H. J., Hama, E., Sekine-Aizawa, Y. et al. (2000). Identification of the major Abeta1-42-degrading catabolic pathway in brain parenchyma: suppression leads to biochemical and pathological deposition. *Nat Med* 6, 143-50.

Jager, J., Gremeaux, T., Cormont, M., Le Marchand-Brustel, Y. and Tanti, J. F. (2007). Interleukin-1beta-induced insulin resistance in adipocytes through down-regulation of insulin receptor substrate-1 expression. *Endocrinology* 148, 241-51.

Jagust, W. J., Seab, J. P., Huesman, R. H., Valk, P. E., Mathis, C. A., Reed, B. R., Coxson, P. G. and Budinger, T. F. (1991). Diminished glucose transport in Alzheimer's disease: dynamic PET studies. *J Cereb Blood Flow Metab* 11, 323-30.

Jiang, Q., Heneka, M. and Landreth, G. E. (2008). The role of peroxisome proliferator-activated receptor-gamma (PPARgamma) in Alzheimer's disease: therapeutic implications. *CNS Drugs* 22, 1-14.

Johnston, A. M., Pirola, L. and Van Obberghen, E. (2003). Molecular mechanisms of insulin receptor substrate protein-mediated modulation of insulin signalling. *FEBS Lett* 546, 32-6.

Jones, A., Kulozik, P., Ostertag, A. and Herzig, S. (2009). Common pathological processes and transcriptional pathways in Alzheimer's disease and type 2 diabetes. *J Alzheimers Dis* 16, 787-808.

Kern, W., Born, J., Schreiber, H. and Fehm, H. L. (1999). Central nervous system effects of intranasally administered insulin during euglycemia in men. *Diabetes* 48, 557-63.

Kitamura, T., Kitamura, Y., Kuroda, S., Hino, Y., Ando, M., Kotani, K., Konishi, H., Matsuzaki, H., Kikkawa, U., Ogawa, W. et al. (1999). Insulin-induced phosphorylation and activation of cyclic nucleotide phosphodiesterase 3B by the serine-threonine kinase Akt. *Mol Cell Biol* 19, 6286-96.

Kojima, M., Hosoda, H., Date, Y., Nakazato, M., Matsuo, H. and Kangawa, K. (1999). Ghrelin is a growth-hormone-releasing acylated peptide from stomach. *Nature* 402, 656-60.

Kopf, S. R. and Baratti, C. M. (1999). Effects of posttraining administration of insulin on retention of a habituation response in mice: participation of a central cholinergic mechanism. *Neurobiol Learn Mem* 71, 50-61.

Krogh-Madsen, R., Plomgaard, P., Keller, P., Keller, C. and Pedersen, B. K. (2004). Insulin stimulates interleukin-6 and tumor necrosis factor-alpha gene expression in human subcutaneous adipose tissue. *Am J Physiol Endocrinol Metab* 286, E234-8.

Lehmann, D. J., Cortina-Borja, M., Warden, D. R., Smith, A. D., Sleegers, K., Prince, J. A., van Duijn, C. M. and Kehoe, P. G. (2005). Large meta-analysis establishes the ACE insertion-deletion polymorphism as a marker of Alzheimer's disease. *Am J Epidemiol* 162, 305-17.

Lesort, M. and Johnson, G. V. (2000). Insulin-like growth factor-1 and insulin mediate transient site-selective increases in tau phosphorylation in primary cortical neurons. *Neuroscience* 99, 305-16.

Lesort, M., Jope, R. S. and Johnson, G. V. (1999). Insulin transiently increases tau phosphorylation: involvement of glycogen synthase kinase-3beta and Fyn tyrosine kinase. *J Neurochem* 72, 576-84.

Li, Y., Barger, S. W., Liu, L., Mrak, R. E. and Griffin, W. S. (2000). S100beta induction of the proinflammatory cytokine interleukin-6 in neurons. *J Neurochem* 74, 143-50.

Liu, F., Grundke-Iqbal, I., Iqbal, K. and Gong, C. X. (2005). Contributions of protein phosphatases PP1, PP2A, PP2B and PP5 to the regulation of tau phosphorylation. *Eur J Neurosci* 22, 1942-50.

Lizcano, J. M. and Alessi, D. R. (2002). The insulin signalling pathway. *Curr Biol* 12, R236-8.

Luchsinger, J. A., Tang, M. X., Shea, S. and Mayeux, R. (2004). Hyperinsulinemia and risk of Alzheimer disease. *Neurology* 63, 1187-92.

Maccioni, R. B., Farias, G., Morales, I. and Navarrete, L. (2010). The revitalized tau hypothesis on Alzheimer's disease. *Arch Med Res* 41, 226-31.

Man, H. Y., Lin, J. W., Ju, W. H., Ahmadian, G., Liu, L., Becker, L. E., Sheng, M. and Wang, Y. T. (2000). Regulation of AMPA receptor-mediated synaptic transmission by clathrin-dependent receptor internalization. *Neuron* 25, 649-62.

Markesbery, W. R. and Carney, J. M. (1999). Oxidative alterations in Alzheimer's disease. *Brain Pathol* 9, 133-46.

McGeer, E. G. and McGeer, P. L. (2003). Inflammatory processes in Alzheimer's disease. *Prog Neuropsychopharmacol Biol Psychiatry* 27, 741-9.

Mecocci, P., MacGarvey, U. and Beal, M. F. (1994). Oxidative damage to mitochondrial DNA is increased in Alzheimer's disease. *Ann Neurol* 36, 747-51.

Messier, C. and White, N. M. (1987). Memory improvement by glucose, fructose, and two glucose analogs: a possible effect on peripheral glucose transport. *Behav Neural Biol* 48, 104-27.

Moon, M., Choi, J. G., Nam, D. W., Hong, H. S., Choi, Y. J., Oh, M. S. and Mook-Jung, I. (2011). Ghrelin ameliorates cognitive dysfunction and neurodegeneration in intrahippocampal amyloid-beta1-42 oligomer-injected mice. *J Alzheimers Dis* 23,147-59.

Morishima-Kawashima, M., Hasegawa, M., Takio, K., Suzuki, M., Yoshida, H., Titani, K. and Ihara, Y. (1995). Proline-directed and non-proline-directed phosphorylation of PHF-tau. *J Biol Chem* 270, 823-9.

Nalivaeva, N. N., Fisk, L. R., Belyaev, N. D. and Turner, A. J. (2008). Amyloid-degrading enzymes as therapeutic targets in Alzheimer's disease. *Curr Alzheimer Res* 5, 212-24.

Neumann, K. F., Rojo, L., Navarrete, L. P., Farias, G., Reyes, P. and Maccioni, R. B. (2008). Insulin resistance and Alzheimer's disease: molecular links & clinical implications. *Curr Alzheimer Res* 5, 438-47.

Nunomura, A., Perry, G., Aliev, G., Hirai, K., Takeda, A., Balraj, E. K., Jones, P. K., Ghanbari, H., Wataya, T., Shimohama, S. et al. (2001). Oxidative damage is the earliest event in Alzheimer disease. *J Neuropathol Exp Neurol* 60, 759-67.

Nunomura, A., Perry, G., Pappolla, M. A., Wade, R., Hirai, K., Chiba, S. and Smith, M. A. (1999). RNA oxidation is a prominent feature of vulnerable neurons in Alzheimer's disease. *J Neurosci* 19, 1959-64.

Ott, A., Stolk, R. P., Hofman, A., van Harskamp, F., Grobbee, D. E. and Breteler, M. M. (1996). Association of diabetes mellitus and dementia: the Rotterdam Study. *Diabetologia* 39, 1392-7.

Ott, A., Stolk, R. P., van Harskamp, F., Pols, H. A., Hofman, A. and Breteler, M. M. (1999). Diabetes mellitus and the risk of dementia: The Rotterdam Study. *Neurology* 53,1937-42.

Ozcan, U., Cao, Q., Yilmaz, E., Lee, A. H., Iwakoshi, N. N., Ozdelen, E., Tuncman, G., Gorgun, C., Glimcher, L. H. and Hotamisligil, G. S. (2004). Endoplasmic reticulum stress links obesity, insulin action, and type 2 diabetes. *Science* 306, 457-61.

Papassotiropoulos, A., Hock, C. and Nitsch, R. M. (2001). Genetics of interleukin 6: implications for Alzheimer's disease. *Neurobiol Aging* 22, 863-71.

Park, C. R., Seeley, R. J., Craft, S. and Woods, S. C. (2000). Intracerebroventricular insulin enhances memory in a passive-avoidance task. *Physiol Behav* 68, 509-14.

Pedersen, W. A., McMillan, P. J., Kulstad, J. J., Leverenz, J. B., Craft, S. and Haynatzki, G. R. (2006). Rosiglitazone attenuates learning and memory deficits in Tg2576 Alzheimer mice. *Exp Neurol* 199, 265-73.

Peters, A. (2011). The selfish brain: Competition for energy resources. *Am J Hum Biol* 23, 29-34.

Phiel, C. J., Wilson, C. A., Lee, V. M. and Klein, P. S. (2003). GSK-3alpha regulates production of Alzheimer's disease amyloid-beta peptides. *Nature* 423, 435-9.

Plum, L., Schubert, M. and Bruning, J. C. (2005). The role of insulin receptor signaling in the brain. *Trends Endocrinol Metab* 16, 59-65.

Pritchard, S. M., Dolan, P. J., Vitkus, A. and Johnson, G. V. (2011). The Toxicity of Tau in Alzheimer Disease: Turnover, Targets and Potential Therapeutics. *J Cell Mol Med.*

Profenno, L. A., Porsteinsson, A. P. and Faraone, S. V. (2010). Meta-analysis of Alzheimer's disease risk with obesity, diabetes, and related disorders. *Biol Psychiatry* 67, 505-12.

Proud, C. G. (2006). Regulation of protein synthesis by insulin. *Biochem Soc Trans* 34, 213-6.

Puglielli, L., Ellis, B. C., Saunders, A. J. and Kovacs, D. M. (2003). Ceramide stabilizes beta-site amyloid precursor protein-cleaving enzyme 1 and promotes amyloid beta-peptide biogenesis. *J Biol Chem* 278, 19777-83.

Qiu, W. Q. and Folstein, M. F. (2006). Insulin, insulin-degrading enzyme and amyloid-beta peptide in Alzheimer's disease: review and hypothesis. *Neurobiol Aging* 27, 190-8.

Rasmussen, M. H., Hvidberg, A., Juul, A., Main, K. M., Gotfredsen, A., Skakkebaek, N. E., Hilsted, J. and Skakkebae, N. E. (1995). Massive weight loss restores 24-hour growth hormone release profiles and serum insulin-like growth factor-I levels in obese subjects. *J Clin Endocrinol Metab* 80, 1407-15.

Reger, M. A., Watson, G. S., Green, P. S., Wilkinson, C. W., Baker, L. D., Cholerton, B., Fishel, M. A., Plymate, S. R., Breitner, J. C., DeGroodt, W. et al. (2008). Intranasal insulin improves cognition and modulates beta-amyloid in early AD. *Neurology* 70, 440-8.

Risner, M. E., Saunders, A. M., Altman, J. F., Ormandy, G. C., Craft, S., Foley, I. M., Zvartau-Hind, M. E., Hosford, D. A. and Roses, A. D. (2006). Efficacy of rosiglitazone in a genetically defined population with mild-to-moderate Alzheimer's disease. *Pharmacogenomics J* 6, 246-54.

Roden, M., Price, T. B., Perseghin, G., Petersen, K. F., Rothman, D. L., Cline, G. W. and Shulman, G. I. (1996). Mechanism of free fatty acid-induced insulin resistance in humans. *J Clin Invest* 97, 2859-65.

Rogers, J. and Lue, L. F. (2001). Microglial chemotaxis, activation, and phagocytosis of amyloid beta-peptide as linked phenomena in Alzheimer's disease. *Neurochem Int* 39, 333-40.

Rojo, L. E., Fernandez, J. A., Maccioni, A. A., Jimenez, J. M. and Maccioni, R. B. (2008). Neuroinflammation: implications for the pathogenesis and molecular diagnosis of Alzheimer's disease. *Arch Med Res* 39, 1-16.

Ronnemaa, E., Zethelius, B., Sundelof, J., Sundstrom, J., Degerman-Gunnarsson, M., Berne, C., Lannfelt, L. and Kilander, L. (2008). Impaired insulin secretion increases the risk of Alzheimer disease. *Neurology* 71, 1065-71.

Rulifson, E. J., Kim, S. K. and Nusse, R. (2002). Ablation of insulin-producing neurons in flies: growth and diabetic phenotypes. *Science* 296, 1118-20.

Saltiel, A. R. and Kahn, C. R. (2001). Insulin signalling and the regulation of glucose and lipid metabolism. *Nature* 414, 799-806.

Saltiel, A. R. and Pessin, J. E. (2002). Insulin signaling pathways in time and space. *Trends Cell Biol* 12, 65-71.

Sastre, M., Dewachter, I., Landreth, G. E., Willson, T. M., Klockgether, T., van Leuven, F. and Heneka, M. T. (2003). Nonsteroidal anti-inflammatory drugs and peroxisome proliferator-activated receptor-gamma agonists modulate immunostimulated processing of amyloid precursor protein through regulation of beta-secretase. *J Neurosci* 23, 9796-804.

Sato, R. (2010). Sterol metabolism and SREBP activation. *Arch Biochem Biophys* 501, 177-81.

Sato, T., Hanyu, H., Hirao, K., Kanetaka, H., Sakurai, H. and Iwamoto, T. (2009). Efficacy of PPAR-gamma agonist pioglitazone in mild Alzheimer disease. *Neurobiol Aging*.

Sayre, L. M., Zelasko, D. A., Harris, P. L., Perry, G., Salomon, R. G. and Smith, M. A. (1997). 4-Hydroxynonenal-derived advanced lipid peroxidation end products are increased in Alzheimer's disease. *J Neurochem* 68, 2092-7.

Scherer, T., O'Hare, J., Diggs-Andrews, K., Schweiger, M., Cheng, B., Lindtner, C., Zielinski, E., Vempati, P., Su, K., Dighe, S. et al. (2011). Brain insulin controls adipose tissue lipolysis and lipogenesis. *Cell Metab* 13, 183-94.

Schinner, S., Scherbaum, W. A., Bornstein, S. R. and Barthel, A. (2005). Molecular mechanisms of insulin resistance. *Diabet Med* 22, 674-82.

Schrijvers, E. M., Witteman, J. C., Sijbrands, E. J., Hofman, A., Koudstaal, P. J. and Breteler, M. M. (2010). Insulin metabolism and the risk of Alzheimer disease: the Rotterdam Study. *Neurology* 75, 1982-7.

Schubert, M., Brazil, D. P., Burks, D. J., Kushner, J. A., Ye, J., Flint, C. L., Farhang-Fallah, J., Dikkes, P., Warot, X. M., Rio, C. et al. (2003). Insulin receptor substrate-2 deficiency impairs brain growth and promotes tau phosphorylation. *J Neurosci* 23, 7084-92.

Schubert, M., Gautam, D., Surjo, D., Ueki, K., Baudler, S., Schubert, D., Kondo, T., Alber, J., Galldiks, N., Kustermann, E. et al. (2004). Role for neuronal insulin resistance in neurodegenerative diseases. *Proc Natl Acad Sci U S A* 101, 3100-5.

Schulingkamp, R. J., Pagano, T. C., Hung, D. and Raffa, R. B. (2000). Insulin receptors and insulin action in the brain: review and clinical implications. *Neurosci Biobehav Rev* 24, 855-72.

Shen, C., Chen, Y., Liu, H., Zhang, K., Zhang, T., Lin, A. and Jing, N. (2008). Hydrogen peroxide promotes Abeta production through JNK-dependent activation of gamma-secretase. *J Biol Chem* 283, 17721-30.

Shibata, M., Yamada, S., Kumar, S. R., Calero, M., Bading, J., Frangione, B., Holtzman, D. M., Miller, C. A., Strickland, D. K., Ghiso, J. et al. (2000). Clearance of Alzheimer's amyloid-ss(1-40) peptide from brain by LDL receptor-related protein-1 at the blood-brain barrier. *J Clin Invest* 106, 1489-99.

Shimomura, I., Bashmakov, Y., Ikemoto, S., Horton, J. D., Brown, M. S. and Goldstein, J. L. (1999). Insulin selectively increases SREBP-1c mRNA in the livers of rats with streptozotocin-induced diabetes. *Proc Natl Acad Sci U S A* 96, 13656-61.

Smith, C. D., Carney, J. M., Starke-Reed, P. E., Oliver, C. N., Stadtman, E. R., Floyd, R. A. and Markesbery, W. R. (1991). Excess brain protein oxidation and enzyme dysfunction in normal aging and in Alzheimer disease. *Proc Natl Acad Sci U S A* 88, 10540-3.

Smith, M. A., Perry, G., Richey, P. L., Sayre, L. M., Anderson, V. E., Beal, M. F. and Kowall, N. (1996). Oxidative damage in Alzheimer's. *Nature* 382, 120-1.

Smits, H. A., Rijsmus, A., van Loon, J. H., Wat, J. W., Verhoef, J., Boven, L. A. and Nottet, H. S. (2002). Amyloid-beta-induced chemokine production in primary human macrophages and astrocytes. *J Neuroimmunol* 127, 160-8.

Soop, M., Duxbury, H., Agwunobi, A. O., Gibson, J. M., Hopkins, S. J., Childs, C., Cooper, R. G., Maycock, P., Little, R. A. and Carlson, G. L. (2002). Euglycemic hyperinsulinemia augments the cytokine and endocrine responses to endotoxin in humans. *Am J Physiol Endocrinol Metab* 282, E1276-85.

Sotthibundhu, A., Sykes, A. M., Fox, B., Underwood, C. K., Thangnipon, W. and Coulson, E. J. (2008). Beta-amyloid(1-42) induces neuronal death through the p75 neurotrophin receptor. *J Neurosci* 28, 3941-6.

Squire, L. R. (1986). Mechanisms of memory. *Science* 232, 1612-9.

Steen, E., Terry, B. M., Rivera, E. J., Cannon, J. L., Neely, T. R., Tavares, R., Xu, X. J., Wands, J. R. and de la Monte, S. M. (2005). Impaired insulin and insulin-like growth factor expression and signaling mechanisms in Alzheimer's disease--is this type 3 diabetes? *J Alzheimers Dis* 7, 63-80.

Strachan, M. W., Deary, I. J., Ewing, F. M. and Frier, B. M. (1997). Is type II diabetes associated with an increased risk of cognitive dysfunction? A critical review of published studies. *Diabetes Care* 20, 438-45.

Tansey, M. G., McCoy, M. K. and Frank-Cannon, T. C. (2007). Neuroinflammatory mechanisms in Parkinson's disease: potential environmental triggers, pathways, and targets for early therapeutic intervention. *Exp Neurol* 208, 1-25.

Tchelingerian, J. L., Le Saux, F. and Jacque, C. (1996). Identification and topography of neuronal cell populations expressing TNF alpha and IL-1 alpha in response to hippocampal lesion. *J Neurosci Res* 43, 99-106.

Twickler, M. T., Cramer, M. J. and Koppeschaar, H. P. (2003). Unraveling Reaven's syndrome X: serum insulin-like growth factor-I and cardiovascular disease. *Circulation* 107, e190-2; author reply e190-2.

van der Heide, L. P., Kamal, A., Artola, A., Gispen, W. H. and Ramakers, G. M. (2005). Insulin modulates hippocampal activity-dependent synaptic plasticity in a N-methyl-d-aspartate receptor and phosphatidyl-inositol-3-kinase-dependent manner. *J Neurochem* 94, 1158-66.

Van Obberghen, E., Baron, V., Delahaye, L., Emanuelli, B., Filippa, N., Giorgetti-Peraldi, S., Lebrun, P., Mothe-Satney, I., Peraldi, P., Rocchi, S. et al. (2001). Surfing the insulin signaling web. *Eur J Clin Invest* 31, 966-77.

Vassar, R., Bennett, B. D., Babu-Khan, S., Kahn, S., Mendiaz, E. A., Denis, P., Teplow, D. B., Ross, S., Amarante, P., Loeloff, R. et al. (1999). Beta-secretase cleavage of Alzheimer's amyloid precursor protein by the transmembrane aspartic protease BACE. *Science* 286, 735-41.

Vuorinen-Markkola, H. and Yki-Jarvinen, H. (1994). Hyperuricemia and insulin resistance. *J Clin Endocrinol Metab* 78, 25-9.

Wang, S., Wang, R., Chen, L., Bennett, D. A., Dickson, D. W. and Wang, D. S. (2010). Expression and functional profiling of neprilysin, insulin-degrading enzyme, and endothelin-converting enzyme in prospectively studied elderly and Alzheimer's brain. *J Neurochem* 115, 47-57.

Wang, Y. T. and Linden, D. J. (2000). Expression of cerebellar long-term depression requires postsynaptic clathrin-mediated endocytosis. *Neuron* 25, 635-47.

Watson, G. S., Cholerton, B. A., Reger, M. A., Baker, L. D., Plymate, S. R., Asthana, S., Fishel, M. A., Kulstad, J. J., Green, P. S., Cook, D. G. et al. (2005). Preserved cognition in patients with early Alzheimer disease and amnestic mild cognitive impairment during treatment with rosiglitazone: a preliminary study. *Am J Geriatr Psychiatry* 13, 950-8.

Watson, G. S. and Craft, S. (2003). The role of insulin resistance in the pathogenesis of Alzheimer's disease: implications for treatment. *CNS Drugs* 17, 27-45.

Xie, L., Helmerhorst, E., Taddei, K., Plewright, B., Van Bronswijk, W. and Martins, R. (2002). Alzheimer's beta-amyloid peptides compete for insulin binding to the insulin receptor. *J Neurosci* 22, RC221.

Yaar, M., Zhai, S., Pilch, P. F., Doyle, S. M., Eisenhauer, P. B., Fine, R. E. and Gilchrest, B. A. (1997). Binding of beta-amyloid to the p75 neurotrophin receptor induces apoptosis. A possible mechanism for Alzheimer's disease. *J Clin Invest* 100, 2333-40.

Yoon, S. Y., Park, J. S., Choi, J. E., Choi, J. M., Lee, W. J., Kim, S. W. and Kim, D. H. (2010). Rosiglitazone reduces tau phosphorylation via JNK inhibition in the hippocampus of rats with type 2 diabetes and tau transfected SH-SY5Y cells.*Neurobiol Dis* 40, 449-55.

Yu, J. X., Bradt, B. M. and Cooper, N. R. (2002). Constitutive expression of proinflammatory complement components by subsets of neurons in the central nervous system. *J Neuroimmunol* 123, 91-101.

Zhang, H., Gao, Y., Dai, Z., Meng, T., Tu, S. and Yan, Y. (2011). IGF-1 reduces BACE-1 expression in PC12 cells via activation of PI3-K/Akt and MAPK/ERK1/2 signaling pathways. *Neurochem Res* 36, 49-57.

Zhao, L., Teter, B., Morihara, T., Lim, G. P., Ambegaokar, S. S., Ubeda, O. J., Frautschy, S. A. and Cole, G. M. (2004). Insulin-degrading enzyme as a downstream target of insulin receptor signaling cascade: implications for Alzheimer's disease intervention. *J Neurosci* 24, 11120-6.

Zhao, W., Chen, H., Xu, H., Moore, E., Meiri, N., Quon, M. J. and Alkon, D. L. (1999). Brain insulin receptors and spatial memory. Correlated changes in gene expression, tyrosine phosphorylation, and signaling molecules in the hippocampus of water maze trained rats. *J Biol Chem* 274, 34893-902.

Zhao, W. Q., De Felice, F. G., Fernandez, S., Chen, H., Lambert, M. P., Quon, M. J., Krafft, G. A. and Klein, W. L. (2008). Amyloid beta oligomers induce impairment of neuronal insulin receptors. *FASEB J* 22, 246-60.

Part 2

Novel Treatments

4

Incretin-Based Treatment Strategy - GLP-1 Receptor Agonists (GLP-1R) or So-Called Incretin Mimetics

Jindra Perusicova and Klara Owen
Charles University, Prague,
Czech Republic

1. Introduction

The pharmacotherapy of Type 2 Diabetes Mellitus (T2DM) has, in the past 60 years, been developing in unison with the advances in our understanding of diabetes pathophysiology. As our knowledge developed and changed, so did appear new drugs which better and in more targeted fashion rectified the pathological processes leading to the development of diabetes.

If we look into the history of T2DM treatment, the first antidiabetic medicine was insulin - a hormone. Insulin is without a doubt the most important hormone in regulation of glycaemia. The secretion of insulin in response to increasing glucose levels in the bloodstream postprandially is influenced by several mechanisms in three stages:

- Neuronal (cephalic) phase
- Gastro-enteral phase (in response to gastrointestinal hormones)
- Nutritional phase (beta cell stimulation in response to nutrients - glucose, aminoacids, FFA)

The gastro-enteral phase has been described many years ago as entero-insular axis. This description has been based on observation that the same glucose load administered orally stimulates higher insulin response than when administered intravenously. The difference has been described as an 'incretin effect'.

However, for decades to come, oral antidiabetics have never been able to capitalise on this mechanisms and took the route of influencing glucose homeostasis via peripheral insulin resistance, endogenous hepatic glucose production, or direct stimulation of beta cells.

Currently, it is understood that glucose homeostasis is governed by complex interaction of several hormones: Insulin, amylin, incretins (GLP-1, GIP and possibly others) in balance with the contraregulatory hormones that include glucagon, cortisol, catecholamines and GH with IGF-1. Our understanding of diabetes pathophysiology has developed from dual basis of insulin resistance (IR) and insulin deficiency (ID), via trio of IR in skeletal muscle, ID in beta cell and increased hepatic gluconeogensis, all the way to DeFronzo's (2009) 'Ominous Octet' of muscle, liver, and β-cell dysfunction, and additionally, fat cell pathology (accelerated lipolysis), gastrointestinal tract (incretin deficiency/resistance), α-cell (hyperglucagonemia), kidney (increased glucose reabsorption), and brain (insulin resistance) disorders.

Such advances in the understanding of the pathological basis of diabetes led, after a long time, to development of new drugs to treat hyperglycaemia of diabetes, notably three quite unique antidiabetics, approved by the FDA (Food and Drug Administration) for clinical use:

- Pramlintide in March 2005
- Exenatide in April 2005, and
- Sitagliptin in October 2006

First experiences with these new drugs were quite varied, ranging from almost euphoria in some authors regarding their ability to lower glycaemia, to quite open scepticism and urging to use the new medicines only to those not reaching adequate diabetic compensation with traditional medication, which is much cheaper and with well documented long term efficacy and safety data.

However, over time new strategies for treatment of DM2T have been developed, with some amendments to treatment guidelines to incorporate the new drugs (ADA 2011) and according to expectations, pharmaceutical companies introduced a host of new molecules, notably in the classes of incretin therapy - incretin enhancers (gliptins) and incretin mimetics (analogues of glucagon-like peptide 1) or, more accurately, agonists of GLP-1 receptor.

We therefore have another hormonal treatment option, apart from insulin, based on the GLP-1 hormone. GLP-1 has been selected as a target for therapeutic intervention due to the fact that it has been demonstrated that Type 2 diabetics have got lower level of GLP-1 in their bloodstream and are somewhat resistant to its action, compared to same-weight same-age nondiabetic individuals. Secondly, GLP-1 is the most potent of known incretins, in stimulation of postprandial insulin secretion.

GLP-1 is a peptide with 30-31 aminoacids, produced from proglucagon in L cells of distal ileum and proximal colon. Its target tissue is in pancreas; it stimulates insulin secretion in beta cells and inhibits glucagon secretion in alpha cells. Its bloodstream level rises 5-10times postprandially, with half-life of just 2 minutes and it exerts its action by binding to a specific receptor. It is excreted by kidney via glomerular filtration and tubular catabolism. Specific receptors for GLP-1 are present not only in the membrane of beta and alpha cells of the pancreas, but throughout the body - in the liver, central and peripheral nervous tissues, in the heart, lungs, kidneys and the gastrointestinal tract (Martin, 2011) A fine tuned cooperation of tissues and organs is needed to achieve normoglycaemia (Table 1.)

Due to GLP-1 action on the suppression of glucagon secretion, and its effect on delaying gastric emptying, it exerts multiple effects on glucose homeostasis: it increases the feeling if satiety, reduces hunger and can lead to a moderate weight loss. It plays a substantial role in DM2T, and the disruption in GLP-1 production and action can lead to impaired glucose tolerance.

In the pancreas, GLP-1 not only influences the production and secretion of insulin in the beta cell, but can also stimulate proliferation and neogenesis of beta cells and was shown to delay their apoptosis (Keating, 2005).

As was noted earlier, Type 2 diabetics suffer from decreased GLP-1 production, have decreased GLP-1 levels in the bloodstream and decreased sensitivity to GLP-1 after it binds to its receptor. The decreased sensitivity of beta cells can be overcome by supraphysiological (pharmacological) doses of GLP-1 receptor agonists. This was demonstrated in vivo by GLP-1 infusion to Type 2 diabetics. However, due to the short half life of GLP-1, which is immediately cleaved by dipeptidylpeptidase-IV enzymes, native GLP-1 is unsuitable for subcutaneous administration.

Pancreas	
	Increase in glucose stimulated insulin secretion
	Increase in insulin gene transcription
	Decrease in glucagon secretion
	Increase in somatostatin secretion
	Increased beta cells responsiveness to glucose
	Neogenesis and proliferation of beta cells
Gastrointestinal tract	
	Delayed gastric emptying
	Decrease in gastric acid production
Cardiovascular system	
	Modest decrease in blood pressure
Central nervous system	
	Reduction in appetite
	Increased production of TSH, LH and corticoids
Fat tissue	
	Increase in insulin mediated glucose uptake in fat cells
Muscle and liver	
	Increase in glycogen production

Table 1. Biological actions of GLP-1

Understanding the production, the promising effects and the pathway of degradation of GLP-1, lead to the development of two classes of drugs. Firstly, drugs that would 'mime' the effect of native GLP-1 and activate the processes following its binding to specific receptor, whilst being resistant to enzymatic cleavage, the incretin mimetics, which act very much like GLP-1, and vary from native GLP-1 only in the substitution in some of its aminoacids. This substitution prevents DPP-IV from binding to the molecule and allows for the GLP-1 like effect to last many hours (Burcelin, 2008).

Secondly, GLP-1 levels in Type 2 diabetics can be increased by reversible inhibition of DPP-IV action, which can be achieved by the other class of incretin-based therapies, the incretin enhancers, also known as gliptins.

In 2008, one of the first reviews of incretin therapy was published by Girard. Let us continue the journey and examine the recent history. GLP-1 is one example how modern diabetology ignored important pathways in regulation of glucose metabolism, notably:

- The action of entero-insular axis,
- Designating DM2T as bi-hormonal disease.

Entero-insular axis, in terms of enhanced insulin response in reaction to orally administered glucose in comparison to intravenous administration, has been discussed earlier.

Unger and Orci, in 1975, proposed a theory of Type 2 diabetes as a bi-hormonal disease, with the crucial role of insulin-glucagon interplay, or more exactly beta and alpha cells interaction, rather than just a disruption in insulin secretion and action, as thought previously.

If we administer insulin to a patient with absolute insulin deficiency, as in Type 1 diabetes, we perform a substitution therapy which leads, to a large degree to a normalisation of physiological functions. Type 2 diabetes, however, is marked by only relative insulin

deficiency where insulin administration only rectifies the pathophysiological processes and re-establishes new equilibrium between insulin sensitivity and insulin levels by overcoming, or compensating insulin resistance. We now know, that type 2 diabetics have got disturbances in the incretin effect produced by gut hormones. After meal stimulation T2 diabetics produce moderately less of the active GLP-1, with relatively preserved action. Moreover, chronic hyperglycaemia of diabetes increases the production and activity of DPP-IV enzymes, increasing the cleavage of active GLP-1 (Perušičová 2009, Asmar 2009) These two mechanisms are probably responsible for the decrease in GLP-1 action in T2 diabetics. Such observation is very important for treatment strategy.
GLP-1 analogues are available for clinical use for 6 years in the US, and for 4 years in Europe. During this time we have been flooded with new data on their action, safety and efficacy in humans. One recent review summarised the most important information known so far thus:

- Confirmed observations
  - GLP-1 stimulates insulin secretion in glucose-dependent manner
  - It increases beta cell proliferation and delays its apoptosis.
- New observations
  - The action of GLP-1 is not limited to only pancreatic islet cells, but regulates the function of many other organs
  - GLP-1 has got marked beneficial effect on the brain and cardiovascular system

These new observations open the way to possible therapeutic use of incretins in the treatment of cardiovascular disease (as is already being investigated for instance by a prospective, randomised 5 year study of liraglutide LEADER: *Liraglutide* Effect and Action in Diabetes: Evaluation of cardiovascular outcome) and obesity (Asmar, 2010).

2. Incretin mimetics

Incretin mimetics are the first class of hypoglycaemic drugs that influence glycaemia not only by modifying insulin secretion and action, but also by lowering increased glucagon levels.
All currently available GLP-1 analogues show the same multiple effects as native GLP-1:

- Increase in insulin secretion
- Increase in proinsulin synthesis in beta cells
- Suppression in glucagon secretion from alpha cells
- Slower gastric emptying
- Increased feeling of satiety, decrease in food intake
- Increase in proliferation and delay in apoptosis of pancreatic cells.

Especially the generally supportive and nutritive effect of GLP-1 on pancreatic islet cell mass is subject to intense study and scrutiny. If was believe, that DM2T can only manifest itself in the presence of the dual defect of insulin resistance and insulin deficiency, then this unique action of this class of antidiabetics could play a crucial role in treatment strategy of Type 2 diabetics.
Experimental studies in vitro on isolated beta cells and in vivo on animals have confirmed the stimulating effect of GLP-1 on beta cell proliferation as well as on their neogenesis. The observed increase in beta cell mass in these studies is also due to the delayed apoptosis which is, in diabetics, mainly increased due to glucotoxicity and lipotoxicity.

Apart from increase in insulin levels, GLP-1 is equally responsible for a significant decrease in glucagon levels. In higher doses GLP-1 leads to delayed gastric emptying and an increase in the feeling of satiety, which is extremely beneficial in weight management of obese DM2T patients. Whether these mechanisms of antidiabetic action of incretin hormones are sufficient to delay or prevent the onset of DM2T remains to be elucidated by valid and long term studies. To date we have the longest experience with exenatide, the first GLP-1 analogue on the market, and its short and long term effects are summarised in Table 2.

Acute administration	Chronic administration
Increase in glucose dependent insulin secretion	Decrease in food intake
Return to bi-phasic insulin response	Decrease in body weight
Suppression of increased glucagon production	Increase in insulin sensitivity
Delayed gastric emptying	Increase in proinsulin synthesis

Table 2. Immediate and chronic effects of exenatide in DM 2T

Every treatment option interests us not only from the viewpoint of efficacy in reducing hyperglycemia, but also in terms of added value, most notably in preventing the development of cardiovascular complications of diabetes. Many experimental and clinical studies investigated potential beneficial effects of GLP-1 and its analogues, demonstrating that such effect really exists, both indirectly, due to decrease in glycaemia, lipid levels and BMI, but more importantly directly, through the effects of:

- GLP-1 binding to brain centres regulating blood pressure and heart rate
- Positive influence on action and survival of cardiomyocytes

In view of available data, many authors conclude that it is highly likely that GLP-1 has positive protective effects on beta cells, neurones and cardiac myocytes (Gautier 2008, Holmes 2009). GLP-1 mimetics can also play a significant role in ameliorating endothelial dysfunction and protecting ischemic myocardial cells. Nathanson (2010) published 13-year observation study of 294 subjects with normal glucose tolerance who developed ischemic heart disease. They found direct link between impaired GLP-1 levels and the development of IGT, but not with DM2T. Also, there didn't seem to be any predictive value of GLP-1 levels in terms of subsequent ischemic heart disease.

Systematic meta-analysis of all published data on incretin-based therapies has been conducted in 2007 by Amori (2007). It reviewed 355 available papers from MEDLINE and Cochrane database to include 29 studies which fulfilled the entry criteria. The authors conclude that GLP-1 analogues:

- Lower HbA1c on average by 0.97% (range -1.13 to -0.81%)
- Lower weight on average by 1.4kg compared to placebo and -4.8kg compared to insulin
- Side effects include nausea (RR 2.9, range 2.0-4.2) and vomiting (RR3.2, range 2.5-4.4)

The effects of GLP-1 and it analogues also excited significant attention of researchers and clinicians. The role of GLP-1 in delayed gastric emptying and suppression of hunger suggest that disruptions to GLP-1 production or action could play an important role in the pathogenesis of obesity.

Such theory has been investigated by a study from 2004 (Lugari et al.), measuring the changes in postprandial levels of GLP-1 and DPP-IV activity which is responsible for the quick cleavage of native GLP-1. The subjects were 22 morbidly obese nondiabetics (BMI 47.5+-1.8 kg/m2) and 9 healthy, age-matched controls. A standard mixed meal of 700kcal has been administered, and the levels of glucose, insulin, GLP-1, and the DPP-IV activity have been measured 4times in the 120minutes postprandially. Furthermore, the same test has been carried out in formerly morbidly obese patients who underwent billiopancreatic diversion (BPD) and have lost at least 5% of their excess weight (BMI 33.8+-1.1 kg/m2). The authors conclude:

- Morbid obesity is at least in part responsible for the accelerated inactivation of GLP-1. Decreased levels of GLP-1 in turn lead to a decrease in the feeling of satiety postprandially, contributing to the abnormal eating patterns of the obese.
- Plasma hyperactivity of DPP-IV does not seem to be influenced by the degree of obesity. The BPD patients showed short increase in GLP-1 levels post-operatively, but this was probably due to the gut manipulation during surgery.

If accelerated cleavage of GLP-1 in obesity is confirmed in further studies, it could present a useful target for treatment of obesity with selective DPP-IV inhibitors.

Long term effects of incretin based therapies (in case of DM longer than 5 years), are not confirmed yet and we have to wait for the results of currently running trials or the acquisition of our own clinical experience.

Most authors welcomed the development of other classes of drugs, GLP-1 mimetics and DPP-IV inhibitors, however, many questions regarding their long-term efficacy, safety, duration of hypoglycaemic effects, and significance of some of their side effects remain to be answered (Penfornis, 2008; Olansky 2010).

On the other hand, many authors advocate the early use of incretin based therapies, not only DPP-IV inhibitors but also GLP-1 agonists, as first line treatment, or as an early add-on in single metformin failure, as they do not pose the risk of hypoglycaemia and have no or beneficial effects on body weight (Henquin, 2008). If a patient follows a majority of lifestyle recommendations, and in the absence of clear insulin deficiency as measured by low C-peptide, it indeed seems to be prudent to prefer rectifying the underlying pathophysiology and improve, via GLP-1 receptor stimulation, the alpha and beta cell crosstalk, and stimulate insulin secretion in glycaemia dependent manner whilst suppressing glucagon production. One question remains, and that is of the durability of such effects.

It has been newly confirmed, that L cells of intestinal epithelium, producing glucagon, GLP-1 and GLP-2 are not the single source of incretins and that the glucagon gene is present not only in the gut, but in neurons and brainstem cells. Glucagon is produced in alpha cells of pancreatic islets from proglucagon, with chain of 160 aminocids. After the cleavage, two probably inactive fragments remain PG1-30 and PG 72-158. In the L-cells of distal ileum, proglucagon is cleaved to give rise to:

- GLP-1 (PG 7-107 amide), potent incretin regulating insulin secretion, glucagon secretion, gastric motility and appetite,
- GLP-2 (PG126-158), significant regulator of growth and mucosal integrity, and
- Glicentin (PG 1-69), whose function is unknown

All three hormones are eliminated mainly by the kidneys, but significant proportion of GLP-2 and some GLP-1 are cleaved and rendered inactive locally and in liver due to DPP-IV action. This would suggest a more paracrine role of GLP-1 rather than classic endocrine one, and there are significant gaps in our understanding of expression of glucagon genes and tissue specific processes that would help us grasp the whole process (Holst 2010).

3. Incretin-based therapy and cardiovascular risk

GLP-1 improves glycaemia and lowers body weight. Both these effects are significant in lowering the increased cardiovascular risk of DM2T. But we are in possession of many more results and studies targeting this issue. There is evidence that native GLP-1 as well as GLP-1 agonists improve the markers of subclinical inflammation as measured by C-reactive protein (Pannaciulli, 2002). GLP-1 could also improve the production of VEGF (vascular endothelial growth factor), which contributes to improvement of EPCs (endothelial progenitor cells) biological function. Circulating EPCs play an important role in preserving endohelium's integrity by aiding neovascularization and reendothelization after injury (Xiao-Yun X, 2011). A clinical studies in diabetic volunteers confirmed that GLP-1 effect on insulin secretion is accompanied by endothelium protective effect, possibly glycaemia related, by decreasing the circulating markers of oxidative stress (Ceriello, 2011).
Other possible beneficial effects on cardiovascular system have been noted in the role of GLP-1 in renal sodium excretion. Double blind, placebo controlled study in 15 healthy nonobese men and 16 obese men monitored the effect of 3-hour GLP-1 infusion on sodium excretion and glomerular filtration after intravenous administration of 9.9g of NaCl. Infusion of GLP-1 lead to statistically significant increase in sodium excretion in the nonobese from 74±8 to 143±18mmol/180 minutes. In the obese sodium excretion increased from 59 to 96 mmol/180 minutes and the hydrogen excretion decreased from 1,1 to 0,3 pmol/180 minutes. At the same time, glomerular filtration decreased from 151 to 142 ml/min in the obese. Authors conclude, that GLP-1 potentially has renoprotective effects, thanks to its action in the proximal tubulus (Gutzwiller, 2004).

4. GLP-1 receptor agonists

4.1 Exenatide

Exenatide was the first GLP-1 receptor agonists introduced into clinical practice. The evaluation of it efficacy and safety in the phase III of clinical trials showed, that as an add-on to sulphonylureas, metformin, thiazolidinediones or their combinations (Buse, 2004; Kendall, 2005) exenatide can achieve the decrease in A1c of 0.8–1.0 percentage points. Moreover, exenatide lead to the significant decrease in weight, by 1.5–3 kg in the first 30 weeks of trials, which continued in the extension of up to 80 weeks, reaching the average 4–5 kg. At the same time, depending on the weight loss achieved, the parameters of cardiovascular factors improved. A decrease in blood pressure, triglyceride levels and an increase in HDL cholesterol levels have been noted, at 30 weeks not statistically significant, but at 3.5 years of follow-up reaching statistical significance. In preclinical trials, exenatide infusion showed beneficial effects not only on beta cells, but also on alpha cells of pancreatic islets, as measured by the insulin/proinsulin ratio and the glucagon levels.
These three pivotal (randomised, placebo controlled and double blind) studies, that have been twice extended, are the *cornerstone of introducing GLP-1 analogues into clinical practice.*
These results also make exenatide one of hypoglycaemic drugs that have the potential to improve atherosclerosis risk factors and thus it has been studied to confirm the possible beneficial influence of incretin-based therapies on cardiovascular system.
It has been confirmed that, similarly to native GLP-1, exenatide can influence other clinical parameters, which in turn can change glucose tolerance of the patient:
- Regulation of satiety and gastric emptying,
- Regulation of water and electrolyte balance

4.1.1 Mechanism of action

Exenatide acts as a replacement of insufficient native GLP-1 level. However, as it is administered in non-physiological route, subcutaneously into peripheral circulation, the circulating levels reach into pharmacological, i.e. significantly higher than physiological amounts of endogenous GLP-1. Such substitution treatment is warranted as the lower GLP-1 levels are found already at the time of DM2T diagnosis, partly due to the hyperglycaemia induced hyperactivity of DPP-IV enzymes. If, after hyperglycaemia is reduced due to improved lifestyle or due to metformin administration, and reduced GLP-1 levels persist, the administration of GLP-1 analogues is a natural next step.

However, in the current clinical practice we cannot measure GLP-1 levels, and therefore we have to wait for the results of clinical studies that would help us identify the patients who would benefit the most from GLP-1 administration.

4.1.2 Tolerability

Exenatide tolerability remains problematic in ca 10-40% patients, where gastrointestinal side effects -nausea, vomiting, and diarrhoea- lead to treatment discontinuation in part of the patients. It has transpired, however, that correct timing of injections in relation to meals, coupled with reassurance about transience of these unwanted effects can significantly modify the numbers of treatment withdrawals by patients.

4.1.3 Safety

All experimental, preclinical and first clinical studies sufficiently demonstrated the safety of exenatide. After few years of clinical use in DM2T, sporadic cases of acute (even hemorrhagic) pancreatitis have been reported, where the connection with exenatide treatment cannot be ruled out. So far, the reports have been confined to individual case-studies, similar to some pancreatitis reports in treatment with DPP-IV inhibitor, sitagliptin (Anderson SL, 2010). *We will refer to the safety issues in detail in the chapter Side-effects.*

4.1.4 Indication and contraindications

Exenatide is a new drug, whose exact place within the range of antidiabetic medication will no doubt change over time. At the moment, exenatide is recommended as a second line treatment in obese DM2T patients with metformin failure, or in patients failing to reach targets on dual OAD therapy.

Contraindications are end stage renal disease and severe gastrointestinal disease in history, including severe hepatic failure and possibly history of acute pancreatitis.

4.1.5 Dosage, combinations, excretion

Exenatide (Byetta) is available in 5 or 10 microgram per dose pre-filled pens. It is recommended to start with 5ug dose twice daily for the first 1 moth of treatment, increasing to 10ug subsequently. Administration sites are identical to insulin's – stomach, thighs or upper arms subcutaneously, 60 minutes before breakfast or dinner.

Exenatide can be combined with all other classes of OAD's. When administering sulphonylureas and exenatide at the same time, higher risk of hypoglycaemia is present. The risk of hypoglycaemia can be minimised by lowering the dose of sulphonylurea. Exenatide is not licensed for concomitant use with insulin.

Exenatide in monotherapy does not lead to hypoglycaemia in diabetics or in healthy subjects.

The maximum levels of exenatide in bloodstream are reached 2 hours after administration. It is primarily excreted by the kidneys.

4.1.6 Side effects

4.1.6.1 Gastrointestinal

As was mentioned repeatedly earlier, gastrointestinal side-effects have been the most common in exenatide - firstly nausea, often very unpleasant and protracted, sometimes coupled with vomiting or diarrhoea. Such unwanted side-effects are present, according to different authors, in 15-50% of patients in the first days to weeks of treatment, and lead to treatment discontinuation in approximately 6-10% of patients. In the remaining patients, these side effects improve and disappear in 3-5 weeks. Nausea was originally suspected to be driving the weight loss, but this assumption has been abandoned due to the two observations:

- Those who lost weight were both from the group with nausea and other GI side effects, and from the group without;
- The decrease in weight is not present only in conjunction with GI side effects, but is longer lasting and progressive (up to 3 years according to current recorded data).

4.1.6.2 Antibodies production

Exenatide is peptide, and therefore capable of inducing antibodies production, according to studies in ca 40-50% of patients, but their effect on safety and efficacy is deemed minimal. It is however possible, that in small minority of patients with high titres of antibodies, exenatide will not be as effective as in others (Russell-Jones, 2010).

4.1.6.3 Acute pancreatitis

From a clinical point of view, acute pancreatitis is a serious adverse event. In 2007, FDA issued a warning about possible link between exenatide use and acute pancreatitis. By 2008, 6 cases of acute hemorrhagic pancreatitis have been reported, 2 of which were fatal. This lead to a host of studies examining the link.

Results have been equivocal. Experimental studies in rats (N=10) who were given exenatide for 75 days, compared to controls (n=10) showed greater degree of acinar inflammation, more pycnotic nuclei, higher lipase concentrations in bloodstream and smaller pancreatic mass in exenatide treated rats compared to controls. (Nachnani, 2010; Ayoub, 2010).

In contrast, studies in mice showed that activation of GLP-1 receptors increases pancreatic mass and selectively modulates expression of genes active in pancreatitis, however, activation or elimination of GLP-1R signal pathway had no effect on the severity of pancreatitis (Koehler, 2009).

To elucidate this, Dore analysed the shared database of commercial medical insurers in the US in 2005-200 for instances of acute pancreatitis in exenatide- or sitagliptin-treated compared to metformin- or glyburide/glibenclamide- treated patients. Evaluation was carried out in 27 996 exenatide treated and 16 276 sitagliptin treated patients. During prospective follow-up of 1 year, 0.13 % patients of exenatide and 0.12% patients on sitagliptin have been hospitalised for acute pancreatitis. This number was no different compared to long known and used OAD treatments, metformin or glyburide/glibenclamide (Dore, 2009).

It is therefore important to remind us, that obesity is a known risk factor for chronic pancreatitis and for acute attacks, regardless of DM2T status (Olansky, 2010).

Anderson (2010) reviewed MEDLINE, internet pages of FDA (Food and Drug Administration) and data from Amylin Pharmaceuticals, the producers of Byetta (exenatide). They found 8 cases of acute pancreatitis during phase II and III of clinical testing, and 36 postmarketing reports, 6 of which have been cases of hemorrhagic pancreatitis. Two cases resulted in death. In case of liraglutide, 3 patients have been reported to develop acute, one chronic pancreatitis. According to the authors, these reports may give rise to clinical suspicion; however, more studies are needed to verify causality.

Gallwitz (2010) also cites recent reviews of this serious complication, and arrives to conclusion that exenatide does not increase the risk compared to other glucose lowering agents (RR 1.0: 95% CI 0.6; 1.7).

Finally, in November 2010, a retrospective analysis was published of 786656 DM2T patients treated with sitagliptin, exenatide or other therapy and control group of non-diabetics. The incidence of acute pancreatitis was 1.9 in non-diabetics, 5,6 in diabetic without incretin based therapy, 5.6 in diabetics on sitagliptin and 5.7 cases per 1000 patient years in diabetics on exenatide. The study demonstrated increased incidence of acute pancreatitis in diabetic versus nondiabetic patients but did not find an association between the use of exenatide or sitagliptin and acute pancreatitis (Garg, 2010).

4.1.7 Other demonstrated and disputed effects of exenatide

Preclinical experience with exenatide, as well as with liraglutide, showed improved endothelial function. Both molecules also improve sodium excretion, myocardial function and recovery from ischemic injury in animals. In humans, GLP-1 agonists seem to decrease blood pressure regardless of weight loss.

Further experimental data in mice showed significant decrease in intimal thickening after vascular injury. The question remains, whether such effect is mediated by exendin-4 induced suppression of platelet-derived growth factor-induced smooth muscle cells proliferation, or other direct or indirect effects (Okerson &Yan, 2010; Goto, 2011).

The question of cardiovascular risk influence, in the current absence of prospective randomised studies, can only be answered by retrospective reviews. Best, in 2010 analysed retrospective data from LifeLink database in 2005-2009. Patients without the history of myocardial infarction, ischemic stroke, or coronary revascularization procedure in the past 9 months were assigned to the exenatide-initiated or non-exenatide-initiated cohorts. Exenatide group had more obesity, dyslipoproteinemia, hypertension or ischemic heart disease in their history. After exenatide initiation, this group showed smaller incidence of CV events compared to other diabetes therapy group.

Contrary to expectations, large prospective studies (ACCORD, VADT) did not demonstrate superiority of aggressive treatment of hyperglycaemia in lowering CV risk. The reason for this, repeatedly discussed at EASD in 2009 and 2010, is suspected to be the increased incidence of unknown hypoglycemia, triggering a cardiovascular event. Regardless of what the final conclusion will be, it is important to note that incretin mimetics do not cause hypoglycemia by themselves.

Brixner published a study rounding up all metabolic effects of exenatide as followed up in regular outpatient practice. It evaluated 1709 subjects fulfilling entry criteria. The results (Table 3.) are summarised in Table 3. Authors conclude that the proclaimed effects of exenatide in rigorous clinical studies do translate to regular practice (Brixner, 2009).

Decrease after 6 months of exenatide treatment		
HbA_{1c} (%; DCCT)	-0.8 (0.05)	(p<0.001)
weight (kg)	-3.2 (0.14)	(p<0.001)
systolic BP (mmHg)	-1.9 (0.46)	(p<0.001)
diastolic BP (mmHg)	-0.5 (0.27)	(p<0.078)
LDL-cholesterol (mg/dl)	-7.4 (1.7)	(p<0.001)
triglycerides (mg/dl)	-23.2 (6.7)	(p=0.001)
Increase after 6 months of exenatide treatment		
HDL-cholesterol (mg/dl)	+0.87 (0.33)	(p<0.012)

Table 3. 6-month follow up of exenatide added to metformin and sulphonylurea combination in regular outpatient practice.

Apart from other complex metabolic influence of exenatide, we have repeatedly mentioned the delayed gastric emptying as one of the mechanisms of improved glucose metabolism in treatment with GLP-1 agonists. One Swedish paper on experimental animals as well as in healthy volunteers lists other effects of GLP-1 analogues in gastrointestinal tract, notably in intestines: decrease in intestinal motility and antispasmodic effect (Hellström, 2010).

Therefore, when considering other effects of treatment rather than the pure and simple decrease in glycaemia as reflected in A1c levels, where GLP-1 agonists seem to be on par with other hypoglycaemic agents, exenatide is superior to other classes of drugs due to is significant and lasting effect on body weight decrease (DeFronzo, 2005; Buse, 2004; Kendall, 2005).

Such beneficial effect lead to examination of the place for exenatide in relation to combination with insulin. To ascertain which treatment option is more beneficial in rectifying the parameters of glucose and metabolic homeostasis, Davies, 2009 studied Type 2 diabetics with BMI over 27kg/m^2, with increased cardiovascular risk and not reaching their targets of glycaemic control on two or three OADs. Average age of the 235 subjects was 56.5 years, BMI 34,1 kg/m^2 and HbA_{1c} 8.65 % (exenatide subgroup) and 8.48 % (glargine subgroup). More than half, 58.5% of the subjects were using double OAD therapy at the beginning of the 26-week study. There was no difference between exenatide or glargine as an add-on to current therapy in terms for A1c improvement. There was, however, statistically significant difference in weight change: exenatide lead to a weight decrease of 2.73kg and glargine to an increase of 2.98kg. The researchers concluded that exenatide as an add-on therapy in obese diabetics lead to slightly better improvement in A1c, coupled with significant improvement in weight, compared to glargine add-on.

Combination of exenatide and insulin can be somewhat difficult to advocate, and from the patient's point of view hard to sell due to the necessity to juggle two injectable medicines, but, with clear clinical benefits as demonstrated by Yoon (2009) and shown in Table 4. In many countries, such combination is still off-label. However, there is accumulating evidence as to the benefit of such combination. Bunck et al. studied 69 metformin-treated DM2T patients into two groups, exenatide add-on and insulin add-on. Exenatide group showed unequivocal improvement in postprandial glycaemia as well as lipaemia, coupled with improvement in oxidative stress markers, when compared with the glargine-treated group after 52 weeks duration (Bunck, 2010).

Duration (months)	HbA_{1c} (%)	weight (kg)	change in insulin dose/day (units)
0–6	-0.66	-2.4	-18.0
6–12	-0.55	-4.3	-14.8
12–18	-0.54	-6.2	NS
18–27	-0.54	-5.5	NS

NB: all changes vs. baseline statistically significant

Table 4. Metabolic compensation with exenatide added on to insulin

There are already some data available on safety and efficacy of these two medicines used concomitantly. MEDLINE search of all results of such treatment were reviewed by Tzefos and colleagues. Despite their reservations, mainly due to the limited number of studies published, they conclude that such combination is indeed safe in Type 2 diabetics. For selected subgroup of patients (obese with high doses of insulin) is such combination more than promising in terms of reducing the necessary doses of insulin whilst achieving clinically significant weight loss (Tzefos, 2010).

Others confirmed, that exenatide treatment added to insulin leads to significant decrease in body weight and decrease in required insulin doses. In another study, insulin doses dropped significantly (mean at baseline to 51 +/- 37 U/day at 12 months). In 25% of the original subjects of this study, insulin has been discontinued altogether after 3 months. Whilst the data regarding weight and insulin doses were more than impressive, the changes in A1c between the groups were minimal (Nayak, 2010).

Our own national and still ongoing follow-up of basic parameters in 359 Type 2 diabetics treated with exenatide, in co-operation with 24 diabetes specialists, showed the following results:

- Gradual, and progressive weight loss, in at least 12 months duration, as shown in BMI decrease (Fig. 1)
- The best effect on A1c lowering in the first months of treatment, after which the improvement tapers off (Fig.2)

4.2 Liraglutide

4.2.1 Structure

The other currently marketed GLP-1 receptor agonist is liraglutide. It has been modified from native GLP-1 by exchanging arginine for lysine at position 34 of the peptide and by attaching glutamic acid to the chain. Liraglutide is therefore 98% homologous with native GLP-1. This molecule binds to serum albumin, extending its half-life, whilst being resistant to cleavage action of DPP-IV. Liraglutide is administered subcutaneously as a isotonic solution which is slowly absorbed into the bloodstream with half-life of 13 hours, allowing it to be administered once daily.

Due to the fact that liraglutide and exenatide both act through the same receptor pathway, the following chapter will highlight only differences between the two compounds, therefore unless stated, both drugs can be deemed clinically very similar.

4.2.2 Excretion

Liraglutide is excreted by both kidneys and liver. Thus in the situation where impaired renal functions often complicate our treatment plan, it allows for liraglutide to be administered to patients with up to moderate degree of renal failure (Jacobsen, 2009).

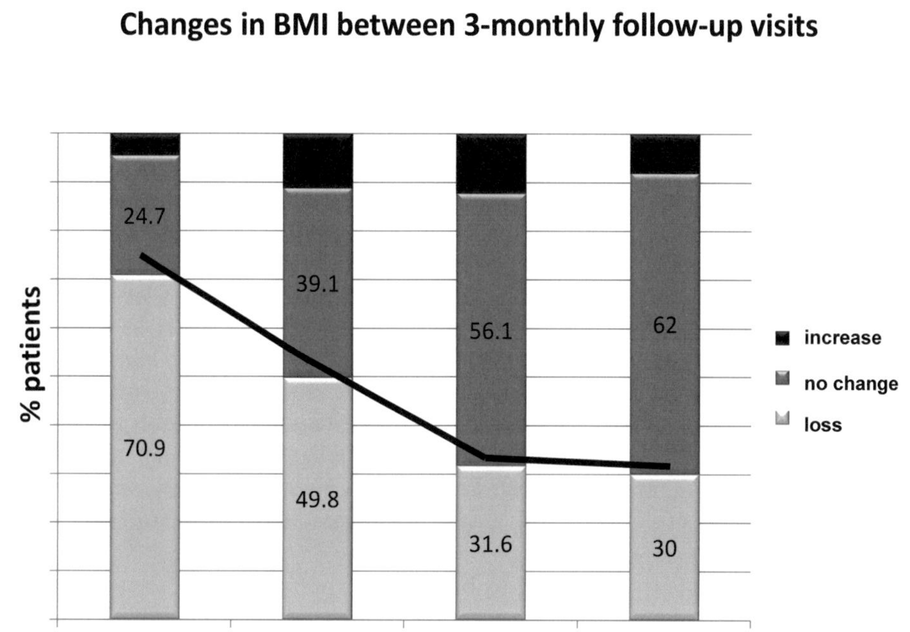

Fig. 1. Changes in BMI after exenatide.

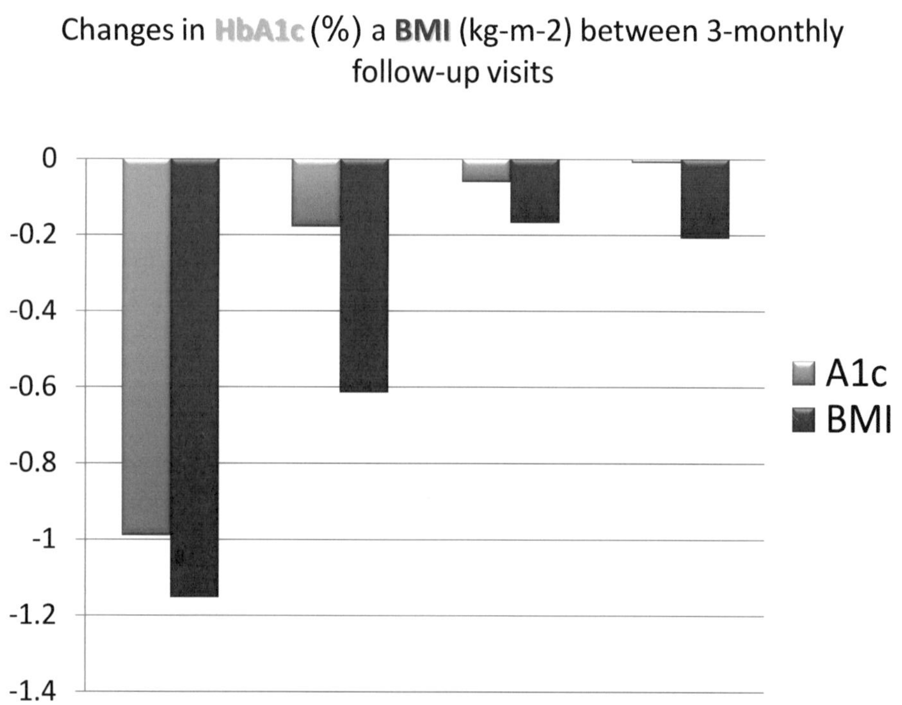

Fig. 2. Changes in A1c and BMI after exenatide.

4.2.3 Safety

First, data from studies in rats and mice suggested that liraglutide was associated with an increased risk of thyroid C-cell focal hyperplasia and C-cell tumours at doses that resulted in plasma drug levels similar to those seen in humans at the approved doses (Bjere Knudsen, 2010). However, the incidence of liraglutide-induced medullary thyroid cancer did not affect the overall survival rate among either rats or mice. The relevance of these findings to humans is unknown. The incidence of medullary thyroid cancer is too low to allow for direct comparison with liraglutide exposed group of patients. The only way how to assess potential risk is by monitoring calcitonin. Serum calcitonin levels below 10 pg/ml are consistent with the absence of medullary thyroid cancer, whereas levels above 100 pg per millilitre are highly predictive of medullary thyroid cancer. In trials, calcitonin levels increased slightly more often with liraglutide than in control patients; but were still within normal ranges. Furthermore, data from a long-term study did not reveal any notable difference in mean calcitonin levels between liraglutide and control groups over 2 years of follow-up (Hegedüs, 2011). As it is very difficult to translate animal data to humans, although FDA was satisfied that liraglutide poses no known safety concern at the moment, as a precautionary measure it ordered 15-year long monitoring of medullary carcinoma in liraglutide-treated patients.

Second, liraglutide, similarly to exenatide, has been suspected in inducing acute pancreatitis in patients receiving it, due to postmarketing reports to FDA regarding exenatide and sitagliptin, because liraglutide acts through the same GLP-1 pathway. The FDA-ordered evaluation of such possible risk from data in Phase II and III studies with liraglutide revealed seven cases of pancreatitis reported among the 4257 patients treated with liraglutide and one case in the 2381 patients in the comparator group. After adjustment for more patient-years of exposure to liraglutide, this finding of pancreatitis represented a 4:1 imbalance between the liraglutide and comparator groups. This lead to suggested change in labelling for all incretin-based therapies, about persistent or severe nausea and vomiting which may be early manifestations of pancreatitis and therefore warrant prompt discontinuation of treatment (Parks, 2010).

4.2.4 Efficacy

4.2.4.1 Glycemic control

The series of Phase III trials establishing the role of liraglutide in monotherapy as well as in combination with other antidiabetic medications was called LEAD (Liraglutide Effect and Action in Diabetes). Overall, the studies demonstrated dose dependent effect of liraglutide on glycemic control and body weight. Earlier published studies showed the A1c decrease of 0.33-0.75% and weight reduction of 1.2-1.9kg in doses up to 0.75mg daily, later studies with dosage escalation up to 1.9mg per day showed A1c decrease of up to 1.7% and weight loss of up to 3 kg in longer duration of studies (14 weeks vs. 8-12 in earlier studies). In normal doses (in many countries the maximum approved dose is 1.2mg per day, not the highest 1.8mg/day), liraglutide is not more effective than glimepiride in glycemic control, but its effect if more durable than either glimepiride or glibenclamide. Liraglutide also improves pancreatic cell function with minimal risk of hypoglycaemia (Croom, 2009).

LEAD programme demonstrated that liraglutide administration (Garber, 2008):

- leads to weight loss; the weight loss is greater with greater baseline BMI
- protects beta cells as assessed by HOMA-B model

- improves glycemic control via both improvements in fasting and postprandial glycaemia and HbA1c
- carries virtually no risk of hypoglycaemia
- lowers triglyceride levels
- lowers systolic blood pressure

The overview of all LEAD Studies is provided in Table 5. Other studies also confirm significant improvements in HbA1c levels, significant improvement in BMI and improved beta cell function in monotherapy as well as in combination with metformin, glimepiride or rosiglitazone. It also lowered systolic blood pressure (Drab, 2009).

	N	Duration (months)	Extension (months)	Entry medication	Comparator	δHbA_{1c} (%) [a] liragl.	δHbA_{1c} (%) comp.	δm (kg)[a] liragl.	δm (kg)[a] comp.
LEAD1	1041	6	0	Glimepiride	Rosiglitazon or placebo	−1.1	−0.4	−0.2	+2.1
LEAD2	1091	6	48	Metformin	Glimepirid or placebo	−1.0	−0.7	−2.8	+1.0
LEAD3	746	12	60	none	Glimepirid	−1.1	−0.5	−2.5	+1.1
LEAD4	533	6	0	Metformin + rosiglitazone	Placebo	−1.5	−0.5	−2.0	+0.6
LEAD5	533	6	0	Metformin + glimepiride	Glargine or placebo	−1.3	−1.1	−1.8	+1.6
LEAD6	464	6	3	Metformin and/or glimepirid	Exenatide	−1.1	−0.8	−3.2	−2.9

Table 5. Overview of LEAD trials. Based on Hansen, 2010.
HbA1c at entry was 8.2-8.5%. [a]on 1.8 mg liraglutide

The metaanalysis of published GLP-1 receptor agonists randomised controlled (with active comparator or placebo) studies (total of 21, out of which 6 have only been partially published) of exenatide and liraglutide, evaluated data on 5429 and 3053 patients respectively. The analysis showed significant improvement in glycemic control as measured by improvement in HbA_{1c} (-1.1; -0.8 %) with very low risk of hypoglycaemia. Authors conclude that liraglutide once daily is as efficacious and safe, with comparable tolerability, as exenatide twice daily (Monami, 2009).

4.2.4.2 Effects on body weight

Significant dose-dependent weight loss was demonstrated in all of the LEAD studies. In the monotherapy study (LEAD 3), absolute weight loss was 2.5 kg at the 1.8 mg dose and 2.1 kg at the 1.2 mg dose. Weight loss was greatest in combination with metformin: 2.8 kg with the 1.8 mg dose and 2.6 kg with the 1.2 mg dose (Nauck, 2009). In LEAD 5, the difference between insulin glargine and liraglutide as an add-on to metformin was 3.4kg, as treatment with insulin glargine increased weight by 1.6 kg, whereas liraglutide decreased weight by 1.8 kg (Russell-Jones, 2009). In LEAD 6, a head-to-head comparison with exenatide, liraglutide at the 1.8 mg dose was superior to exenatide in inducing weight loss of 3.2 kg compared with 2.9 kg in the exenatide group (Buse, 2009). The reduction of body weight with liraglutide is confirmed to result from a reduction in body fat (Jendle, 2009). Overall, liraglutide induces the maximum weight loss in metformin-treated patients, but also appears to offset the weight gain of sulfonylurea, thiazolidinediones, or insulin treatment.

A potential role of liraglutide as a weight loss treatment is emerging. In a recently reported trial of 20 weeks duration, 564 obese individuals with BMI 30–40 kg/m^2 were randomly assigned to one of 4 doses of liraglutide (1.2, 1.8, 2.4, or 3.0 mg), placebo, or orlistat. All subjects were instructed to decrease their calorie intake by 500 a day and to increase their physical activity. Subjects on liraglutide lost significantly more weight than did those on placebo and orlistat. Mean weight loss with these 4 doses of liraglutide was 4.8, 5.5, 6.3, and 7.2 kg vs. 2.8 kg in the placebo group and 4.1 kg in the orlistat group. About 76% of individuals lost more than 5% weight with liraglutide 3.0 mg compared with 30% in the placebo or 44% in the orlistat groups (Astrup, 2009).

4.2.4.3 Effects on cardiovascular risk modification

First concern with any newly developed drug should be its safety. Regarding liraglutide, FDA approved the drug before new guidelines have been published regarding the assessment of safety whereby comparing the incidence of cardiovascular events in the group receiving the agent under investigation with that in comparator groups have to demonstrate that the upper bound of the two-sided 95% confidence interval for the estimated risk ratio was less than 1.8. Analyses of cardiovascular events from the combined phase II and phase III trials showed that liraglutide met the standard for ruling out an unacceptable increase in cardiovascular risk. The overall rates of cardiovascular events in the preapproval clinical trials were low, however, and the FDA is therefore requiring a postapproval study of cardiovascular safety (Parks, 2010).

A welcome and consistent effect of liraglutide in the LEAD programme was the modest reduction of blood pressure, ranging from 2.1 to 6.7 mm Hg (Nauck, 2009, Buse, 2009, Zinman, 2009, Russell-Jones, 2009). GLP-1 has been reported to have a natriuretic effect, which might explain its effect on blood pressure (Gutzwiller, 2004). Compared to exenatide, the effect on blood pressure was slightly more pronounced, but coupled with slight increase in heart rate. (Hattori, 2010; Jackson, 2010; Okerson, 2010).

In terms of actual cardiovascular risk reduction in DM2T, the initial results with liraglutide are promising. Liraglutide lowers the low-grade inflammation of vascular endothelium via:

- Increased production of nitrous oxide,
- Suppression of NF-kB activation, and
- Partially through AMP kinase activation

These effects seem to explain the vasoprotective action of liraglutide, which can, in the longer run, translate to cardiovascular risk factor modification. This, coupled with results of metaanalysis of LEAD studies showing decrease in PAI-1 and CRP levels, and primary improvement in endothelial function by improved vascular wall relaxation, make liraglutide a molecule interesting not only to diabetologists but to cardiologists, too.

Recent experimental work of Noyan-Ashraf, 2009, in mice, showed that liraglutide administration activates cytoprotective mechanisms in myocardium of non-diabetic as well as diabetic animals, and improves survival after acute myocardial infarction.
Poor control of diabetes leads to accelerated development of atherosclerosis, leading to cardiovascular complications. Sullivan and colleagues applied the diabetic model CORE to valid epidemiologic data on morbidity and mortality in clinical studies and simulated the effects on cardiovascular events based on LEAD 1 data, comparing addition of rosiglitazone or liraglutide to glimepiride. The findings in hypothetical 5000 patients slightly favoured liraglutide in terms of survival, when compared to rosiglitazone. However, these are hypothetical results and we have to expect long term safety and efficacy information from postmarketing data (Sullivan, 2009).

4.2.5 Conclusion

Although liraglutide and exenatide act through the same GLP-1 receptor, their different structure leads to some differences in action. This favours liraglutide in allowing once daily administration, irrespective of meal time, at any time of a day. Also, the head to head comparison of liraglutide with exenatide in LEAD 6 suggests that liraglutide is somewhat more effective than exenatide in lowering the blood glucose and HbA_{1c} levels. Liraglutide seems to be more consistent in lowering blood pressure (Pinckney, 2010). Moreover, in terms of tolerability, despite both drugs being well tolerated (again with some shift towards shorter duration of side effects in liraglutide), liraglutide should be less likely to cause hypoglycaemia, and there is no allergy or antibody development, due to higher structural homology to native GLP-1.
All these factors could become unimportant, when new molecules or new formulations become available. The pipeline is in brief discussed in the following chapter.

5. New compounds and formulations in the pipeline

Incretin-based therapies are undoubtedly the fastest developing area of Type 2 diabetes treatment. After the halting of taspoglutide during Phase III studies mainly due to adverse allergic reactions, two molecules are still significantly advanced in the pipeline to be of potential clinical interest. First, extended release exenatide, to be marketed under the name Bydureon, and albiglutide, modified GLP-1 receptor agonist bound with human recombinant albumin, to be marketed under the brand name Syncria.

5.1 Exenatide LAR

In this extended release formulation, exenatide is encapsulated in microspheres made of poly (D,L lactic-co-glycolic acid), a biodegradable polymer, that breaks down over time and allows a controlled rate of drug delivery. In terms of safety, drug interactions and possible combinations with other hypoglycemic therapies, there seems to be little difference between exenatide twice daily and once weekly. We therefore present only studies concerning the differences in efficacy between these two formulations of the same compound.

5.1.1 Efficacy

Our knowledge on the clinical efficacy and safety of exenatide LAR comes, similarly to the LEAD battery of studies for liraglutide, from the group of DURATION 1-5 (Diabetes

Therapy Utilization: Researching Changes in A1C, Weight and Other Factors Through Intervention with Exenatide Once Weekly) studies. We review the results, with the exception of DURATION 4, which, according to the clinical trials website (www.clinicaltrials.gov), has not reported any results yet.

DURATION 1 (Drucker, 2008) was designed as a non-inferiority study of exenatide LAR compared to exenatide BID in patients drug naive, on single or multiple OADs. Long acting exenatide (2 mg once weekly) was found to cause a greater reduction in HbA1c than exenatide 10 µg twice daily (-1.9% vs. -1.5%, mean difference 0.40 (95% CI: 0.12, 0.68), p = 0.005). However, exenatide BID was superior to the once weekly 2 mg regimen in controlling PPG. Exenatide LAR led to greater reduction in TC (-0.31 vs. -0.10) and LDL (-0.13 vs. +0.03) than twice daily exenatide. The study found no difference in weight loss or the percentage of participants losing weight (76% with exenatide once weekly versus 79% with exenatide twice daily). A significantly greater proportion of LAR patients achieved target HbA1c levels of 7.0% or less (77%vs 61% of evaluable patients, p=0.0039). Weight decreased in participants who reported no episodes of nausea throughout the study (70%). Nausea and vomiting were less frequent with once weekly exenatide compared with twice daily exenatide.

This study has been extended to 52 weeks with sustained effects on diabetes control and weight loss maintenance. Patients on exenatide LAR maintained A1C improvements through 52 weeks (-2.0% [95% CI -2.1 to -1.8%]). Patients switching from exenatide BID to exenatide QW achieved further A1C improvements, ‚catching up' those on LAR formulation and achieving same mean A1C (6.6%) at week 52. At week 52, 71 and 54% of all patients achieved A1C <7.0% and <or=6.5%, respectively. In both treatment arms, fasting plasma glucose was reduced by >40 mg/dl, and body weight was reduced by >4 kg after 52 weeks (Buse, 2010).

DURATION 2 studied exenatide LAR as an add-on therapy for patients failing on metformin. This study was designed as randomised, double-blind, double-dummy, superiority trial, comparing exenatide once weekly in combination with oral placebo against sitagliptin 100mg/day and injectable placebo or pioglitazone 45mg/day and injectable placebo. Treatment with exenatide reduced HbA1c (-1.5%, 95% CI -1.7 to -1.4) significantly more than did sitagliptin (-0.9%, -1.1 to -0.7) or pioglitazone (-1.2%, -1.4 to -1.0). Weight loss in the treatment arm containing exenatide (-2.3 kg, 95% CI-2.9 to -1.7) was statistically significantly greater than in the treatment arm containing sitagliptin (difference -1.5 kg, 95% CI -2.4 to -0.7, p=0.0002) or indeed pioglitazone (difference -5.1 kg, -5.9 to -4.3, p<0.0001) (Bergenstal, 2010).

DURATION 3 compared exenatide LAR with insulin glargine (titrated to glycemia of 4.0-5.5mmol/l) in adults with type 2 diabetes with suboptimal control on maximum tolerated doses of OADs (single metformin 70%, metformin + sulphonylurea 30%) for at least 3 months. Exenatide 2 mg once weekly led to slightly greater reduction in TC and LDL than glargine (-0.12 vs. -0.04 mmol/l TC; -0.05 vs. +0.04 mmol/l LDL). There was no difference in triglyceride levels. Change in HbA(1c) at 26 weeks was greater in patients taking exenatide (n=228; -1.5%, SE 0.05) than in those taking insulin glargine (n=220; -1.3%, 0.06; treatment difference -0.16%, 0.07, 95% CI -0.29 to -0.03). Slightly higher number of exenatide LAR patients dropped out of the study (5% vs 1%, p=0.012) due to adverse events (Diamant, 2010).

DURATION 4 was designed to test the hypothesis that exenatide once weekly is superior to metformin, sitagliptin, and pioglitazone in HbA1c reduction at 26 weeks compared to baseline, in drug-naive patients with type 2 diabetes who are inadequately treated with diet and exercise. To our knowledge, the results of this trial have not yet been reported in the scientific press.

DURATION 5 (Blevins, 2011) was designed as head to head comparison of exenatide LAR and exenatide BID in drug naive (19% of the study population), on single OAD (47%) and on multiple OADs (35%). The results again showed greater efficacy of LAR formulation in lowering HbA1c (-1.6 ± 0.1% vs. -0.9 ± 0.1%; P < 0.0001) and fasting plasma glucose (-35 ± 5 mg/dl vs. -12 ± 5 mg/dl; P = 0.0008). The difference in mean body weight reductions was likewise not statistically significant (-2.3 ± 0.4 kg and -1.4 ± 0.4 kg). The mild and transient nausea, well known in the currently available exenatide formulation, was less common in LAR (14%) than with BID formulation (35%). Injection-site reactions were genrally fairly infrequent, but more common in exenatide LAR.

5.2 Albiglutide

There is paucity of published data on albiglutide, as this molecule is not available anywhere in the world and has not yet been filed for approval, so the majority of the following data is cited from an article by Rosenstock and Stewart, 2010.

5.2.1 Structure

Albiglutide is a GLP-1 receptor agonist macromolecule comprised of two copies of a 30-amino-acid sequence of human GLP-1(7-36) (as a tandem repeat) coupled to recombinant human albumin (rHA). A single substitution (Ala→Gly) at the DPP IV cleavage site confers resistance to degradation, while retaining 97% homology with native GLP-1. The half-life of albiglutide is 5 days, and can be administered at weekly or less frequent intervals.

5.2.2 Side effects

Nausea and vomiting correlated with albiglutide exposure. Compared with biweekly and monthly dosing, weekly dosing of albiglutide had the lowest peak:trough ratio, and also the lowest incidence of GI events (Rosenstock 2009).

There was no increase in documented hypoglycemia with albiglutide (0-3.1%) compared with placebo (3.9%) or exenatide (2.9%). Antialbiglutide antibodies were detected in only 2.5% patients; however, the appearance of antibodies was mainly transient, the antibodies were non-neutralizing, and of low titer. There was no evidence of an association between albiglutide antibodies and efficacy or safety.

5.2.3 Efficacy

There was consistent weight loss in the albiglutide groups (–1.1 to –1.7 kg for patients receiving the highest dose in each schedule) compared with the placebo group (–0.7 kg). The weight loss with albiglutide was numerically less than that observed with exenatide (–2.4 kg) but there were weight differences at baseline between the groups. Albiglutide provided dose-dependent HbA1c reductions within each dosing schedule of the 16-week phase IIb study. In patients receiving the highest dose in each treatment schedule, HbA1c reductions were –0.87%, –0.79% and –0.87%, respectively, from baseline HbA1c of 8.0%, 7.9% and 8.1%, respectively, for 30 mg weekly, 50 mg biweekly and 100 mg monthly, compared with exenatide –0.54% and placebo –0.17% from baselines of 7.8% and 8.0%, respectively. Decreases in both systolic and diastolic blood pressure were also observed, with the group receiving albiglutide 30 mg weekly experiencing a decrease of –5.8 mmHg and –1.9 mmHg, respectively, for systolic and diastolic blood pressure.

5.2.4 Future

The Phase III HARMONY program will provide the first long-term blinded comparative data on a GLP-1 receptor agonists in clinically meaningful range of combinations whilst also extensively examining positioning of albiglutide in respect to active comparators.

6. GLP-1 summary

Type 2 diabetes mellitus is a well-established risk factor for cardiovascular disease. Therefore all therapeutic modalities used in diabetes have to be evaluated with regard to cardiovascular effects. Incretin-based therapies, and notably GLP-1 receptor agonists are therefore a promising class of antidiabetic drugs.

Sufficient data supports beneficial effects of GLP-1 receptor agonists on: *glycemia, weight, blood pressure* and the circulating levels of *CRP, triglycerides and free fatty acids.*

GLP-1 analogues seem to have beneficial effects on beta cell function (Wang, 2011), protecting beta cells from the harmful effects of *lipotoxicity*. There is, however, a question of timing for GLP-1 analogues in the *natural course of DM2T*, most likely in combination with metformin (Cho, 2011). They can play crucial role in preserving beta cell function. Later in the course, when insulin deficiency prevails, substitution therapy with insulin is warranted.

GLP-1 analogues (GLP-1 receptor agonists) possess unique characteristics and are at the moment the only therapeutic class that influences multiple pathologies inherent to DM2T:

- hyperglycemia;
- beta cell dysfunction;
- alimentary obesity;
- insulin resistance;
- hypertension and dyslipidemia.

6.1 Overall comparison of two first GLP-1 analogues

In general, there seem to be very little clinical difference between the two currently available molecules of GLP-1 receptor agonists, exenatide and liraglutide. Overall, Shyangdan, 2010, provides us with most up to date review and meta-analysis of these two drugs, in comparison between each other and with other classes of oral antidiabetics:

Diabetes control (glycated haemoglobin)

Liraglutide daily was superior to glargine, rosiglitazone, sitagliptin and exenatide BD.

Exenatide twice daily was equivalent to both insulin and rosiglitazone twice daily, taking differences in HbA1c of less than 0.5% as being not clinically significant.

Weight loss

Exenatide and liraglutide caused greater weight loss than all active comparators (oral agents and insulin) - most of which led to weight gain. Weight loss was independent of nausea.

Hypoglycaemia and adverse events

The incidence of hypoglycaemia in combination with metformin is very low. Hypoglycaemia was seen most often when GLP-1 analogues were used in combination with sulphonylureas.

The most commonly reported adverse events with both GLP-1 agonists were gastrointestinal (nausea, vomiting and diarrhoea).

7. References

Amori RE, Lau J, Pittas AG. Efficacy and safety of incretin therapy in type 2 diabetes: systematic review and meta-analysis. JAMA. 2007 Jul 11;298(2):194-206. ISSN 0098-7484

Anderson SL, Trujillo JM. Association of pancreatitis with glucagon-like peptide-1 agonist use. Ann Pharmacother 44, 5: 904–909, 2010. ISSN 1060-0280

Asmar M, Højberg PV, Deacon CF. et al. Pancreatic beta-cell responses to GLP-1 after near-normalization of blood glucose in patients with type 2 diabetes. Regul Pept 160, 1–3: 175–180, 2009. ISSN 0167-0115

Asmar M, Holst JJ. GLP-1 and glucose-dependent insulinotropic polypeptide: new advances. Curr Opin Endocrinol Diabetes Obes 17, 1: 57–62, 2010. ISSN 1752-296X

Astrup A, Rossner S, Van Gaal L, et al. Effects of liraglutide in the treatment of obesity: a randomised, double-blind, placebo-controlled study. Lancet. 2009;374(9701):1606–1616. ISSN 0140-6736

Ayoub WA, Kumar AA, Naguib HS, et al. Exenatide-induced acute pancreatitis. Endocr Pract 16, 1: 80–83, 2010. ISSN 1530-891X

Bergenstal RM, Wysham C, Macconell L, et al. Efficacy and safety of exenatide once weekly versus sitagliptin or pioglitazone as an adjunct to metformin for treatment of type 2 diabetes (DURATION-2): a randomised trial. Lancet. 2010 Aug 7;376(9739):431-9. ISSN 0140-6736

Best JH, Hoogwerf BJ, Herman WH, et al: Risk of Cardiovascular Disease Events in Patients with Type 2 Diabetes Prescribed the GLP-1 Receptor Agonist Exenatide Twice Daily or Other Glucose-Lowering Therapies: A Retrospective Analysis of the LifeLinkTM Database. Diabetes Care. 2011 Jan;34(1):90-5.. ISSN 0149-5992

Bjerre Knudsen L, Madsen LW, Andersen S, et al. Glucagon-like Peptide-1 receptor agonists activate rodent thyroid C-cells causing calcitonin release and C-cell proliferation. Endocrinology. 2010 Apr;151(4):1473-86. ISSN 0013-7227

Blevins T, Pullman J, Malloy J, et al. DURATION-5: Exenatide Once Weekly Resulted in Greater Improvements in Glycemic Control Compared with Exenatide Twice Daily in Patients with Type 2 Diabetes. J Clin Endocrinol Metab. 2011 Feb 9. [Epub ahead of print] ISSN 0021-972X

Brixner DI, McAdam-Marx C, Ye X. et al. Six-month outcomes on A1C and cardiovascular risk factors in patients with type 2 diabetes treated with exenatide in an ambulatory care setting. Diabetes Obes Metab 11, 12: 1122–1130, 2009. ISSN 1462-8902

Bunck MC, Cornér A, Eliasson B, et al: One-year treatment with exenatide vs. Insulin Glargine: Effects on postprandial glycemia, lipid profiles, and oxidative stress. Atherosclerosis. 2010 Sep;212(1):223-9. Epub 2010 Apr 29. ISSN 0021-9150

Burcelin R.; EuCSGLP-1. What is known, new and controversial about GLP-1? Minutes of the 1st European GLP-1 Club Meeting. Diabetes Metab 34, 6 Pt 1: 627–630, 2008. ISSN 1262-3636

Buse JB, Drucker DJ, Taylor KL, et al. DURATION-1: exenatide once weekly produces sustained glycemic control and weight loss over 52 weeks. Diabetes Care 2010 Jun; 33(6):1255-61. ISSN 0149-5992

Buse JB, Rosenstock J, Sesti G, et al. Liraglutide once a day versus exenatide twice a day for type 2 diabetes: a 26-week randomised, parallel-group, multinational, open-label trial (LEAD-6). Lancet 2009; 374(9683):39–47. ISSN 0140-6736

Buse JB, Henry RR, Han J. et al.; Exenatide-113 Clinical Study Group. Effects of exenatide (exendin-4) on glycemic control over 30 weeks in sulfonylurea-treated patients with type 2 diabetes. Diabetes Care 27, 11: 2628–2635, 2004. ISSN 0149-5992

Ceriello A, Esposito K, Testa R, et al. The possible protective role of glucagon-like peptide 1 on endothelium during the meal and evidence for an "endothelial resistance" to glucagon-like peptide 1 in diabetes. Diabetes Care. 2011 Mar; 34(3):697-702. ISSN 0149-5992

Croom KF, McCormack PL. Liraglutide: a review of its use in type 2 diabetes mellitus. Drugs 69, 14: 1985–2004, 2009. ISSN 0012-6667

Davies MJ, Donnelly R, Barnett AH, et al. Exenatide compared with long-acting insulin to achieve glycaemic control with minimal weight gain in patients with type 2 diabetes: results of the Helping Evaluate Exenatide in patients with diabetes compared with Long-Acting insulin (HEELA) study. Diabetes Obes Metab 11, 12: 1153–1162, 2009. ISSN 1462-8902

Defronzo RA. Banting Lecture. From the triumvirate to the ominous octet: a new paradigm for the treatment of type 2 diabetes mellitus. Diabetes 2009 Apr;58(4):773-95. ISSN 0012-1797

DeFronzo RA, Ratner RE, Han J. et al. Effects of exenatide (exendin-4) on glycemic control and weight over 30 weeks in metformin-treated patients with type 2 diabetes. Diabetes Care 28, 5: 1092–1100, 2005. ISSN 0149-5992

Diamant M, Van Gaal L, Stranks S, et al.Once weekly exenatide compared with insulin glargine titrated to target in patients with type 2 diabetes (DURATION-3): an open-label randomised trial. Lancet. 2010 Jun 26; 375(9733):2234-43. ISSN 0140-6736

Dore DD, Seeger JD, Arnold Chan K. Use of a claims-based active drug safety surveillance system to assess the risk of acute pancreatitis with exenatide or sitagliptin compared to metformin or glyburide. Curr Med Res Opin 25, 4: 1019–1027, 2009. ISSN 0300-7995

Drab SR. Clinical studies of liraglutide, a novel, once-daily human glucagon-like peptide-1 analog for improved management of type 2 diabetes mellitus. Pharmacotherapy 29, 12 Pt2: 43S–54S, 2009. ISSN 0277-0008

Drucker DJ, Buse JB, Taylor K, et al. Exenatide once weekly versus twice daily for the treatment of type 2 diabetes: a randomised, open-label, non-inferiority study. Lancet. 2008 Oct 4;372(9645):1240-50. ISSN 0140-6736

Fineman MS, Bicsak TA, Shen LZ, et al. Effect on glycemic control of exenatide (synthetic exendin-4) additive to existing metformin and/or sulfonylurea treatment in patients with type 2 diabetes. Diabetes Care 26, 8: 2370–2377, 2003. ISSN 0149-5992

Gallwitz B. Benefit-risk assessment of exenatide in the therapy of type 2 diabetes mellitus. Drug Saf 33, 2: 87–100, 2010. ISSN 0114-5916

Garber A, Henry R, Ratner R, et al. Liraglutid versus glimepiride monotherapy for type 2 diabetes (LEAD-3): a randomised , 52-week, phase III, double-blind, paralell-treatment trial. Lancet 373, 9662: 473–481, 2009. ISSN 0140-6736

Garg SK. The role of basal insulin and glucagon-like peptide-1 agonists in the therapeutic management of type 2 diabetes – a comprehensive review. Diabetes Technol Ther 12, 1: 11–24, 2010. ISSN 1520-9156

Gautier JF, Choukem SP, Girard J. Physiology of incretins (GIP and GLP-1) and abnormalities in type 2 diabetes. Diab Metab. 2008 Feb; 34 Suppl 2:S65-72. ISSN 1262-3636

Girard J.The incretins: from the concept to their use in the treatment of type 2 diabetes. Part A: incretins: concept and physiological functions.Diabetes Metab. 2008 Dec;34(6 Pt 1):550-9. ISSN 1262-3636

Goto H, Nomiyama T, Mita T, et al.Exendin-4, a glucagon-like peptide-1 receptor agonist, reduces intimal thickening after vascular injury. Biochem Biophys Res Commun. 2011 Feb 4;405(1):79-84. ISSN 0006-291X

Gutzwiller JP, Tschopp S, Bock A, et al. Glucagon-like peptide 1 induces natriuresis in healthy subjects and in insulin-resistant obese men. J Clin Endocrinol Metab 2004;89(6):3055–3061. ISSN 0021-972X

Hansen KB, Vilsbøll T, Knop FK. Incretin mimetics: a novel therapeutic option for patients with type 2 diabetes – a review. Diab Metab Syndr Obes. 2010; 3: 155–163. ISSN 1178-7007

Hattori Y, Jojima T, Tomizawa A, et al: A glucagon-like peptide-1 (GLP-1) analogue, liraglutide, upregulates nitric oxide production and exerts anti-inflammatory action in endothelial cells. Diabetologia. 2010 Oct;53(10):2256-63. ISSN 0012-186X

Hegedüs L, Moses AC, Zdravkovic M, et al: GLP-1 and Calcitonin Concentration in Humans: Lack of Evidence of Calcitonin Release from Sequential Screening in over 5000 Subjects with Type 2 Diabetes or Nondiabetic Obese Subjects Treated with the Human GLP-1 Analog, Liraglutide. J Clin Endocrinol Metab. 2011 Mar;96(3):853-60. ISSN 0021-972X

Hellström PM.: GLP-1 playing the role of a gut regulatory compound. Acta Physiol (Oxf). 2011 Jan;201(1):151-6. ISSN 1748-1708

Henquin JC, Cerasi E, Efendic S, et al. Pancreatic beta-cell mass or beta-cell function? That is the question! Diabetes Obes Metab. 2008 Nov;10 Suppl 4:1-4. ISSN 1462-8902

Holmes GM, Browning KN, Tong M, et al. Vagally mediated effects of GLP-1: in vitro and in vivo gastric actions. J Physiol. 2009 Oct 1;587(Pt 19):4749-59. ISSN 0022-3751

Holst JJ. Glucagon and glucagon-like peptides 1 and 2. Results Probl Cell Differ 2010;50:121-35. ISSN 0080-1844

Jackson SH, Martin TS, Jones JD, et al. Liraglutide (Victoza): the first once-daily incretin mimetic injection for type-2 diabetes. P T. 2010 Sep;35(9):498-529. ISSN 1052-1372

Jacobsen LV. Hindsberger C, Robson R, et al.. Effect of renal impairment on the pharmacokinetics of the GLP-1 analogue liraglutide. Br J Clin Pharmacol 68, 6: 898–905, 2009. ISSN 0306-5251

Jendle J, Nauck MA, Matthews DR. et al.; LEAD-2 and LEAD-3 Study Groups. Weight loss with liraglutide, a once-daily human glucagon-like peptide-1 analogue for type 2 diabetes treatment as monotherapy or added to metformin, is primarily as a result of a reduction in fat tissue. Diabetes Obes Metab 11, 12: 1163–1172, 2009. ISSN 1462-8902

Keating GM. Exenatide. Drugs. 2005;65(12):1681-92. ISSN 0012-6667

Kendall DM, Riddle MC, Rosenstock J. et al. Effects of exenatide (exendin-4) on glycemic control over 30 weeks in patients with type 2 diabetes treated with metformin and a sulfonylurea. Diabetes Care 28, 5: 1083–1091, 2005. ISSN 0149-5992

Koehler JA, Baggio LL, Lamont BJ. et al. Glucagon-like peptide-1 receptor activation modulates pancreatitis-associated gene expression but does not modify the susceptibility to experimental pancreatitis in mice. Diabetes 58, 9: 2148–2161, 2009. ISSN 0012-1797

Lugari, R., Dei Cas, A., Ugolotti, D. et al. GLP-1 secretion and plasma DPP-IV activity in morbidly obese undergoing BPD. Horm Metab Res 36, 2: 111–115, 2004. ISSN 0018-5043

Martin JH, Deacon CF, Gorrell MD, Prins JB. Incretin-based therapies- review of the physiology, pharmacology and emerging clinical experience. Intern Med J. 2011 Apr;41(4):299-307.. ISSN 1444-0903

Martin TS, Jones JD, et al: Liraglutide (victoza): the first once-daily incretin mimetic injection for type-2 diabetes. P T. 2010 Sep;35(9):498-529. ISSN 1052-1372

McAdam-Marx C, Gaebler JA, Bellows BK, et al.: Contemporary management of patients with Type 2 diabetes. Expert Rev Cardiovasc Ther. 2010 Jun;8(6):767-70. ISSN 1477-9072

Monami M, Marchionni N, Mannucci E. GLP-1 receptor agonists in type 2 diabetes: a meta-analysis of randomized clinical trials. Eur J Endocrinol 160, 6: 909–917, 2009. ISSN 0804-4643

Nachnani JS, Bulchandani DG, Nookala A. et al. Biochemical and histological effects of exendin-4 (exenatide) on the rat pancreas. Diabetologia 53, 1: 153–159, 2010. ISSN 0012-186X Nathanson D, Zethelius B, Berne C, et al. Reduced plasma levels of glucagon-like peptide-1 in elderly men are associated with impaired glucose tolerance but not with coronary heart disease. Diabetologia. 2010 Feb;53(2):277-80. ISSN 0012-186X

Nauck M, Frid A, Hermansen K, et al. Efficacy and safety comparison of liraglutide, glimepiride, and placebo, all in combination with metformin, in type 2 diabetes: the LEAD-2 study. Diabetes Care. 2009;32(1):84–90. ISSN 0149-5992

Nayak UA, Govindan J, Baskar V, et al: Exenatide therapy in insulin-treated type 2 diabetes and obesity. QJM. 2010 Jul 12. ISSN 1460-2725

Noyan-Ashraf MH, Momen MA, Ban K. et al. GLP-1R agonist liraglutide activates cytoprotective pathways and improves outcomes after experimental myocardial infartion in mice. Diabetes 58, 4: 975–983, 2009. ISSN 0012-1797

Okerson T, Chilton RJ.: The Cardiovascular Effects of GLP-1 Receptor Agonists. Cardiovasc Ther. 2010 Dec 19. doi: 10.1111/j.1755-5922.2010.00256.x. ISSN 1755-5914

Okerson T, Yan P, Stonehouse A, Brodows R. Effects of exenatide on systolic blood pressure in subjects with Type 2 diabetes. Am. J. Hypertens.23(3), 334-339 (2010). ISSN 0895-7061.

Olansky L. Do incretin-based therapies cause acute pancreatitis? J Diabetes Sci Technol 4, 1: 228–229, 2010. ISSN 1932-2968

Pannacciulli N, De Pergola G, Giorgino F, et al. A family history of Type 2 diabetes is associated with increased plasma levels of C-reactive protein in non-smoking healthy adult women. Diabet Med. 2002 Aug;19(8):689-92. ISSN 0742-3071

Parks M, Rosebraugh C.Weighing risks and benefits of liraglutide--the FDA's review of a new antidiabetic therapy. N Engl J Med. 2010 Mar 4;362(9):774-7. ISSN 0028-4793

Penfornis, A., Borot, S., Raccah, D. Therapeutic approach of type 2 diabetes mellitus with GLP-1 based therapies. Diabetes Metab 34, Suppl. 2: S78–S90, 2008. ISSN 1262-3636

Perušičová J. Inkretinová mimetika v léčbě diabetes mellitus 2. typu. In: Perušičová, J. (ed). Léčba inzulínem a DM 2. typu. Brno: Facta Medica, 2009; 179–192. ISBN 978-80-904260-3-0

Pinkney J, Fox T, Ranganath L.Selecting GLP-1 agonists in the management of type 2 diabetes: differential pharmacology and therapeutic benefits of liraglutide and exenatide. Ther Clin Risk Manag. 2010 Sep 7;6:401-11. ISSN 1176-6336

Rosenstock J, Stewart M. Albiglutide. Drugs of the Future 2010, 35(9):701-712. ISSN 0377-8282

Rosenstock J, Reusch J, Bush M, et al. The potential of albiglutide, a long-acting GLP-1 receptor agonist, in type 2 diabetes: A randomized controlled trial exploring weekly, biweekly, and monthly dosing. Diabetes Care 2009, 32(10): 1880-6. ISSN 0149-5992

Russell-Jones D, Vaag A, Schmitz O, et al. Liraglutide vs insulin glargine and placebo in combination with metformin and sulfonylurea therapy in type 2 diabetes mellitus (LEAD-5): a randomised controlled trial. Diabetologia. 2009;52(10):2046–2055. ISSN 0012-186X

Russell-Jones D.The safety and tolerability of GLP-1 receptor agonists in the treatment of type-2 diabetes. Int J Clin Pract. 2010 Sep;64(10):1402-14. ISSN 1368-5031

Sullivan SD, Alfonso-Cristancho R, Conner C, et al. Long-term outcomes in patients with type 2 diabetes receiving glimepiride combined with liraglutide or rosiglitazone. Cardiovasc Diabetol. 2009 Feb 26;8:12. ISSN 1475-2840

Tzefos M, Olin JL.:Glucagon-like peptide-1 analog and insulin combination therapy in the management of adults with type 2 diabetes mellitus. Ann Pharmacother. 2010 Jul-Aug;44(7-8):1294-300. ISSN 1060-0280

Unger RH, Orci I: The essential role of glucagon in the pathogenesis of diabetes mellitus. Lancet 1, 7897: 14–16, 1975. ISSN 0140-6736

Xiao-Yun X, Zhao-Hui M, Ke C, et al. Glucagon-like peptide-1 improves proliferation and differentiation of endothelial progenitor cells via upregulating VEGF generation. Med Sci Monit. 2011 Feb;17(2):BR35-41. ISSN 1234-1010

Yoon NM, Cavaghan MK, Brunelle RL, et al. Exenatide added to insulin therapy: a retrospective review of clinical practice over two years in an academic endocrinology outpatient setting. Clin Ther 31, 7: 1511–1523, 2009. ISSN 0149-2918

Zinman B, Gerich J, Buse JB, et al. Efficacy and safety of the human glucagon-like peptide-1 analog liraglutide in combination with metformin and thiazolidinedione in patients with type 2 diabetes mellitus (LEAD-4). Diabetes Care 32, 7: 1224–1230, 2009. ISSN 0149-5992

5

Carbohydrate Derivatives and Glycomimetic Compounds in Established and Investigational Therapies of Type 2 Diabetes Mellitus

László Somsák, Éva Bokor, Katalin Czifrák,
László Juhász and Marietta Tóth
Department of Organic Chemistry, University of Debrecen
Hungary

1. Introduction

Diabetes mellitus is characterized by chronically elevated serum glucose levels resulting in damage of several tissues (e. g. retina, kidney, nerves) due to higher protein glycation, retardation of wound healing, impaired insulin secretion, enhanced insulin resistance, cell apoptosis, and increased oxidative stress. Type 2 diabetes (T2DM), representing 90-95 % of all diabetic cases, is a multifactorial disease where impaired insulin secretion and the development of insulin resistance ultimately leads to hyperglycemia (Hengesh, 1995). The end of the 20th century has witnessed a dramatic increase in the number of patients diagnosed with diabetes worldwide. The predicted number for the year 2025 is well over 300 million representing a 4-5 % yearly increase of the population above 20 years of age (Treadway et al., 2001). This striking prevalence can even be an underestimate due to methodological uncertainties as well as undiagnosed cases (Green et al., 2003). The highest increases are expected in the developing countries of Africa, Asia, and South America, while European populations seem to be less affected (Diamond, 2003). T2DM has been considered as the adult- or late-onset variant, however, the recent decade has seen the appearance and spreading of the disease among young people including children: this forecasts severe economic and health service burdens in the near future (Alberti et al., 2004; Ehtisham & Barrett, 2004).
The epidemic of T2DM is in conjunction with genetic susceptibility: evidence for a genetic component to the disease are accumulating, and the potential of these factors in the treatment and prevention of diabetes has been reviewed (Barroso, 2005; Bonnefond et al., 2010; Sladek et al., 2007; Toye & Gauguier, 2003). A similarly high contribution to this epidemic may originate from behavioral factors such as sedentary lifestyle, overly rich nutrition, and obesity (Bloomgarden, 2004).
Especially due to its long term complications (Brownlee, 2001) like retinopathy, neuropathy, nephropathy, and in particular cardiovascular diseases, as well as significantly higher risk of myocardial infarction, stroke, gangrene, and limb amputation diabetes has become one of the largest contributors to disability and mortality. Although several pathomechanisms (Lowell & Shulman, 2005; Panunti et al., 2004; Stumvoll et al., 2005) are under investigation, no firm understanding of the molecular origins (Ross et al., 2004) of the disease exists.

Thereby, all available and investigational treatments are symptomatic. As the complications can first of all be attributed to the high blood glucose levels, current antidiabetic therapies (Table 1) aim at reaching normoglycemia. However, most of the applied oral hypoglycemic agents (Cheng & Fantus, 2005; Krentz & Bailey, 2005; Mizuno et al., 2008; Padwal et al., 2005; Rendell, 2004; Uwaifo & Ratner, 2005) have several side effects and are inadequate for 30-40 % of the patients (Wagman & Nuss, 2001). On the other hand, their efficacy is lost over the time, and several concerns exist regarding their safety (Israili, 2011).

Drug type	Molecular target	Site of action	Adverse effects
Insulin sensitizers			
Metformin (biguanides)	Unknown	Liver, intestine, pancreas	Gastrointestinal intolerance (diarrhea, nausea), lactic acidosis, decreased vitamin B_{12} level
Thiazolidinediones (glitazones)	PPARγ	Liver, adipose tissue, skeletal muscle	Weight gain, ankle edema, sodium and fluid retention, possible bone loss
Insulin secretagogues			
Sulfonylureas	Sulfonylurea receptor	Pancreas	Weight gain, hypoglycemia, hyperinsulinemia, hypoglycemia-provoked ischemia and arrhythmia, progressive decline in β-cell function
Meglitinides	K-ATP channel	Pancreas	Weight gain, hypoglycemia, hypoglycemia-provoked ischemia and arrhythmia
GLP-1 analogues and mimetics	GLP-1 receptor	Pancreas	Nausea, vomiting, diarrhea
DPP-4 inhibitors (glinides)	DPP-4	Intestine, pancreas	Gastrointestinal intolerance, nasopharyngitis, upper respiratory infection, urinary tract infection
Others			
α-Glucosidase inhibitors	α-Glucosidases	Pancreas, small intestine	Gastrointestinal intolerance (flatulence, bloating)
SGLT2-inhibitors (gliflozins)	SGLT2	Kidney	Gastrointestinal intolerance (nausea), urinary tract infection
Insulin	Insulin receptor	Liver, muscles	Weight gain, hypoglycemia

Table 1. Main types of current therapeutic agents for T2DM and their major side effects (Israili, 2011; Moller, 2001)

The complexity of T2DM offers many potential points of intervention for pharmacotherapy for which the main molecular targets and strategies such as insulin secretagogues, insulin sensitizers, hormones, inhibitors of PTP-1B, GSK3, and hepatic glucose production, methods for altering lipid metabolism, combination therapies, etc. have been reviewed in details (Israili, 2011; Morral, 2003; Nourparvar et al., 2004; Wagman et al., 2004).

Among the numerous methods used to treat type 2 diabetes and investigated to find new therapeutic possibilities there are several approaches which apply carbohydrate (especially glucose) derivatives as well as compounds mimicking the properties of sugars. Based on our experience in the chemistry of carbohydrates and glycomimetics, in this survey we summarize the roles of such compounds in combatting type 2 diabetes relying on the review literature and very recent primary scientific papers.

2. Inhibitors of α-glucosidase enzymes

Starch and sucrose are the most important dietary carbohydrates but they are not directly available for the cells. They are digested in the gastrointestinal tract to monosaccharides which can be absorbed to the circulation to raise the serum concentration (Hanhineva et al., 2010). The normal blood glucose level (3.6–5.8 mM) fluctuates throughout the day, is usually lowest in the morning, before the first meal of the day, and rises after meals for an hour or two.

A medically applied treatment of diabetes is to retard the absorption of glucose by inhibition of the carbohydrate hydrolyzing enzymes α-amylase and α-glucosidase in the digestive tract. In humans the digestion of starch, maltodextrins, and maltooligosaccharides includes several stages: degradation of the polymeric substrates results in shorter oligomers which are than cleaved by α-amylase into smaller oligosaccharides. This mixture is broken down to monosaccharides by α-glucosidase from the non-reducing end of the oligosaccharides. By inhibition of these enzymes the rate of glucose production can be reduced that contributes to diminishing the blood glucose levels, too (Tundis et al., 2010). Such inhibitors decrease postprandial hyperglycaemia and hyperinsulinaemia, thereby may improve sensitivity to insulin and release the stress on β-cells (Scheen, 2003).

Glycosidases are a long known and studied class of glycoenzymes for which an enormous number of compounds have been tested as inhibitors (El Ashry et al., 2000a; El Ashry et al., 2000b; El Ashry et al., 2000c; Lillelund et al., 2002). Analogues of monosaccharides in which the ring oxygen is replaced by a nitrogen atom are known as iminosugars (or less properly azasugars) comprising both natural and synthetic molecules (Table 2) which, as the most potent inhibitors of glycosidases, have high pharmacological potential not only in the context of T2DM (Asano, 2009; Compain & Martin, 2007).

The naturally occurring salacinol and analogous sugar mimics with a 4-thiofuranoid type ring (Table 2) belong to a growing class of zwitterionic glycosidase inhibitors, which attract great interest both as synthetic targets and applications for α-glucosidase inhibition (Praly & Vidal, 2010).

The positive charge on the sulfur atom in the thiosugar derivatives and in the iminosugar-based glycosidase inhibitors at physiological pH is facilitating the binding in the active sites of glycosidase enzymes as a mimicry of the charge of the oxocarbeniumion-like transition state formed during hydrolysis of the natural enzyme substrate (Zechel & Withers, 2000). The stabilizing electrostatic interactions between the ammonium (protonated nitrogen) or sulfonium (positively charged sulfur) moieties and an active-site carboxylate residue are considered to be a possible mechanism of action of these inhibitors (Mohan & Pinto, 2007).

Three competitive inhibitors of α-glucosidases: acarbose, miglitol, and voglibose (de Melo et al., 2006) (Table 3) are used as drugs in the treatment of T2DM under various brand names. These compounds are known to inhibit a wide range of glycosidases. In the absence of specificity and because of the known serious side effects, the applications of these first generation iminosugar drugs are limited. Current investigations aim at discovering safer, more specific, and effective iminosugar based derivatives not only as hypoglycemic agents but for several other purposes among others in oncology, as antivirals, and against cystic fibrosis as reviewed in (Home et al., 2011).

IC50/Ki* [μM] (Compain et al., 2007)	Pyrrolidine type		Piperidine type		
	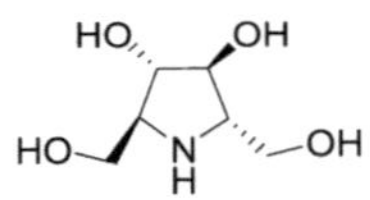	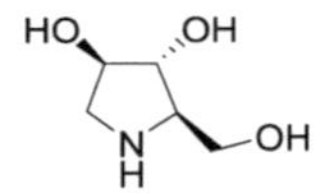 **DAB**	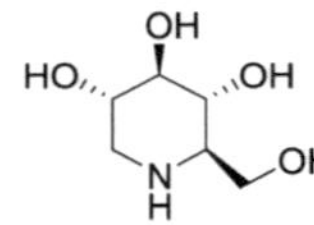 **Deoxy-nojirimycin**	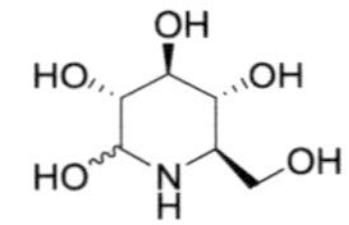 **Nojirimycin**	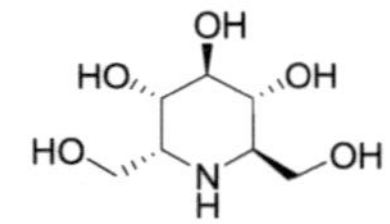 **α-Homonojirimycin**
Rat intestinal sucrase	0.01	16	0.21	0.56 (de Melo et al., 2006)	0.17 (de Melo et al., 2006)
Rat intestinal maltase	1.4	55	0.36	1.7 (de Melo et al., 2006)	0.34* (de Melo et al., 2006)
Rat intestinal isomaltase	0.05	5.8	0.03	0.25 (de Melo et al., 2006)	0.70 (de Melo et al., 2006)
Rat intestinal lactase	-	260	26	-	-

IC50/Ki* [μM] (Compain et al., 2007)	Pyrrolizidine type	Indolizidine type	Nortropane type	Thiosugar type	
	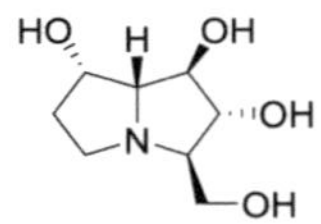 **Australine**	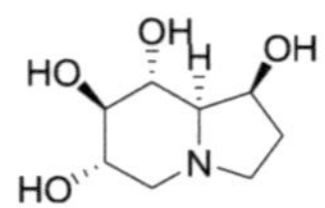 **Castanospermine**	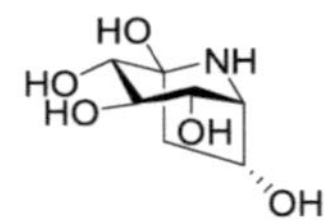 **Calistegin derivative**	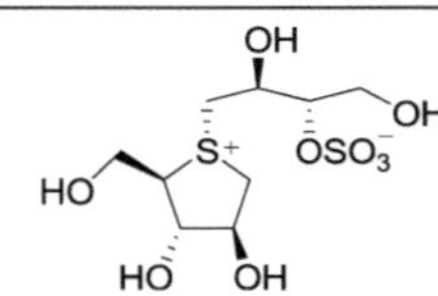 **Salacinol**	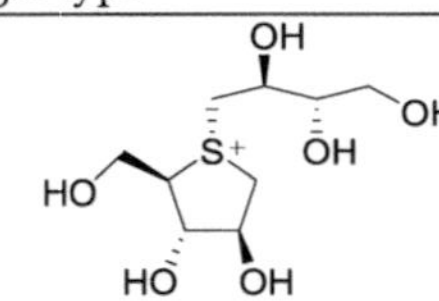 **Neosalacinol**
Rat intestinal sucrase	4.6	0.00055 (de Melo et al., 2006)	160	1.3 (Muraoka et al., 2011) 1.5 (Xie et al., 2011)	2.5 (Muraoka et al., 2011) 1.3
Rat intestinal maltase	24	-	190	6.0 (Muraoka et al., 2011) 5.2 (Xie et al., 2011)	22.2 (Muraoka et al., 2011) 8.0 (Xie et al., 2011)
Rat intestinal isomaltase	97		-	1.3 (Muraoka et al., 2011) 1.5 (Xie et al., 2011)	0.68 (Muraoka et al., 2011) 0.3 (Xie et al., 2011)
Rat intestinal lactase	-		0.38	-	-
Rat intestinal glucoamylase	5.8 (de Melo et al., 2006)	-	-	-	-

Table 2. Select iminosugar and thiosugar type inhibitors and their effect against α-glucosidases originating from mammalian gastrointestinal tract

Name	Structure	Side-effect
Acarbose Approved in 1995	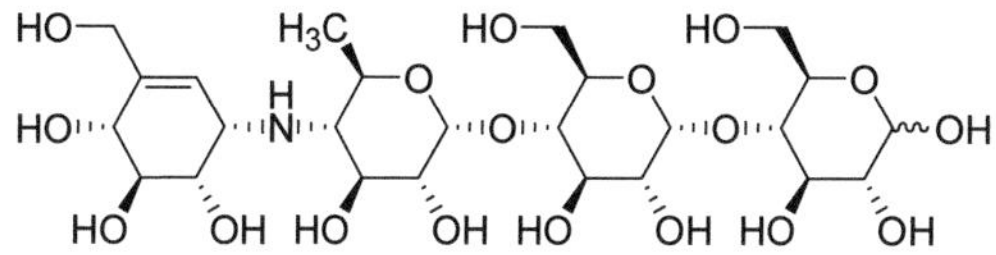	Flatulence (78% of the patients) Diarrhea (14% of the patients)
Miglitol Approved in 1996	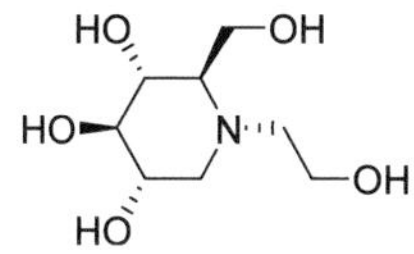	Diarrhea, gas, soft stools, stomach pain
Voglibose Approved in 1997	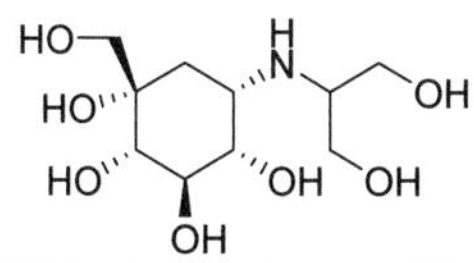	Diarrhea, stool loss, meteorism, upset stomach

Table 3. α-Glucosidase inhibitors in the clinical practice against T2DM

3. Inhibitors of renal sodium-glucose cotransporters

The mammalian kidney plays an important role in the maintenance of energy balance of the organism. In healthy individuals 180 g/day of D-glucose is filtered from plasma through the glomerulus, which is completely reabsorbed in the renal proximal tubules to the bloodstream, thereby preventing the loss of glucose in the urine (Wright, 2001). This reabsorption process is mediated by two sodium dependent glucose cotransporters (SGLTs). SGLT1 is a high-affinity, low-capacity glucose/galactose transporter located predominantly in the small intestine, but is also present in the S3 segment of the proximal tubule in the kidney, as well as in the heart. The primary function of SGLT1 is the absorbtion of dietary glucose in the intestine, however it shares in the renal glucose transport in the kidney and regulates cardiac glucose transport in the heart, as well. SGLT2 is a low affinity, high capacity glucose transporter specifically expressed in the S1 segment of the proximal convoluted tubule. SGLT2 is responsible for ~90 % of renal glucose reabsorption, while SGLT1 plays only an auxiliary role in this process (Boldys & Okopien, 2009; Idris & Donnelly, 2009; Washburn, 2009b). Genetic studies demonstrated that defects of SGLT2 but in a lesser extent of SGLT1 genes had neither adverse effects on kidney function as well as carbohydrate metabolism, nor hypoglycaemia (Handlon, 2005; Santer & Calado, 2010; Wright, 2001).

Nowadays sodium-glucose cotransporters have received remarkable attention as new drug targets for the treatment of diabetes (Bailey, 2011). Considering the exclusive expression of SGLT2 in the kidney and its predominant role in renal glucose recovery, most pharmaceutical investigations have focused primarily on selective SGLT2 inhibition to facilitate benign glucosuria (Santer & Calado, 2010; Washburn, 2009b). In contrast to the currently applied diabetic therapies most of which aim at insulin resistance and insulin deficiency, targeting SGLT2 is an insulin-independent strategy based on enhanced renal glucose excretion and, consequently, lowering plasma glucose levels without severe side effects (Isaji, 2007).

In recent years aromatic, heteroaromatic, and fused aromatic *O*- and *N*-glucopyranosides, *C*-glucopyranosyl derivatives, anomeric spirocycles, as well as their congeners with modified sugar rings have been developed as SGLT2 inhibitors (Handlon, 2005; Idris & Donnelly, 2009; Isaji, 2007; Nomura, 2010; Vaidya & Goyal, 2010; Washburn, 2009a; Washburn, 2009b).

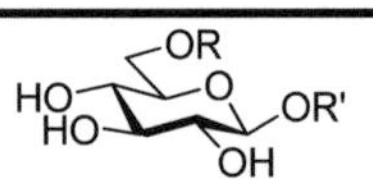

R = H unless indicated otherwise

Entry	R′	Entry	R′	Entry	R′
1.	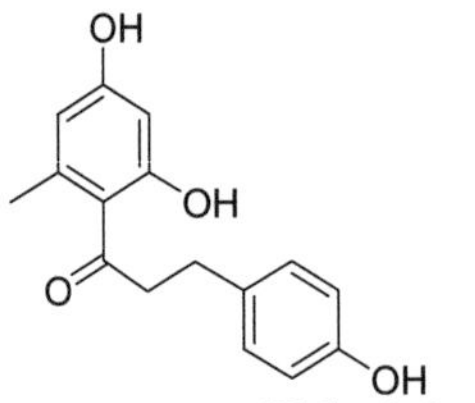 **Phlorizin** 35.6* (Meng et al., 2008) 18.6** (Katsuno et al., 2007)	2.	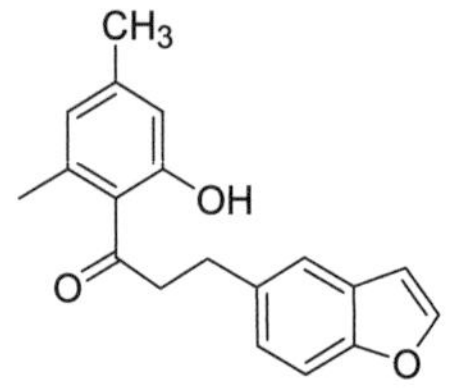 **T-1095** R = COOMe (prodrug form) **T-1095A** R = H (active form) 50 (Handlon, 2005) 6.6* (Meng et al., 2008)	3.	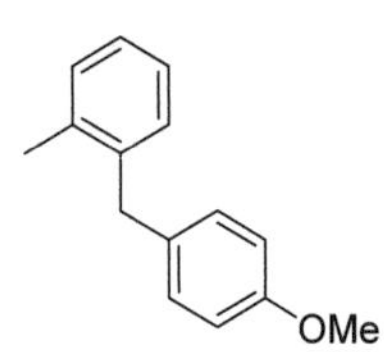 **Sergliflozin** R = COOEt (prodrug form) **Sergliflozin-A** R = H (active form) 9.2* (Meng et al., 2008) 2.39** (Katsuno et al., 2007)
4.	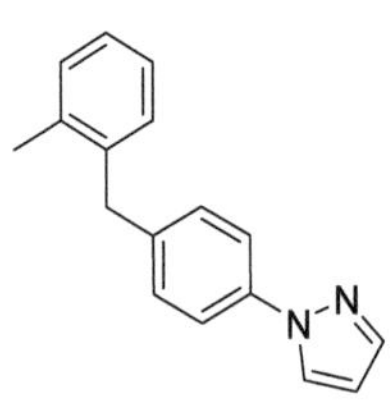 0.1 (Handlon, 2005)	5.	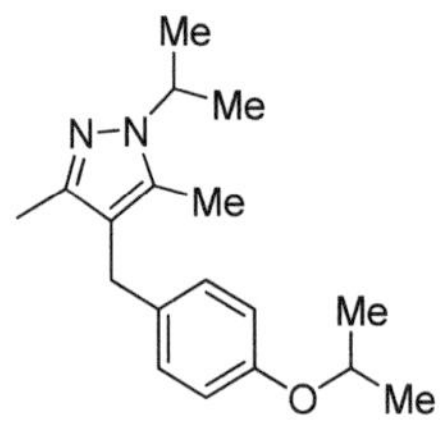 **Remogliflozin etabonate** R = COOEt (prodrug form) **Remogliflozin** R = H (active form) 12.4** (Fujimori et al., 2008)	6.	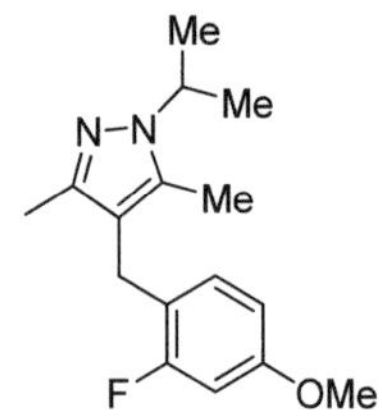 **BI 44847** (Washburn, 2009b)
7.	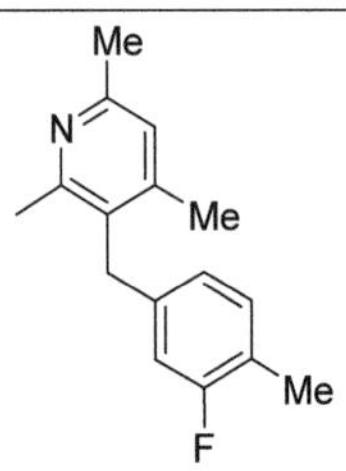 3 (Handlon, 2005)	8.	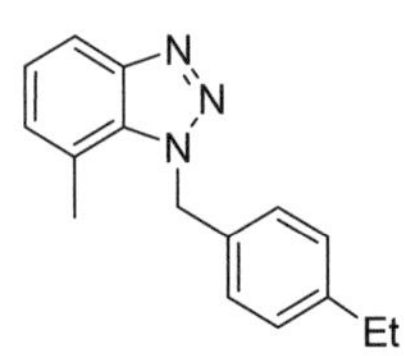 8 (Handlon, 2005)	9.	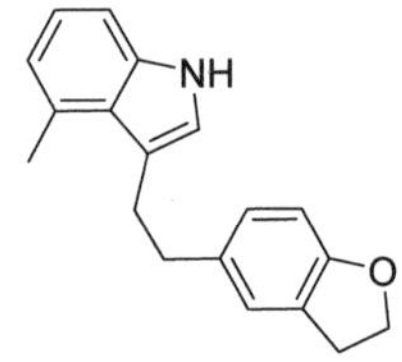 20 (Handlon, 2005)

Table 4. Selected *O*-glucopyranoside type inhibitors of SGLT2 (IC_{50}, EC_{50}^{*}, K_i^{**} values [nM])

The first class of potential SGLT2 inhibitors to be explored was the *O*-glucosides derived from the structure of phlorizin (Table 4, Entry 1) of natural origin isolated from the root bark of the apple tree (Ehrenkranz et al., 2005). Phlorizin lowers plasma glucose levels and improves insulin resistance by increasing renal glucose excretion (Isaji, 2007). However, it is not considered as an antidiabetic drug because of its nonselective inhibition against SGLTs as well as its metabolic instability due to hydrolysis by glucosidase enzymes in the intestinal tract that prevented oral administration (Washburn, 2009a). In addition, enzymatic release of the aglycone phloretin, a micromolar inhibitor of sodium-independent facilitative glucose transporters (GLUTs), could potentially inhibit GLUT-mediated cellular uptake of glucose (Ehrenkranz et al., 2005; Washburn, 2009a). Because of the poor bioavailability and the aforementioned undesirable effects of phlorizin, initial efforts entailed exploring more stable and selective *O*-glucoside analogues of this compound.

T-1095 (Table 4, Entry 2) is a methyl carbonate prodrug which, after oral administration, is rapidly converted to an active metabolite, T-1095A showing high affinity and plausible selectivity against human SGLT2 (Handlon, 2005). Development of T-1095 reached phase II clinical trials but was subsequently discontinued (Isaji, 2007).

The β-D-glucosides in which the aglycone moiety is a phenyl ring substituted in ortho position by a benzyl group represent a promising type of *O*-glucoside candidates (Entries 3 and 4). Sergliflozin (Entry 3), an ethyl carbonate prodrug, emerged from this series to enter clinical trials (Isaji, 2007). According to the *in vitro* assay, its active form is a highly potent and 296-fold more selective inhibitor for human SGLT2 over SGLT1 (Katsuno et al., 2007).

Heteroaromatic *O*-glucosides are the next potent series of SGLT2 inhibitors. Among pyrazole derivatives remogliflozin (Entry 5) showed a reassuring 365-fold selectivity for SGLT2 versus SGLT1 *in vitro* (Fujimori et al., 2008), and reached clinical developments (Isaji, 2007). In addition, an analogue of remogliflozin (Entry 6) presumably entered clinical trials as BI 44847 (Washburn, 2009b). 2-Pyridyl-*O*-glucoside (Entry 7) with a potency of 3 nM against human SGLT2 represent an additional highly active compound of this class (Handlon, 2005).

Efficacy of a series of benzofused heterocyclic derivatives was also investigated and, for example, benzotriazole and indole *O*-glucosides (Entries 8 and 9, respectively) were found to strongly inhibit human SGLT2 (Handlon, 2005).

Susceptibility of *O*-glucosides to enzymatic degradation by glucosidases impacted bioavailability and duration of action (Washburn, 2009b). Therefore, remarkable attention has been paid to metabolically more stable *C*-glucopyranosyl derivatives.

Compounds containing a diarylmethane aglycone represent the first type of this class (Table 5). According to the SAR the benzyl substituent in meta position of the central aryl ring is more favourable compared to the ortho attached derivatives of high activity in case of *O*-glucosides (Washburn, 2009a; Washburn, 2009b). At present, dapagliflozin (Entry 1) with considerable *in vitro* as well as *in vivo* activity is the most advanced SGLT2 inhibitor in phase III clinical trials and has become a leading structure for further inhibitor design (Washburn, 2009a; Washburn, 2009b).

Additional SAR exploration revealed that introduction of an appropriate ortho substituent at the proximal phenyl ring adjacent to the glycosidic bond is beneficial in respect of inhibitory efficiency (Entry 2) (Washburn, 2009a). For example, propargyl ether derivative (Entry 3) exhibited sub-nanomolar activity and a more than 3300-fold selectivity for SGLT2 (Xu et al., 2010).

Replacement of the distal phenyl group with fused rings resulted in a new potent inhibitor type. For example, 1:1 choline complex of azulene (Entry 4) as well as 1:1 L-proline complex of benzothiophene (Entry 5) derivatives appeared as clinical candidates (Washburn, 2009b).

Modification of dapagliflozin by replacing the distal aryl ring by heterocycles led to the discovery of canagliflozin (Entry 6) which obtained the second highest interest in clinical developments (Nomura et al., 2010).

Recently, along this line, the structure of dapagliflozin was modified by other heterocycles such as thiazole (Song et al., 2011), 1,3,4-thiadiazole (Lee et al., 2010b), pyridazine (Kim et al., 2010), and pyrimidine (Lee et al., 2010a) moieties. Among them, the thiazole derivative

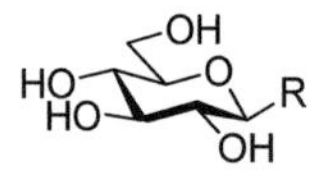

Entry	R	Entry	R	Entry	R
1.	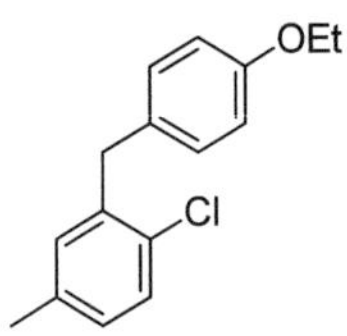 **Dapagliflozin** **BMS-512148** 1.1* (Meng et al., 2008) 0.49 (Song et al., 2011) 6.7 (Xu et al., 2010) 1.4 (Robinson et al., 2010)	2.	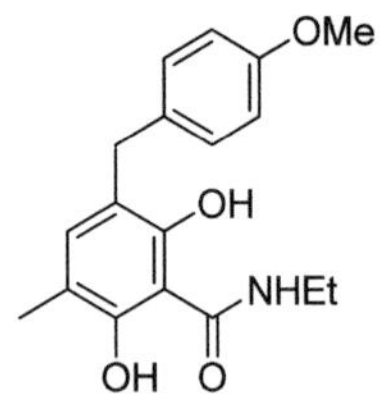 1.3* (Nomura, 2010)	3.	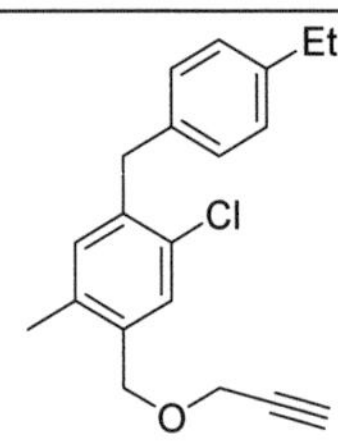 0.3 (Xu et al., 2010)
4.	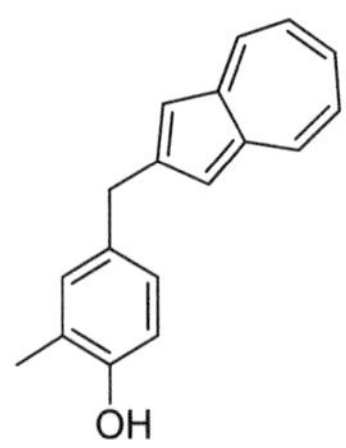 **YM-543** = 1:1 complex with choline 8.9 (Washburn, 2009b)	5.	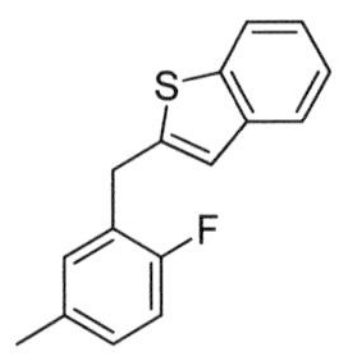 **ASP1941** = 1:1 complex with L-proline 8.4 (Washburn, 2009b)	6.	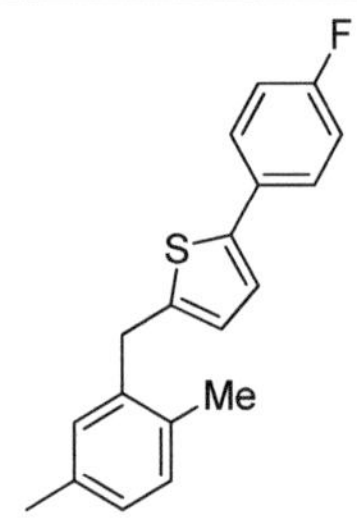 **Canagliflozin** **TA-7284** 2.2 (Nomura et al., 2010)
7.	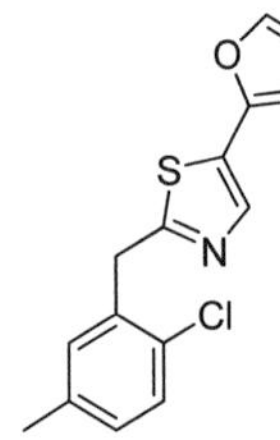 0.72 (Song et al., 2011)	8.	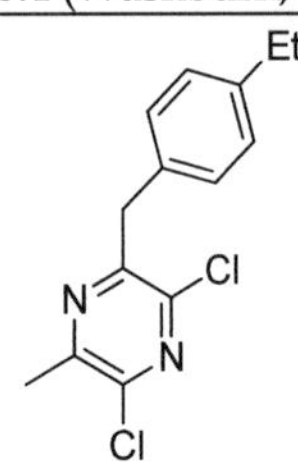 6.5 (Handlon, 2005)	9.	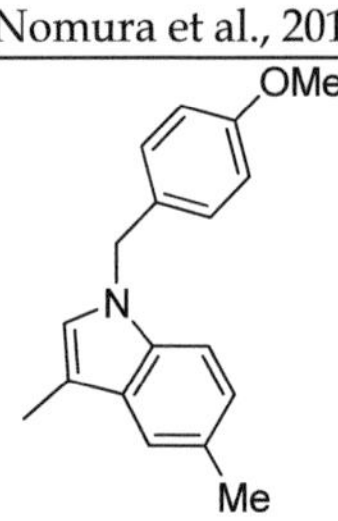 6 (Washburn, 2009b)
10.	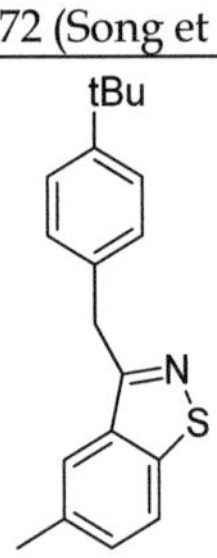 10 (Zhou et al., 2010)	11.	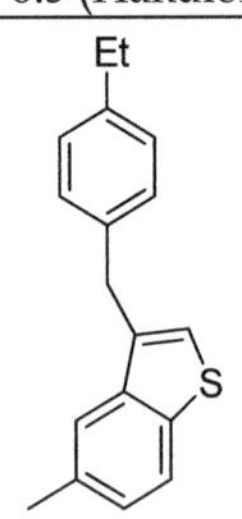 1.4 (Washburn, 2009b)	12.	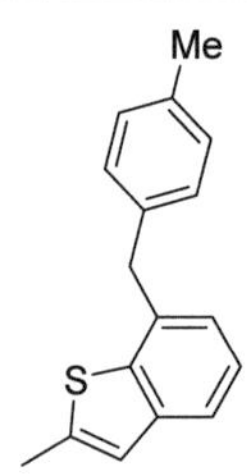 2 (Washburn, 2009b)

Table 5. *C*-glucopyranosyl compounds as SGLT2 inhibitors (IC_{50}, EC_{50}^{*} values [nM])

(Entry 7) displayed the best result, however, according to its *in vitro* (IC_{50} = 0.72 nM) as well as *in vivo* activity, it was less potent than dapagliflozin (IC_{50} = 0.49 nM) (Song et al., 2011).
From *C*-glucosyl hetarenes containing a central heterocyclic ring such as pyrazine, indole, benzisothiazole, and benzothiophenes (Entries 8-12, respectively) the latter two proved most efficient (Washburn, 2009b).
N-Glucopyranosides represent an other series of SGLT2 inhibitors with probably higher metabolic stability as compared to *O*-glucopyranosides. Among these derivatives benzylated aniline-, pyrrole-, and indole *N*-glucosides (Table 6, Entries 1-4, respectively) are potent orally active SGLT2 inhibitors (Washburn, 2009b).
O-Spiroketal *C*-arylglucosides (Entries 5 and 6) which combine the character of both *O*-glucosides and *C*-glucosyl derivatives, show good inhibitory activity (Lv et al., 2009) and high selectivity (Washburn, 2009b) for SGLT2 which can be attributed, in part, to a greater conformational constraint imposed by the spiro-annelated ring system.
In the quest of new candidates for SGLT2 inhibition the modification of the sugar part of the molecules is a further possibility. Replacement of the ring oxygen by a sulfur atom provided new potent 1,5-anhydro-1-thio-D-glucitol derivatives (Table 7, Entries 1-3) (Washburn, 2009b). TS-071 (Entry 1) showed excellent urinary glucose excretion in dogs and is currently undergoing phase II clinical trials (Kakinuma et al., 2010). Modification of the glucose moiety by substituting the hydroxyl groups attached to either C-4 or C-6 with fluorine (Entries 4 and 5) also resulted in effective molecules (Washburn, 2009b). Replacement of the hydroxymethyl side chain of the glucose part with a methyl- or methylsulfanyl group (Entries 6 and 7, respectively) provided molecules with good inhibitory effect, from which LX4211 (Entry 7) is a clinical candidate (Washburn, 2009b). Further transformation of the

Entry		Entry	
1.	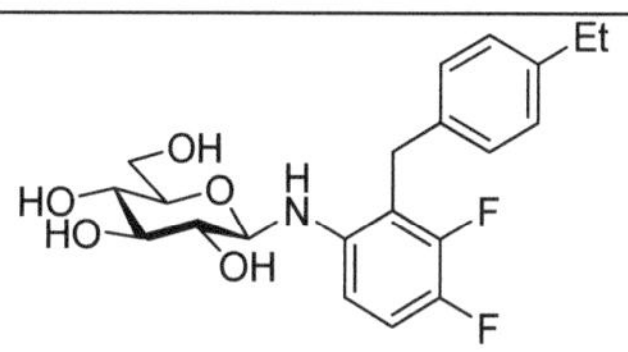 2.9 (Washburn, 2009b)	2.	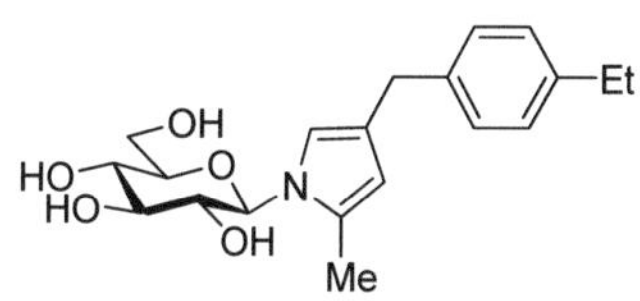 1.1 (Washburn, 2009b)
3.	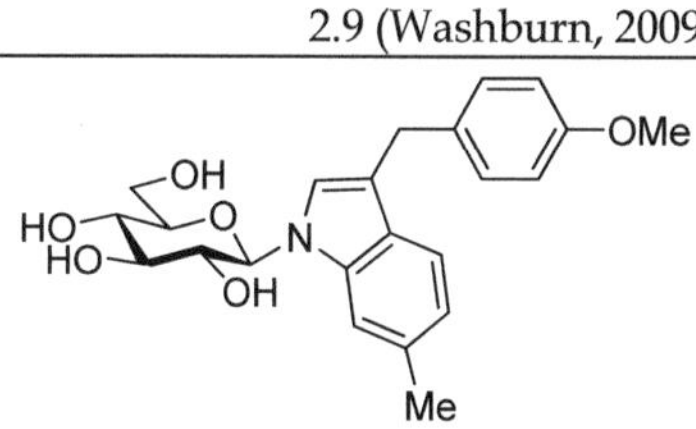 0.9 (Washburn, 2009b)	4.	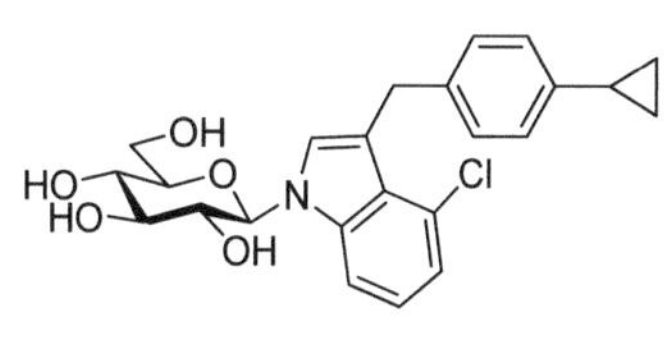 2.3 (Washburn, 2009b)
5.	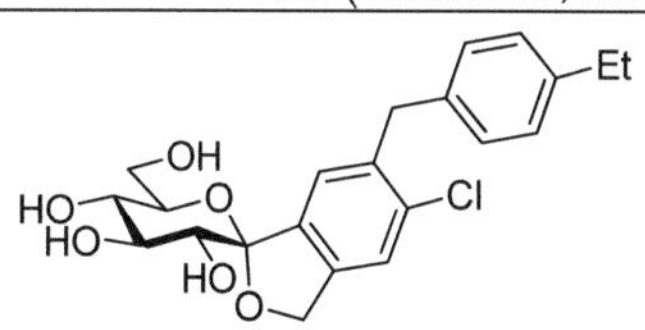 1.5 (Washburn, 2009b)	6.	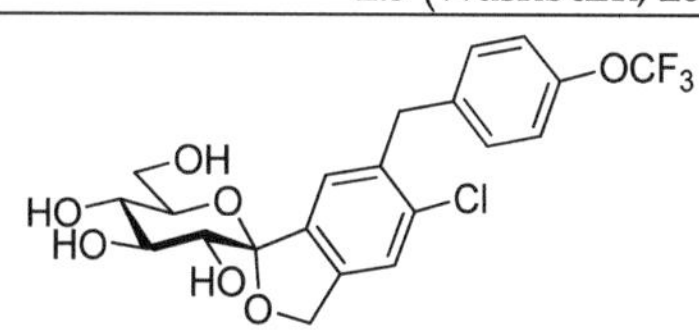 0.3 (Lv et al., 2009)

Table 6. Select compounds of *N*-glucopyranosides, *N*-glucopyranosyl heterocycles, and anomeric spirocycles (IC_{50} [nM])

side chain of the sugar moiety as in the C-5-spirocyclic analogues (Entries 8 and 9) as well as removal of the 4-OH from the glucose ring (Entry 10) furnished compounds exhibiting SGLT2 inhibitory effect in the low nanomolar range (Robinson et al., 2010).

Entry		Entry	
1.	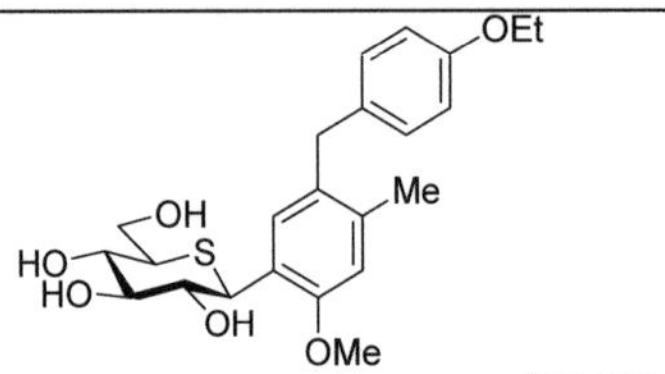 **TS-071** 2.26 (Kakinuma et al., 2010)	2.	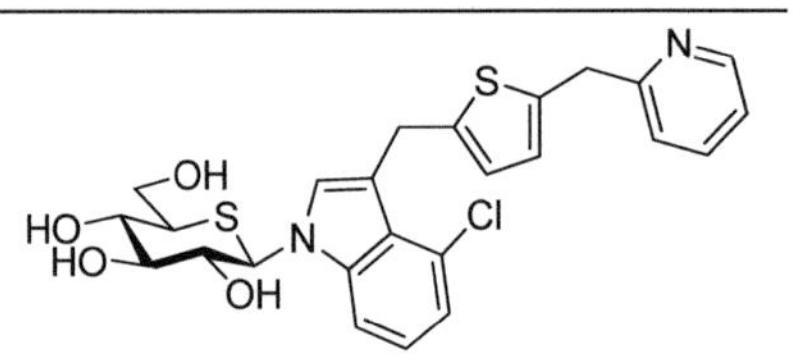 10 (Washburn, 2009b)
3.	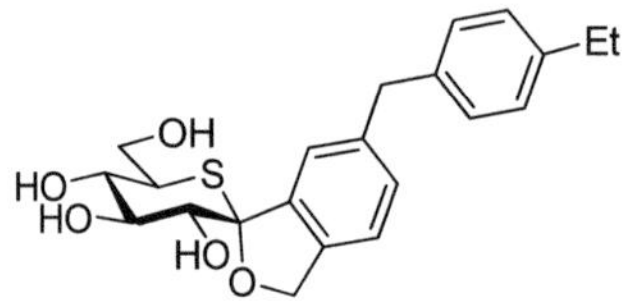 12 (Washburn, 2009b)	4.	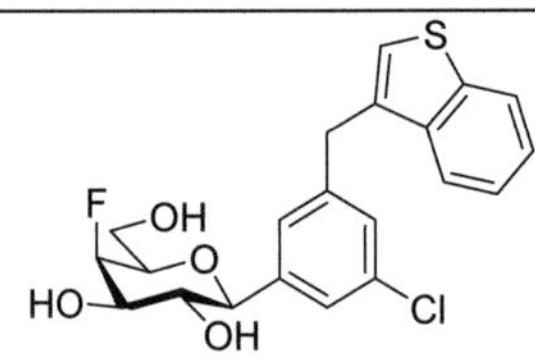 5 (Washburn, 2009b)
5.	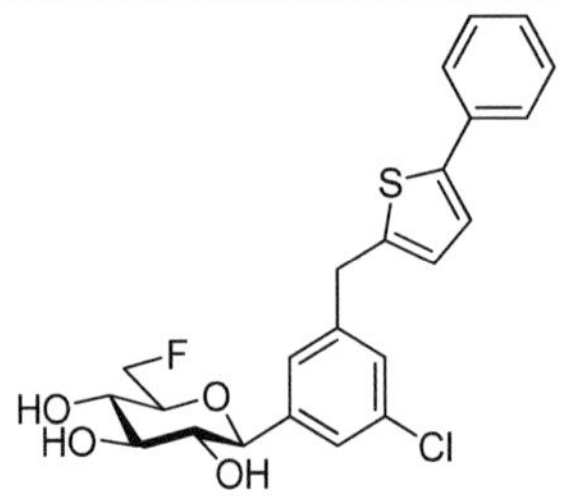 31 (Washburn, 2009b)	6.	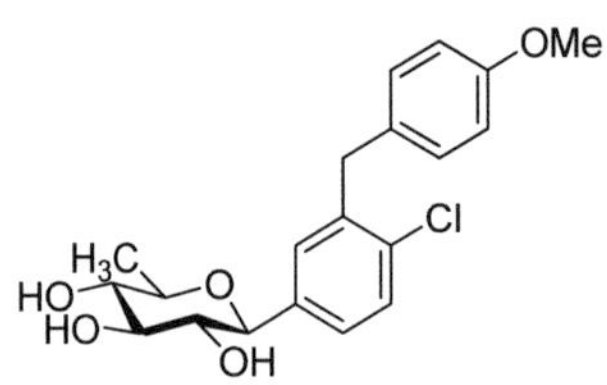 2.4 (Robinson et al., 2010)
7.	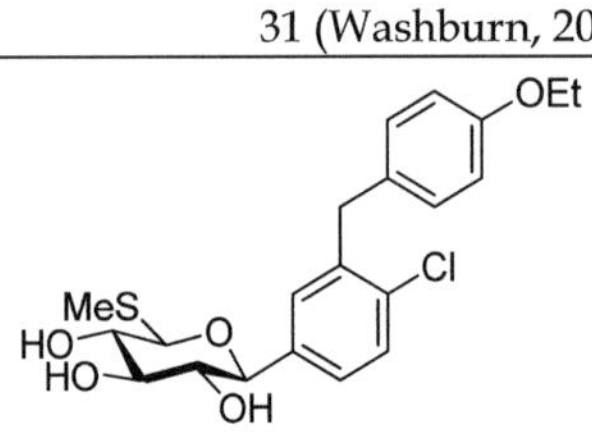 **LX4211** (Washburn, 2009b)	8.	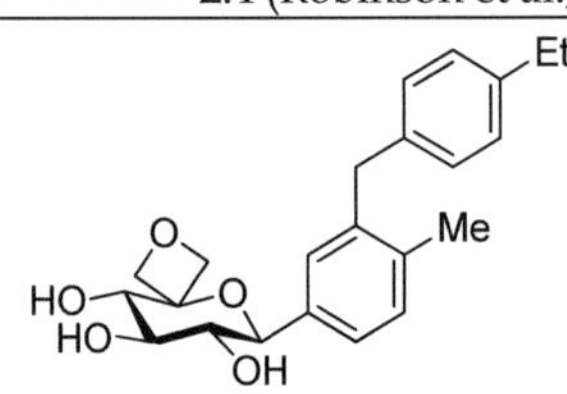 3.4 (Robinson et al., 2010)
9.	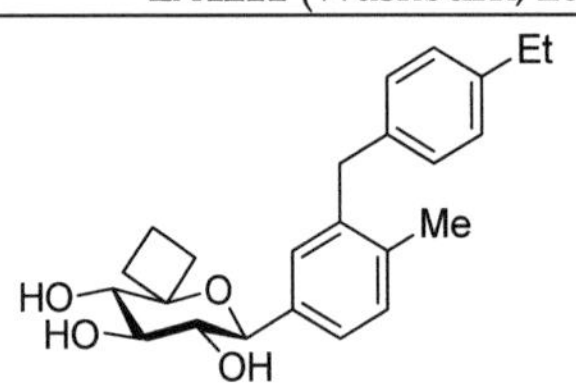 3.0 (Robinson et al., 2010)	10.	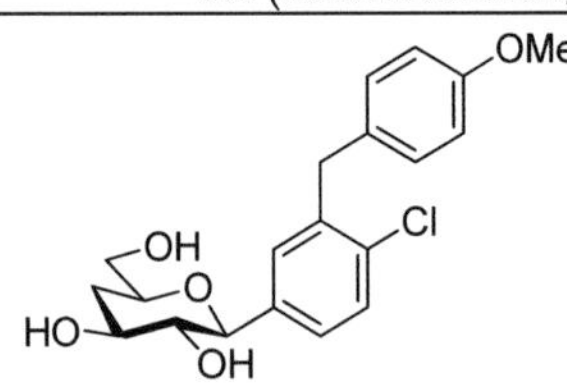 21 (Robinson et al., 2010)

Table 7. Miscalleneous compounds with modifications in the glucose unit as inhibitors of SGLT2 (IC_{50}, [nM])

4. Glucose analogue inhibitors of glycogen phosphorylase

The liver accounts for ~90 % of the body's endogenous glucose production. Hepatic glucose is formed via two pathways: glycogenolysis (release of monomeric glucose from the glycogen polymer storage form) and gluconeogenesis (*de novo* synthesis of glucose from C-3 precursors). Hepatic glucose output is elevated in type 2 diabetic patients, therefore, modulation (mostly inhibition) of one or more of the respective biochemical pathways may contribute to diminishing blood sugar levels. Targets for this can be the glucagon receptor (enhances hepatic glucose output), GCK (catalyzes the first step of glycolysis), 6PF-2-K/F-2,6-P2ase (regulator of glycolytic and gluconeogenic rates through production of F-2,6-P2), G-6-Pase (catalyzes the last step of gluconeogenesis), F-1,6-P2ase (regulates gluconeogenic rates), GSK3 (inhibits glycogen synthase), and glycogen phosphorylase (GP, catalyzes the conversion of glycogen to glucose-1-phosphate monomers) (Morral, 2003). Current evidence indicates that glycogenolysis is an important contributor (~75 %) to the production of glucose by the liver. Furthermore, a substantial portion of glucose formed by gluconeogenesis is cycled through the glycogen pool prior to efflux from the liver cells (Andersen et al., 1999). As GP is the rate determining enzyme of glycogen breakdown (Kurukulasuriya et al., 2003; Ross et al., 2004) its pharmacological inhibition has been regarded as an effective therapeutic approach to treating diseases caused by abnormalities in glycogen metabolism, such as type 2 diabetes (Oikonomakos, 2002; Somsák et al., 2003; Somsák et al., 2005), myocardial ischemia (Tracey, W. et al., 2003; Tracey, W. R. et al., 2004), cerebral ischemia (Sun & Xu, 2010), and tumors (Geschwind et al., 2004; Schnier et al., 2003).

Glycogen phosphorylases (existing as 'muscle', 'brain', or 'liver' isoforms) are allosterically regulated enzymes consisting of a dimeric arrangement of two identical subunits related to each other by a C2 symmetry. Protein crystallographic studies (Chrysina, 2010; Oikonomakos, 2002) revealed the existence of six binding sites in GP (Fig. 1): the catalytic, the inhibitor, the allosteric, the glycogen storage, and the new allosteric sites, as well as the newly discovered benzimidazole site (Chrysina et al., 2005). Each binding site can be targeted by small molecules, and a large variety of inhibitors were tested as described in recent reviews (Loughlin, 2010; Oikonomakos & Somsák, 2008; Somsák et al., 2008).

Physiological investigations with glycogen phosphorylase inhibitors in the context of T2DM have recently been reviewed (Agius, 2010).

Under physiological conditions glucose (Fig. 2) serves as a regulator of GP since the less active T state of the enzyme is stabilized (Board et al., 1995) by its weak binding to the catalytic centre. This has raised the possibility to search for glucose derivatives with much higher affinity to the active site. A large variety of glucose based compounds were synthesized and tested mainly against the prototype of the GP enzymes, the best available rabbit muscle GP (Chrysina, 2010).

For the inhibitory glucose derivatives (Gimisis, 2010; Praly & Vidal, 2010; Somsák, 2011; Somsák et al., 2003; Somsák et al., 2005) protein crystallography showed primary binding to the catalytic site of the enzyme. Some glucose analogues can also occupy the new allosteric site (Oikonomakos et al., 2002), and the benzimidazole-site was evidenced by a 2-(β-D-glucopyranosyl)-benzimidazole (Chrysina et al., 2005).

The studied *O*-, and *S*-glucopyranosides proved very weak inhibitors with K_i values in the 2000-25000 μM and 650-21100 μM, respectively (Somsák et al., 2003; Somsák et al., 2005).

Extensive investigation of *N*-glucopyranosylamide type compounds (Table 8, Entries 1-4) revealed that a) the NHCONHCO linker between the sugar and the aromatic part of the

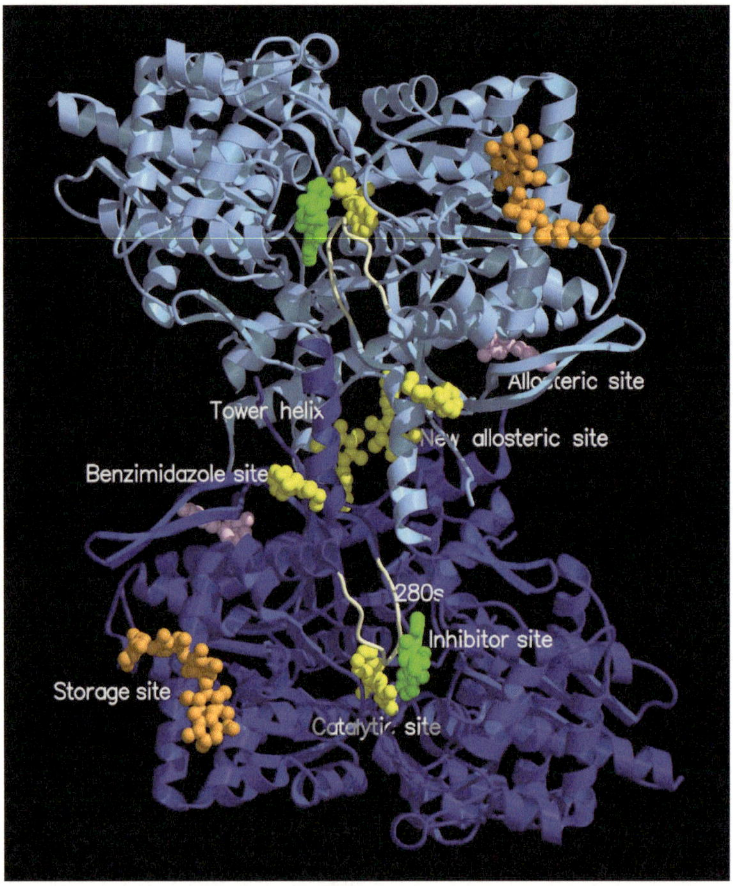

Fig. 1. A schematic diagram of the muscle GPb dimeric molecule viewed down the molecular dyad. (The positions are shown for the catalytic, allosteric, glycogen storage, inhibitor, new allosteric, and benzimidazole sites. The catalytic site, marked by 2-β-D-glucopyranosyl benzimidazole, is buried at the center of the subunit and is accessible to the bulk solvent through a 15 Å-long channel. Binding of the competitive inhibitor benzimidazole promotes the less active T state through stabilization of the closed position of the 280s loop (shown in white). The allosteric site, which binds the activator AMP (indicated in the figure), is situated at the subunit–subunit interface some 30 Å from the catalytic site. The inhibitor site or caffeine binding site, which binds purine compounds such as caffeine and flavopiridol (indicated) is located on the surface of the enzyme some 12 Å from the catalytic site and, in the T state, obstructs the entrance to the catalytic site tunnel. The glycogen storage site (with bound maltopentaose) is on the surface of the molecule some 30 Å from the catalytic site, 40 Å from the allosteric site and 50 Å from the new allosteric inhibitor site. The new allosteric or indole binding site, located inside the central cavity, formed on association of the two subunits, binds indole-2 carboxamide analogs, *N*-benzoyl-*N*′-β-D-glucopyranosyl urea, and benzimidazole (indicated). The novel binding site with bound benzimidazole, also located on the surface of the molecule, is some 31 Å from the catalytic site, 32 Å from the allosteric site, and 32 Å from the indole site. (Figure by courtesy of N. G. Oikonomakos and E. D. Chrysina.)

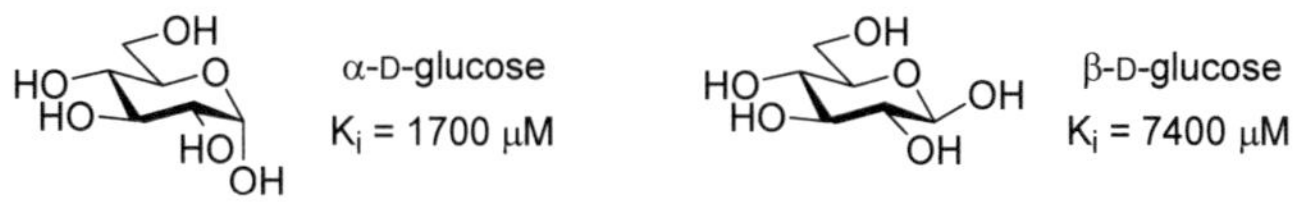

Fig. 2. Structure of α- and β-D-glucose and their inhibition constants with RMGPb.

Entry	Compound	R		
		A	B	C
	(Somsák, 2011; Somsák et al., 2008)		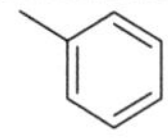	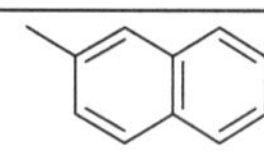
1.	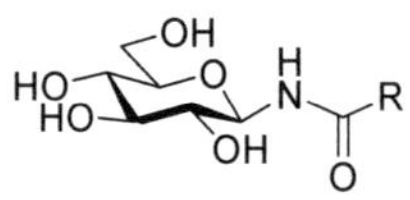	CH_3 32	81	10
2.	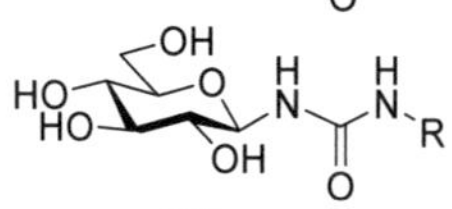	H 140	18	5.2
3.	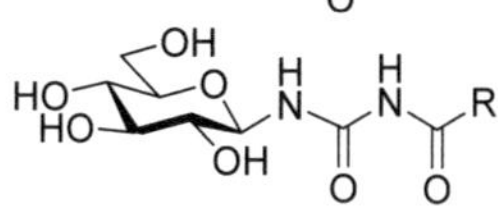	-	4.6	0.35
4.	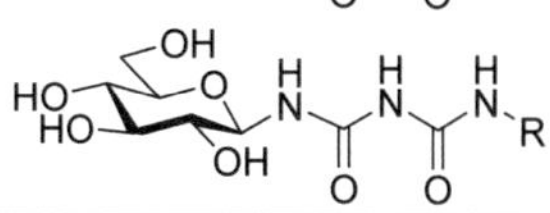	-	21	-
	(Gimisis, 2010)	$-CH_3$	$-(CH_2)_2SCH_3$	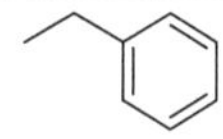
5.	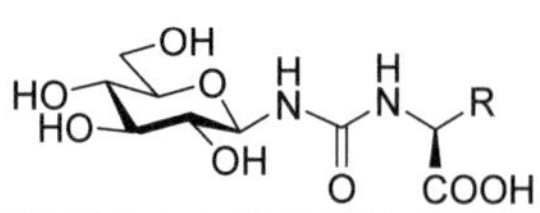	510	1200	350
	(Alexacou et al., 2010; Deleanu et al., 2008)	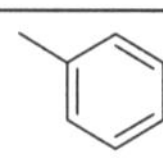	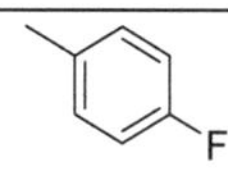	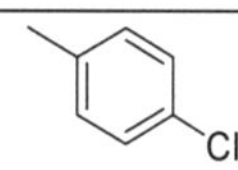
6.	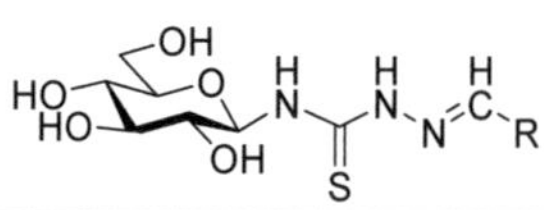	33	5.7	28

Table 8. Inhibition of RMGPb by *N*-glucopyranosidic derivatives (K_i [μM])

compounds and b) a large hydrophobic substituent (compare columns B and C) make the best inhibitor (Entry 3C), actually the first glucose analogue in the nanomolar inhibition range. Other structures, e. g. those in Entries 1-2A, are much less efficient. For further detailed analysis of structure-activity relationships of analogous compounds see (Somsák et al., 2008). *N*-Glucopyranosylamides incorporating natural L-amino acids (Entry 5) proved weaker inhibitors (Gimisis, 2010), although the hydrophobicity of the appendage seems to play an important role in this series, as well (compare Entries 5A and 5B to 5C). Very recently thiosemicarbazone type inhibitors (Entry 6) have been published with inhibitory efficiency in the low micromolar range (Alexacou et al., 2010; Deleanu et al., 2008).

Among 1-glucopyranosyl-1,2,3-triazoles (Table 9, Entries 1-3), which can be regarded as non-classical bioisosteres of *N*-glucopyranosylamides (Table 8, Entry 1), some low micromolar inhibitors were found (Somsák, 2011) which again show the preference for a

Entry	Compound	R	K_i [µM]
	(Somsák, 2011)		
1.	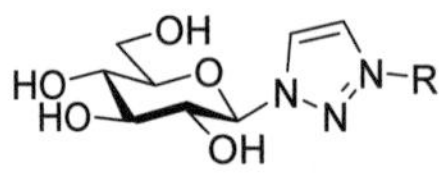	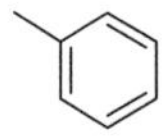	151
2.		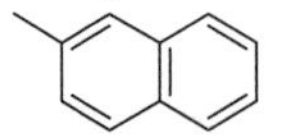	16
3.		$-CH_2OH$	14
	(Gimisis, 2010; Praly & Vidal, 2010)		
4.	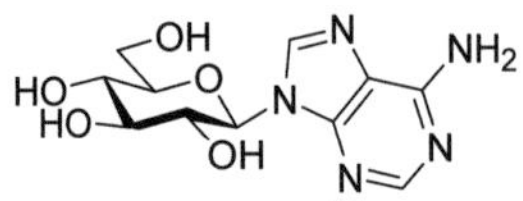		310
5.	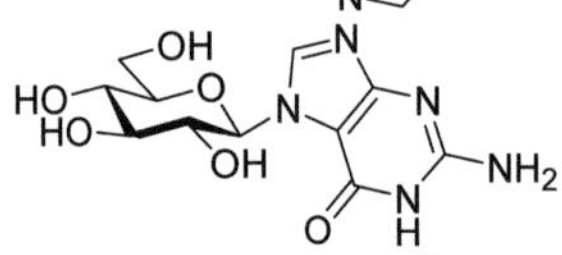		170
6.	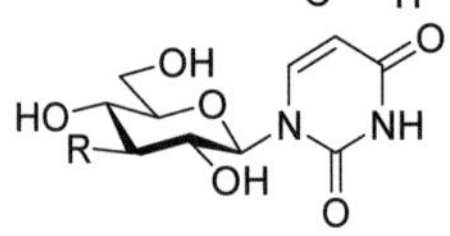	OH	6.1
7.		F	3460
8.	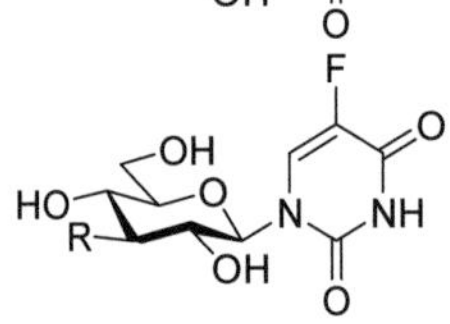	OH	5.5
9.		F	3670
10.	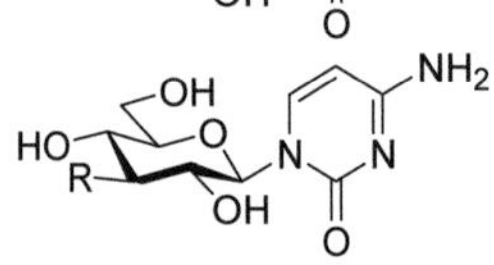	OH	7.7
11.		F	4010
12.	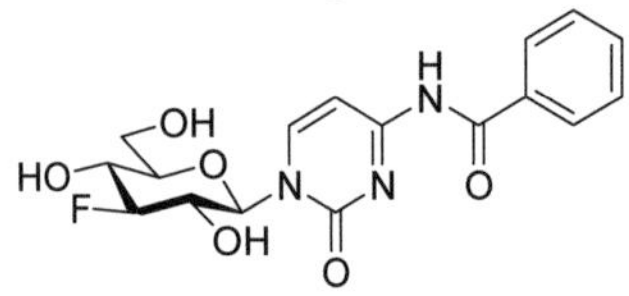		46
13.	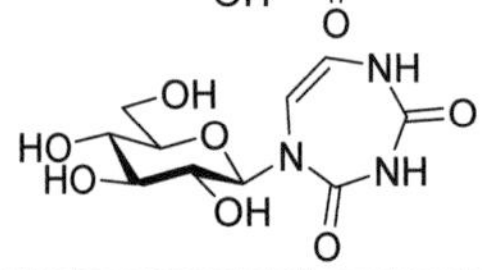		76

Table 9. Inhibition of RMGPb by *N*-glucopyranosyl heterocycles

large aromatic moiety (compare Entries 1 and 2 in Table 9). Interestingly, a polar appendage also led to an inhibitor of similar efficiency (Entry 3). *N*-Glucopyranosyl derivatives of the well known nucleobases were also tested towards GP (Gimisis, 2010): while the purine derivatives (Entries 4 and 5) proved modest inhibitors, pyrimidines in Entries 6, 8, and 10 showed binding in the low micromolar range. Modification of the glucose moiety by replacing the 3-OH of these compounds by fluorine (Entries 7, 9, and 11) weakened the inhibition by a factor of ~600 on an average. On the other hand, introduction of a hydrophobic group (compare Entries 11 and 12) was beneficial in this series, as well, resulting in an almost 100-fold stronger inhibitor. Enlarging the heterocyclic ring to a seven-membered one (Entry 13) gave a weaker inhibitor in comparison to the six-membered pyrimidine derivatives.

Entry	Compound		K_i [μM]
	(Somsák et al., 2003)		
1.	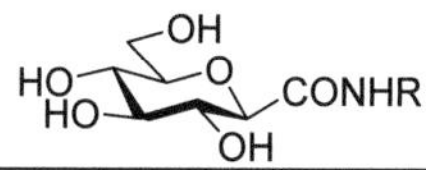	R = H	440
2.		R = CH_3	160
	(Somsák, 2011)		
3.	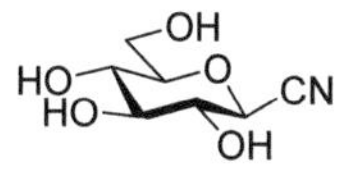		130
4.	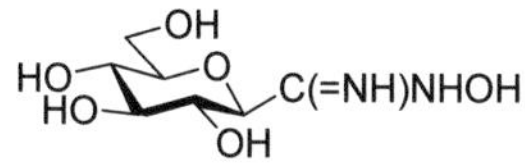		No inhibition
5.	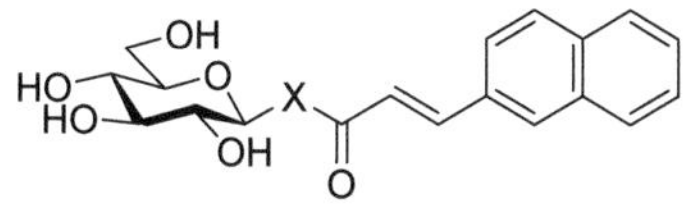	X = CH_2	52 % at 100 μM
6.		X = NH	3.5
7.	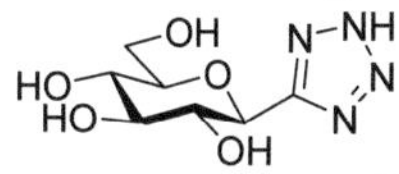		No inhibition
8.	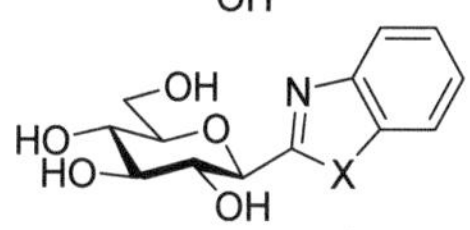	X = S	76
9.		X = NH	9
10.	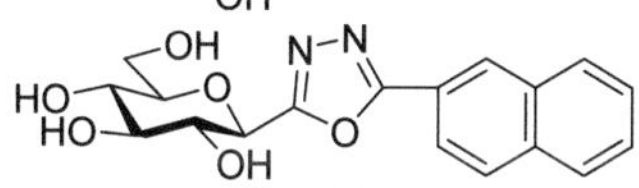		10 % at 625 μM
11.	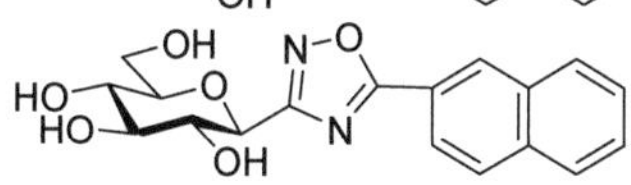		38
12.	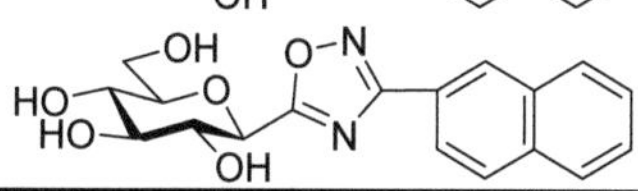		2.4

Table 10. Inhibition of RMGPb by *C*-glucopyranosyl compounds

Glucose derivatives with a substituent attached by a carbon-carbon bond (Table 10, Entries 1-4) showed weak or no inhibition. A comparison of the *C*-glucosyl compound in Entry 5 to the analogous *N*-glucosyl derivative in Entry 6 demonstrates that the more rigid amide type structure binds stronger to GP than its counterpart with the CH_2-group lending more flexibility to the molecule. In a series of *C*-glucopyranosyl heterocycles (Entries 7-12) the size and nature of the heterorings proved very important showing stronger inhibition for the larger ones (compare Entries 7-9), and especially for the benzimidazole in Entry 9. Among oxadiazole derivatives of equal size (Entries 10-12) the constitution of the heterocycle proved decisive to give the low micromolar inhibitor of Entry 12.

The anomeric spiro-hydantoin and -thiohydantoin (Table 11, Entries 1 and 2, respectively) belong to the first efficient compounds of early GP inhibitor design. Changing the sugar part from glucose to xylose (by removal of the CH_2OH substituent, Entries 3 and 4) resulted in complete loss of inhibition. Reversal of the spiro-configuration (compare Entries 1 and 5) as well as spiro-annelation of a six-membered ring (Entry 6) gave compounds with significantly weaker binding (Somsák et al., 2003). Extension of the anomeric spirocycles by further ring-condensations as in Entries 7 and 8 produced practically inefficient structures (Gimisis, 2010). Substitution by aromatic groups in the spiro-isoxazolines (Entries 9 and 11) and spiro-oxathiazoles (Entries 10 and 12) gave good inhibitors and the naphthyl derivatives (Entries 11 and 12) are among the best known glucose derived compounds (Somsák, 2011). Contrary to α-glucosidases, iminosugar type compounds with 5-7 membered rings do not show significant inhibition against GP enzymes: e. g. nojirimicin has no effect, for 1-deoxy-nojirimicin K_i = 55000 μM (for the structures see Table 2) (Compain et al., 2007). There are a few exceptions to this such as DAB and isofagomine derivatives (Fig. 3) (Praly & Vidal, 2010; Somsák et al., 2008; Somsák et al., 2003). A comprehensive tabulation of glycogen phosphorylase inhibition studies with iminosugars can be found in (Compain et al., 2007).

Entry	Compound	X	K_i [μM]
	(Somsák et al., 2003)		
1.	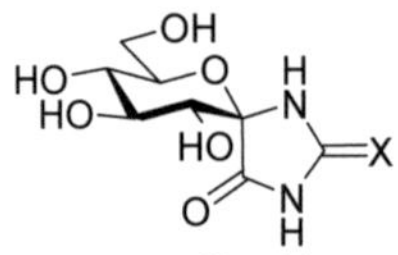	O	3.1
2.		S	5.1
3.	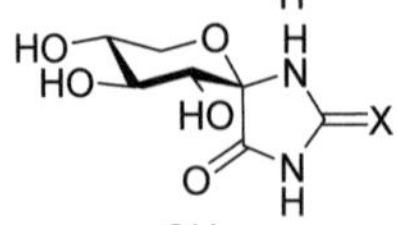	O	No inhibition
4.		S	No inhibition
5.	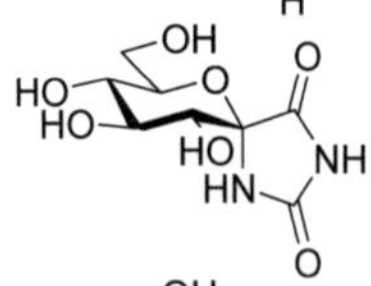		320
6.	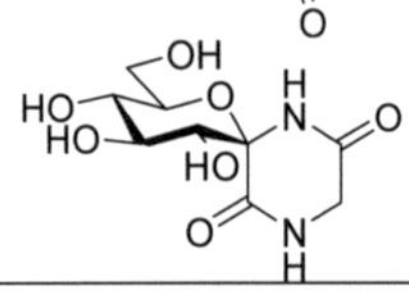		59
	(Gimisis, 2010)		
7.	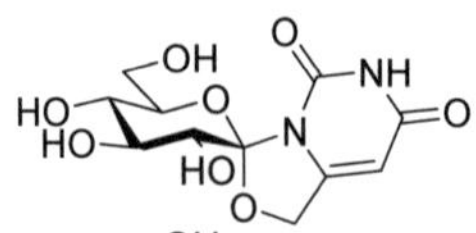		~2100
8.	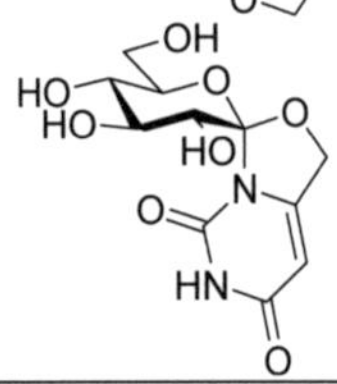		~1700
	(Somsák, 2011)		
9.	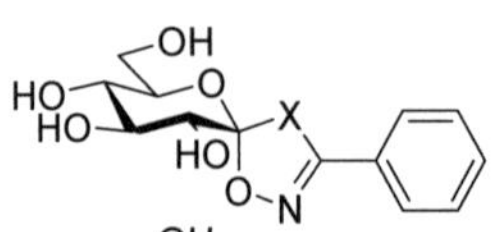	CH_2	19.6
10.		S	26
11.	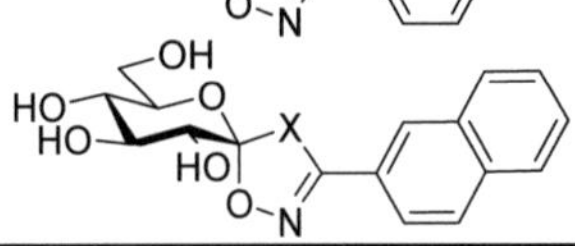	CH_2	0.63
12.		S	0.16

Table 11. Inhibition of RMGPb by anomeric spirocycles

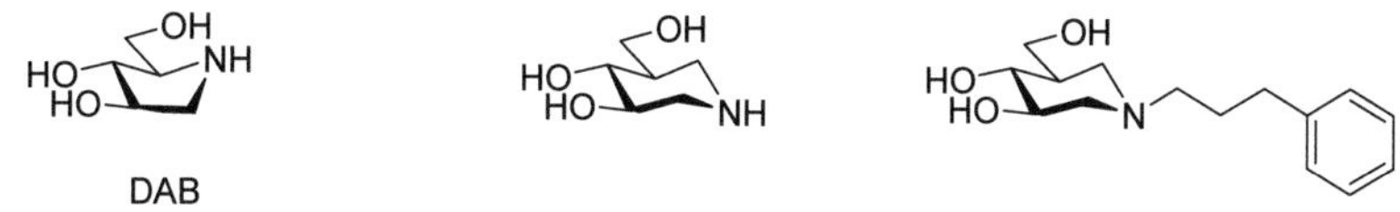

	DAB 1,4-dideoxy-1,4-imino-D-arabinitol	isofagomine	*N*-(3-phenylpropyl)-isofagomine
		IC_{50} [μM]	
RMGPb	0.39	1.21	0.84
RLGPa	0.37	0.68	1.22
PLGPa	0.49	0.67	0.85

Fig. 3. Iminosugar type inhibitors of various GP enzymes

Miscellaneous sugar derivatives including further *O*-, *S*-, and *N*-glucopyranosides, *C*-glucopyranosyl compounds, *S*-glucopyranosyl sulfonamide, homo- and heteromultivalent glucose derivatives, as well as other sugar type compounds with significantly lower efficiency as compared to the above listed ones were also reviewed (Praly & Vidal, 2010; Somsák, 2011; Somsák et al., 2008; Somsák et al., 2003).

While no physiological investigations with glucose analogue inhibitors of GP can be found in the literature, very recently it has been demonstrated that glucopyranosylidene-spiro-thiohydantoin (Table 11, Entry 2) is effective in lowering blood glucose levels and restoring hepatic glycogen content in streptozotocin-induced diabetic rats (Docsa et al., 2011).

5. Conclusion

This survey provided an overview of carbohydrate derivatives and sugar like compounds (glycomimetics) which are employed in current therapies or investigated as potential future medications for type 2 diabetes mellitus. Although these applications and explorations do not exceed the symptomatic level of treatments characteristic of present curing, they promise the possibility of broadening the arsenal of the physician. Together with several other carbohydrate-based therapeutics these drugs and studied molecules pave the way for a more extensive use of saccharides in medicine.

6. Acknowledgment

This work was supported by the Hungarian Scientific Research Fund (OTKA CK 77712) and by the TÁMOP 4.2.1/B-09/1/KONV-2010-0007 project co-financed by the European Union and the European Social Fund.

7. Abbreviations

DPP-4	dipeptidyl-peptidase-4	6PF-2-K	6-phosphofructo-2-kinase
F-1,6-P2ase	fructose-1,6-bisphosphatase	PLGP	pig liver glycogen phosphorylase
F-2,6-P2	fructose-2,6-bisphosphate	PPARγ	peroxisome proliferator-activated receptor γ
G-6-Pase	glucose-6-phosphatase	PTP-1B	protein tyrosin phosphatase-1B
GCK	glucokinase	RLGP	rat liver glycogen phosphorylase
GLP-1	glucagon-like peptide-1	RMGP	rabbit muscle glycogen phosphorylase
GLUT	glucose transporter	SAR	structure-activity relationship
GP	glycogen phosphorylase	SGLT	sodium dependent glucose transporter
GPI	glycogen phosphorylase inhibitor	T2DM	type 2 diabetes mellitus
GSK3	glycogen synthase kinase-3		

8. References

Agius, L. (2010). Physiological control of liver glycogen metabolism: Lessons from novel glycogen phosphorylase inhibitors. *Mini-Reviews in Medicinal Chemistry*, Vol. 10, pp. 1175-1187.

Alberti, G., Zimmet, P., Shaw, J., Bloomgarden, Z., Kaufman, F. & Silink, M. (2004). Type 2 diabetes in the young: The evolving epidemic - The International Diabetes Federation Consensus Workshop. *Diabetes Care*, Vol. 27, pp. 1798-1811.

Alexacou, K. M., Tenchiu, A. C., Chrysina, E. D., Charavgi, M. D., Kostas, I. D., Zographos, S. E., Oikonomakos, N. G. & Leonidas, D. D. (2010). The binding of β-D-glucopyranosyl-thiosemicarbazone derivatives to glycogen phosphorylase: A new class of inhibitors. *Bioorganic & Medicinal Chemistry*, Vol. 18, pp. 7911-7922.

Andersen, B., Rassov, A., Westergaard, N. & Lundgren, K. (1999). Inhibition of glycogenolysis in primary rat hepatocytes by 1,4-dideoxy-1,4-imino-arabinitol. *Biochemical Journal*, Vol. 342, pp. 545-550.

Asano, N. (2009). Sugar-mimicking glycosidase inhibitors: bioactivity and application. *Cellular and Molecular Life Sciences*, Vol. 66, pp. 1479-1492.

Bailey, C. J. (2011). Renal glucose reabsorption inhibitors to treat diabetes. *Trends in Pharmacological Sciences*, Vol. 32, pp. 63-71.

Barroso, I. (2005). Genetics of type 2 diabetes. *Diabetic Medicine*, Vol. 22, pp. 517-535.

Bloomgarden, Z. T. (2004). Type 2 diabetes in the young - The evolving epidemic. *Diabetes Care*, Vol. 27, pp. 998-1010.

Board, M., Hadwen, M. & Johnson, L. N. (1995). Effects of novel analogs of D-glucose on glycogen-phosphorylase activities in crude extracts of liver and skeletal-muscle. *European Journal of Biochemistry*, Vol. 228, pp. 753-761.

Boldys, A. & Okopien, B. (2009). Inhibitors of type 2 sodium glucose co-transporters - a new strategy for diabetes treatment. *Pharmacological Reports*, Vol. 61, pp. 778-784.

Bonnefond, A., Froguel, P. & Vaxillaire, M. (2010). The emerging genetics of type 2 diabetes. *Trends in Molecular Medicine*, Vol. 16, pp. 407-416.

Brownlee, M. (2001). Biochemistry and molecular cell biology of diabetic complications. *Nature*, Vol. 414, pp. 813-820.

Cheng, A. Y. Y. & Fantus, I. G. (2005). Oral antihyperglycemic therapy for type 2 diabetes mellitus. *Canadian Medical Association Journal*, Vol. 172, pp. 213-226.

Chrysina, E. D. (2010). The prototype of glycogen phosphorylase. *Mini-Reviews in Medicinal Chemistry*, Vol. 10, pp. 1093-1101.

Chrysina, E. D., Kosmopolou, M. N., Tiraidis, C., Kardarakis, R., Bischler, N., Leonidas, D. D., Hadady, Z., Somsák, L., Docsa, T., Gergely, P. & Oikonomakos, N. G. (2005). Kinetic and crystallographic studies on 2-(β-D-glucopyranosyl)-5-methyl-1,3,4-oxadiazole, -benzothiazole, and -benzimidazole, inhibitors of muscle glycogen phosphorylase *b*. Evidence for a new binding site. *Protein Science*, Vol. 14, pp. 873-888.

Compain, P., Desvergnes, V., Liautard, V., Pillard, C. & Toumieux, S. (2007). Tables of iminosugars, their biological activities and their potential as therapeutic agents. In: *Iminosugars: From synthesis to therapeutic applications*. Compain, P. & Martin, O. R. (Ed(s).). Chichester, John Wiley & Sons Ltd. pp. 327-455.

Compain, P. & Martin, O. R., Eds. (2007). *Iminosugars: From synthesis to therapeutic applications*. Chichester, John Wiley & Sons Ltd.

de Melo, E. B., Gomes, A. D. & Carvalho, I. (2006). α- and β-Glucosidase inhibitors: chemical structure and biological activity. *Tetrahedron*, Vol. 62, pp. 10277-10302.

Deleanu, A. C., Kostas, I. D., Liratzis, I., Alexacou, K.-M., Leonidas, D. D., Zographos, S. E. & Oikonomakos, N. G. (2008). β-D-Glucopyranosyl-modified thiosemicarbazones as inhibitors of glycogen phosphorylase. *4th Central European Conference Chemistry towards Biology*. Dobogókő, Hungary, September 8-11, 2008. Book of Abstracts p. 80.

Diamond, J. (2003). The double puzzle of diabetes. *Nature*, Vol. 423, pp. 599-602.

Docsa, T., Czifrák, K., Hüse, C., Somsák, L. & Gergely, P. (2011). The effect of glucopyranosylidene-spiro-thiohydantoin on the glycogen metabolism in liver tissues of streptozotocin-induced and obese diabetic rats. *Molecular Medicine Reports*, Vol. 4, pp. 477-481.

Ehrenkranz, J. R. L., Lewis, N. G., Kahn, C. R. & Roth, J. (2005). Phlorizin: a review. *Diabetes-Metabolism Research and Reviews*, Vol. 21, pp. 31-38.

Ehtisham, S. & Barrett, T. G. (2004). The emergence of type 2 diabetes in childhood. *Annals of Clinical Biochemistry*, Vol. 41, pp. 10-16.

El Ashry, E. S. H., Rashed, N. & Shobier, A. H. S. (2000a). Glycosidase inhibitors and their chemotherapeutic value, part 1. *Pharmazie*, Vol. 55, pp. 251-262.

El Ashry, E. S. H., Rashed, N. & Shobier, A. H. S. (2000b). Glycosidase inhibitors and their chemotherapeutic value, part 2. *Pharmazie*, Vol. 55, pp. 331-348.

El Ashry, E. S. H., Rashed, N. & Shobier, A. H. S. (2000c). Glycosidase inhibitors and their chemotherapeutic value, part 3. *Pharmazie*, Vol. 55, pp. 403-415.

Fujimori, Y., Katsuno, K., Nakashima, I., Ishikawa-Takemura, Y., Fujikura, H. & Isaji, M. (2008). Remogliflozin etabonate, in a novel category of selective low-affinity sodium glucose cotransporter (SGLT2) inhibitors, exhibits antidiabetic efficacy in rodent models. *Journal of Pharmacology and Experimental Therapeutics*, Vol. 327, pp. 268-276.

Geschwind, J.-F., Georgiades, C. S., Ko, Y. H. & Pedersen, P. L. (2004). Recently elucidated energy catabolism pathways provide opportunities for novel treatments in hepatocellular carcinoma. *Expert Review of Anticancer Therapy*, Vol. 4, pp. 449-457.

Gimisis, T. (2010). Synthesis of *N*-glucopyranosidic derivatives as potential inhibitors that bind at the catalytic site of glycogen phosphorylase. *Mini-Reviews in Medicinal Chemistry*, Vol. 10, pp. 1127-1138.

Green, A., Hirsch, N. C. & Pramming, S. K. (2003). The changing world demography of type 2 diabetes. *Diabetes-Metabolism Research and Reviews*, Vol. 19, pp. 3-7.

Handlon, A. L. (2005). Sodium glucose co-transporter 2 (SGLT2) inhibitors as potential antidiabetic agents. *Expert Opinion on Therapeutic Patents*, Vol. 15, pp. 1531-1540.

Hanhineva, K., Torronen, R., Bondia-Pons, I., Pekkinen, J., Kolehmainen, M., Mykkanan, H. & Poutanen, K. (2010). Impact of dietary polyphenols on carbohydrate metabolism. *International Journal of Molecular Sciences*, Vol. 11, pp. 1365-1402.

Hengesh, E. J. (1995). Drugs affecting sugar metabolism. In: *Principles of Medicinal Chemistry*. Foye, W. O., Lemke, T. L. & Williams, D. A. (Ed(s).). Baltimore, Williams & Wilkins. pp. 581-600.

Home, G., Wilson, F. X., Tinsley, J., Williams, D. H. & Storer, R. (2011). Iminosugars past, present and future: medicines for tomorrow. *Drug Discovery Today*, Vol. 16, pp. 107-118.

Idris, I. & Donnelly, R. (2009). Sodium-glucose co-transporter-2 inhibitors: an emerging new class of oral antidiabetic drug. *Diabetes Obesity & Metabolism,* Vol. 11, pp. 79-88.

Isaji, M. (2007). Sodium-glucose cotransporter inhibitors for diabetes. *Current Opinion in Investigational Drugs,* Vol. 8, pp. 285-292.

Israili, Z. H. (2011). Advances in the treatment of type 2 diabetes mellitus. *American Journal of Therapeutics,* Vol. 18, pp. 117-152.

Kakinuma, H., Oi, T., Hashimoto-Tsuchiya, Y., Arai, M., Kawakita, Y., Fukasawa, Y., Iida, I., Hagima, N., Takeuchi, H., Chino, Y., Asami, J., Okumura-Kitajima, L., Io, F., Yamamoto, D., Miyata, N., Takahashi, T., Uchida, S. & Yamamoto, K. (2010). (1*S*)-1,5-Anhydro-1-[5-(4-ethoxybenzyl)-2-methoxy-4-methylphenyl]-1-thio-D-glucitol (TS-071) is a potent, selective sodium-dependent glucose cotransporter 2 (SGLT2) inhibitor for type 2 diabetes treatment. *Journal of Medicinal Chemistry,* Vol. 53, pp. 3247-3261.

Katsuno, K., Fujimori, Y., Takemura, Y., Hiratochi, M., Itoh, F., Komatsu, Y., Fujikura, H. & Isaji, M. (2007). Sergliflozin, a novel selective inhibitor of low-affinity sodium glucose cotransporter (SGLT2), validates the critical role of SGLT2 in renal glucose reabsorption and modulates plasma glucose level. *Journal of Pharmacology and Experimental Therapeutics,* Vol. 320, pp. 323-330.

Kim, M. J., Lee, J., Kang, S. Y., Lee, S. H., Son, E. J., Jung, M. E., Lee, S. H., Song, K. S., Lee, M., Han, H. K., Kim, J. & Lee, J. (2010). Novel *C*-aryl glucoside SGLT2 inhibitors as potential antidiabetic agents: pyridazinylmethylphenyl glucoside congeners. *Bioorganic & Medicinal Chemistry Letters,* Vol. 20, pp. 3420-3425.

Krentz, A. J. & Bailey, C. J. (2005). Oral antidiabetic agents - current role in type 2 diabetes mellitus. *Drugs,* Vol. 65, pp. 385-411.

Kurukulasuriya, R., Link, J. T., Madar, D. J., Pei, Z., Richards, S. J., Rohde, J. J., Souers, A. J. & Szczepankiewicz, B. G. (2003). Potential drug targets and progress towards pharmacologic inhibition of hepatic glucose production. *Current Medicinal Chemistry,* Vol. 10, pp. 123-153.

Lee, J., Kim, J. Y., Choi, J., Lee, S. H., Kim, J. & Lee, J. (2010a). Pyrimidinylmethylphenyl glucoside as novel *C*-aryl glucoside SGLT2 inhibitors. *Bioorganic & Medicinal Chemistry Letters,* Vol. 20, pp. 7046-7049.

Lee, J., Lee, S. H., Seo, H. J., Son, E. J., Lee, S. H., Jung, M. E., Lee, M., Han, H. K., Kim, J., Kang, J. & Lee, J. (2010b). Novel *C*-aryl glucoside SGLT2 inhibitors as potential antidiabetic agents: 1,3,4-thiadiazolylmethylphenyl glucoside congeners. *Bioorganic & Medicinal Chemistry,* Vol. 18, pp. 2178-2194.

Lillelund, V. H., Jensen, H. H., Liang, X. & Bols, M. (2002). Recent developments of transition-state analogue glycosidase inhibitors of non-natural product origin. *Chemical Reviews,* Vol. 102, pp. 515-553.

Loughlin, W. A. (2010). Recent advances in the allosteric inhibition of glycogen phosphorylase. *Mini-Reviews in Medicinal Chemistry,* Vol. 10, pp. 1139-1155.

Lowell, B. B. & Shulman, G. I. (2005). Mitochondrial dysfunction and type 2 diabetes. *Science,* Vol. 307, pp. 384-387.

Lv, B. H., Xu, B. H., Feng, Y., Peng, K., Xu, G., Du, J. Y., Zhang, L. L., Zhang, W. B., Zhang, T., Zhu, L. C., Ding, H. F., Sheng, Z. L., Welihinda, A., Seed, B. & Chen, Y. W. (2009). Exploration of *O*-spiroketal *C*-arylglucosides as novel and selective renal sodium-dependent glucose co-transporter 2 (SGLT2) inhibitors. *Bioorganic & Medicinal Chemistry Letters*, Vol. 19, pp. 6877-6881.

Meng, W., Ellsworth, B. A., Nirschl, A. A., McCann, P. J., Patel, M., Girotra, R. N., Wu, G., Sher, P. M., Morrison, E. P., Biller, S. A., Zahler, R., Deshpande, P. P., Pullockaran, A., Hagan, D. L., Morgan, N., Taylor, J. R., Obermeier, M. T., Humphreys, W. G., Khanna, A., Discenza, L., Robertson, J. G., Wang, A., Hang, S., Wetterau, J. R., Janovitz, E. B., Flint, O. P., Whaley, J. M. & Washburn, W. N. (2008). Discovery of dapagliflozin: A potent, selective renal sodium-dependent glucose cotransporter 2 (SGLT2) inhibitor for the treatment of type 2 diabetes. *Journal of Medicinal Chemistry*, Vol. 51, pp. 1145-1149.

Mizuno, C. S., Chittiboyina, A. G., Kurtz, T. W., Pershadsingh, H. A. & Avery, M. A. (2008). Type 2 diabetes and oral antihyperglycemic drugs. *Current Medicinal Chemistry*, Vol. 15, pp. 61-74.

Mohan, S. & Pinto, B. M. (2007). Zwitterionic glycosidase inhibitors: salacinol and related analogues. *Carbohydrate Research*, Vol. 342, pp. 1551-1580.

Moller, D. E. (2001). New drug targets for type 2 diabetes and the metabolic syndrome. *Nature*, Vol. 414, pp. 821-827.

Morral, N. (2003). Novel targets and therapeutic strategies for type 2 diabetes. *Trends in Endocrinology and Metabolism*, Vol. 14, pp. 169-175.

Muraoka, O., Morikawa, T., Miyake, S., Akaki, J., Ninomiya, K., Pongpiriyadacha, Y. & Yoshikawa, M. (2011). Quantitative analysis of neosalacinol and neokotalanol, another two potent alpha-glucosidase inhibitors from Salacia species, by LC-MS with ion pair chromatography. *Journal of Natural Medicines*, Vol. 65, pp. 142-148.

Nomura, S. (2010). Renal sodium-dependent glucose cotransporter 2 (SGLT2) inhibitors for new anti-diabetic agent. *Current Topics in Medicinal Chemistry*, Vol. 10, pp. 411-418.

Nomura, S., Sakamaki, S., Hongu, M., Kawanishi, E., Koga, Y., Sakamoto, T., Yamamoto, Y., Ueta, K., Kimata, H., Nakayama, K. & Tsuda-Tsukimoto, M. (2010). Discovery of canagliflozin, a novel *C*-glucoside with thiophene ring, as sodium-dependent glucose cotransporter 2 inhibitor for the treatment of type 2 diabetes mellitus. *Journal of Medicinal Chemistry*, Vol. 53, pp. 6355-6360.

Nourparvar, A., Bulotta, A., Di Mario, U. & Perfetti, R. (2004). Novel strategies for the pharmacological management of type 2 diabetes. *Trends in Pharmacological Sciences*, Vol. 25, pp. 86-91.

Oikonomakos, N. G. (2002). Glycogen phosphorylase as a molecular target for type 2 diabetes therapy. *Current Protein & Peptide Science*, Vol. 3, pp. 561-586.

Oikonomakos, N. G., Kosmopolou, M., Zographos, S. E., Leonidas, D. D., Somsák, L., Nagy, V., Praly, J.-P., Docsa, T., Tóth, B. & Gergely, P. (2002). Binding of *N*-acetyl-*N'*-β-D-glucopyranosyl urea and *N*-benzoyl-*N'*-β-D-glucopyranosyl urea to glycogen phosphorylase *b*: Kinetic and crystallographic studies. *European Journal of Biochemistry*, Vol. 269, pp. 1684-1696.

Oikonomakos, N. G. & Somsák, L. (2008). Recent advances in glycogen phosphorylase inhibitor design. *Current Opinion in Investigational Drugs*, Vol. 9, pp. 379-395.

Padwal, R., Majumdar, S. R., Johnson, J. A., Varney, J. & McAlister, F. A. (2005). A systematic delay or pre review of drug therapy to delay or prevent type 2 diabetes. *Diabetes Care*, Vol. 28, pp. 736-744.

Panunti, B., Jawa, A. A. & Fonseca, V. A. (2004). Mechanisms and therapeutic targets in type 2 diabetes mellitus. *Drug Discovery Today: Disease Mechanisms*, Vol. 1, pp. 151-157.

Praly, J. P. & Vidal, S. (2010). Inhibition of glycogen phosphorylase in the context of type 2 diabetes, with focus on recent inhibitors bound at the active site. *Mini-Reviews in Medicinal Chemistry*, Vol. 10, pp. 1102-1126.

Rendell, M. (2004). The role of sulphonylureas in the management of type 2 diabetes mellitus. *Drugs*, Vol. 64, pp. 1339-1358.

Robinson, R. P., Mascitti, V., Boustany-Kari, C. M., Carr, C. L., Foley, P. M., Kimoto, E., Leininger, M. T., Lowe, A., Klenotic, M. K., MacDonald, J. I., Maguire, R. J., Masterson, V. M., Maurer, T. S., Miao, Z., Patel, J. D., Preville, C., Reese, M. R., She, L., Steppan, C. M., Thuma, B. A. & Zhu, T. (2010). C-Aryl glycoside inhibitors of SGLT2: exploration of sugar modifications including C-5 spirocyclization. *Bioorganic & Medicinal Chemistry Letters*, Vol. 20, pp. 1569-1572.

Ross, S. A., Gulve, E. A. & Wang, M. H. (2004). Chemistry and biochemistry of type 2 diabetes. *Chemical Reviews*, Vol. 104, pp. 1255-1282.

Santer, R. & Calado, J. (2010). Familial renal glucosuria and SGLT2: From a Mendelian trait to a therapeutic target. *Clinical Journal of the American Society of Nephrology*, Vol. 5, pp. 133-141.

Scheen, A. J. (2003). Is there a role for α-glucosidase inhibitors in the prevention of type 2 diabetes mellitus? *Drugs*, Vol. 63, pp. 933-951.

Schnier, J. B., Nishi, K., Monks, A., Gorin, F. A. & Bradbury, E. M. (2003). Inhibition of glycogen phosphorylase (GP) by CP-91,149 induces growth inhibition correlating with brain GP expression. *Biochemical and Biophysical Research Communications*, Vol. 309, pp. 126-134.

Sladek, R., Rocheleau, G., Rung, J., Dina, C., Lishuang, S., Serre, D., Boutin, P., Vincent, D., Belisle, A., Hadjadj, S., Balkau, B., Heude, B., Charpentier, G., Hudson, T. J., Montpetit, A., Pshezhetsky, A. V., Prentki, M., Posner, B. I., Balding, D. J., Meyre, D., Sladek, R., Rocheleau, G., Rung, J., Dina, C., Shen, L., Serre, D., Boutin, P., Vincent, D., Belisle, A., Hadjadj, S., Balkau, B., Heude, B., Charpentier, G., Hudson, T. J., Montpetit, A., Pshezhetsky, A. V., Prentki, M., Posner, B. I., Balding, D. J., Meyre, D., Polychronakos, C., Sladek, R., Rocheleau, G., Rung, J., Dina, C., Shen, L., Serre, D., Boutin, P., Vincent, D., Belisle, A., Hadjadj, S., Balkau, B., Heude, B., Charpentier, G., Hudson, T. J., Montpetit, A., Pshezhetsky, A. V., Prentki, M., Posner, B. I., Balding, D. J., Meyre, D., Polychronakos, C., Froguel, P., Sladek, R., Rocheleau, G., Rung, J., Dina, C., Shen, L., Serre, D., Boutin, P., Vincent, D., Belisle, A., Hadjadj, S., Balkau, B., Heude, B., Charpentier, G., Hudson, T. J., Montpetit, A., Pshezhetsky, A. V., Prentki, M., Posner, B. I., Balding, D. J., Meyre, D., Polychronakos, C. & Froguel, P. (2007). A genome-wide association study identifies novel risk loci for type 2 diabetes. *Nature*, Vol. 445, pp. 881-885.

Somsák, L. (2011). Glucose derived inhibitors of glycogen phosphorylase. *Comptes Rendus Chimie*, Vol. 14, pp. 211-223.

Somsák, L., Czifrák, K., Tóth, M., Bokor, É., Chrysina, E. D., Alexacou, K. M., Hayes, J. M., Tiraidis, C., Lazoura, E., Leonidas, D. D., Zographos, S. E. & Oikonomakos, N. G. (2008). New inhibitors of glycogen phosphorylase as potential antidiabetic agents. *Current Medicinal Chemistry*, Vol. 15, pp. 2933-2983.

Somsák, L., Nagy, V., Hadady, Z., Docsa, T. & Gergely, P. (2003). Glucose analog inhibitors of glycogen phosphorylases as potential antidiabetic agents: recent developments. *Current Pharmaceutical Design*, Vol. 9, pp. 1177-1189.

Somsák, L., Nagy, V., Hadady, Z., Felföldi, N., Docsa, T. & Gergely, P. (2005). Recent developments in the synthesis and evaluation of glucose analog inhibitors of glycogen phosphorylases as potential antidiabetic agents. In: *Frontiers in Medicinal Chemistry*. Reitz, A. B., Kordik, C. P., Choudhary, M. I. & Rahman, A. u. (Ed(s).). Bentham. pp. 253-272.

Song, K. S., Lee, S. H., Kim, M. J., Seo, H. J., Lee, J., Lee, S. H., Jung, M. E., Son, E. J., Lee, M., Kim, J. & Lee, J. (2011). Synthesis and SAR of thiazolylmethylphenyl glucoside as novel C-aryl glucoside SGLT2 inhibitors. *ACS Medicinal Chemistry Letters*, Vol. 2, pp. 182-187.

Stumvoll, M., Goldstein, B. J. & van Haeften, T. W. (2005). Type 2 diabetes: principles of pathogenesis and therapy. *Lancet*, Vol. 365, pp. 1333-1346.

Sun, H. & Xu, L. (2010). Pharmacological manipulation of brain glycogenolysis as a therapeutic approach to cerebral ischemia. *Mini-Reviews in Medicinal Chemistry*, Vol. 10, pp. 1188-1193.

Toye, A. & Gauguier, D. (2003). Genetics and functional genomics of type 2 diabetes mellitus. *Genome Biology*, Vol. 4, pp. 241.

Tracey, W., Treadway, J., Magee, W., McPherson, R., Levy, C., Wilder, D., Li, Y., Yue, C., Zavadoski, W., Gibbs, E., Smith, A., Flynn, D. & Knight, D. (2003). A novel glycogen phosphorylase inhibitor, CP-368296, reduces myocardial ischemic injury. *Diabetes*, Vol. 52, pp. A135-A135.

Tracey, W. R., Treadway, J. L., Magee, W. P., Sutt, J. C., McPherson, R. K., Levy, C. B., Wilder, D. E., Yu, L. J., Chen, Y., Shanker, R. M., Mutchler, A. K., Smith, A. H., Flynn, D. M. & Knight, D. R. (2004). Cardioprotective effects of ingliforib, a novel glycogen phosphorylase inhibitor. *American Journal of Physiology-Heart and Circulatory Physiology*, Vol. 286, pp. H1177-H1184.

Treadway, J. L., Mendys, P. & Hoover, D. J. (2001). Glycogen phosphorylase inhibitors for treatment of type 2 diabetes mellitus. *Expert Opinion on Investigational Drugs*, Vol. 10, pp. 439-454.

Tundis, R., Loizzo, M. R. & Menichini, F. (2010). Natural products as α-amylase and α-glycosidase inhibitors and their hypoglycaemic potential in the treatment of diabetes: An update. *Mini-Reviews in Medicinal Chemistry, 2010, 10, 315*, Vol. 10, pp. 315-331.

Uwaifo, G. I. & Ratner, R. E. (2005). Novel pharmacologic agents for type 2 diabetes. *Endocrinology and Metabolism Clinics of North America*, Vol. 34, pp. 155-197.

Vaidya, H. B. & Goyal, R. K. (2010). Exploring newer target sodium glucose transporter 2 for the treatment of diabetes mellitus. *Mini-Reviews in Medicinal Chemistry*, Vol. 10, pp. 905-913.

Wagman, A. S., Johnson, K. W. & Bussiere, D. E. (2004). Discovery and development of GSK3 inhibitors for the treatment of type 2 diabetes. *Current Pharmaceutical Design*, Vol. 10, pp. 1105-1137.

Wagman, A. S. & Nuss, J. M. (2001). Current therapies and emerging targets for the treatment of diabetes. *Current Pharmaceutical Design*, Vol. 7, pp. 417-450.

Washburn, W. N. (2009a). Development of the renal glucose reabsorption inhibitors: A new mechanism for the pharmacotherapy of diabetes mellitus type 2. *Journal of Medicinal Chemistry*, Vol. 52, pp. 1785-1794.

Washburn, W. N. (2009b). Evolution of sodium glucose co-transporter 2 inhibitors as anti-diabetic agents. *Expert Opinion on Therapeutic Patents*, Vol. 19, pp. 1485-1499.

Wright, E. M. (2001). Renal Na^+-glucose cotransporters. *American Journal of Physiology-Renal Physiology*, Vol. 280, pp. F10-F18.

Xie, W., Tanabe, G., Akaki, J., Morikawa, T., Ninomiya, K., Minematsu, T., Yoshikawa, M., Wu, X. & Muraoka, O. (2011). Isolation, structure identification and SAR studies on thiosugar sulfonium salts, neosalaprinol and neoponkoranol, as potent [alpha]-glucosidase inhibitors. *Bioorganic & Medicinal Chemistry*, Vol. 19, pp. 2015-2022.

Xu, B. H., Feng, Y., Lv, B. H., Xu, G., Zhang, L. L., Du, J. Y., Peng, K., Xub, M., Dong, J. J., Zhang, W. B., Zhang, T., Zhu, L. C., Ding, H. F., Sheng, Z. L., Welihinda, A., Seed, B. & Chen, Y. W. (2010). ortho-Substituted *C*-aryl glucosides as highly potent and selective renal sodium-dependent glucose co-transporter 2 (SGLT2) inhibitors. *Bioorganic & Medicinal Chemistry*, Vol. 18, pp. 4422-4432.

Zechel, D. L. & Withers, S. G. (2000). Glycosidase mechanisms: Anatomy of a finely tuned catalyst. *Accounts of Chemical Research*, Vol. 33, pp. 11-18.

Zhou, H. Q., Danger, D. P., Dock, S. T., Hawley, L., Roller, S. G., Smith, C. D. & Handlon, A. L. (2010). Synthesis and SAR of benzisothiazole- and indolizine-β-D-glucopyranoside inhibitors of SGLT2. *ACS Medicinal Chemistry Letters*, Vol. 1, pp. 19-23.

6

Effect of Dehydroepiandrosterone on Insulin Sensitivity and Adipocyte Growth in Otsuka Long-Evans Tokushima-Fatty Rats

Tatsuo Ishizuka[1] et al.,*
[1]Departments of General Internal Medicine and [2]Endocrinology and Metabolism, Gifu University Graduate School of Medicine, Gifu 501-1194 Japan

1. Introduction

Dehydroepiandrosterone (DHEA) (1) is the major adrenal androgen of young adults. However, serum concentration of DHEA in 60 year- old men shows a gradual decrease, when compared with young men aged 25-30 years old. This decrease occurs as the incidence of atherosclerosis (2), obesity (3), and diabetes increases (4), suggesting that administration of DHEA may protect against the development of these disorders. Previously, we reported that in vitro DHEA treatment increased glucose uptake and activation of PI 3-kinase in native rat adipocytes (5).

Protein kinase C (PKC) is a family of serine/threonine kinases, which play key functions in cellular signal transduction. Three categories of PKC, conventional, novel, and atypical PKCs, have been described depending on their mechanisms of activation. Moreover, it is known that 3-phosphoinositide-dependent protein kinase-1 (PDK1) is the hub of many signaling pathways, which phosphorylate many downstream kinases of phosphatidylinositol 3-kinase (PI 3-kinase), such as Akt kinase, S6 kinase and PKC. Previous studies suggested that atypical PKC (aPKCζ/λ) isoforms are required for insulin stimulation of glucose uptake (6), and PDK1 is necessary for activation of aPKCs (7).

It has been reported that DHEA treatment reduces fat accumulation and protects against insulin resistance via an increase in PI 3-kinase after immunoprecipitation with insulin receptor substrate-1 (IRS-1) in male rats (8). We have investigated the in-vitro and in-vivo effects of DHEA on insulin-induced glucose uptake in adipocytes of Otsuka Log-Evans Tokushima fatty (OLETF) (9) and LETO rats. Moreover, we have shown the DHEA-induced glucose uptake by activation of PI 3-kinase/atypaical PKC siganlling without association with IRS-1 (10). In vivo treatment with DHEA affects on a decrease of adipose tissue via downregulation of peroxisome proliferator-activated receptor γ (PPARγ) expression (11). Based on above results, we have searched more precise mechanism of DHEA-induced amelioration of insulin sensitivity and clinical application of DHEA in diabetic animal models and human male adults.

---

* Kazuo Kajita[1], Kei Fujioka[1], Takayuki Hanamoto[1], Takahide Ikeda[1], Ichiro Mori, Masahiro Yamauchi[1], Hideyuki Okada[1], Taro Usui[1], Noriko Takahashi[1], Hiroyuki Morita[1], Yoshihiro Uno[1] and Atsushi Miura[2]

Obesity is one of the most important public health problems because of its association with increased risk for diabetes, hypertension, coronary heart disease, and other serious diseases. In addition to the environmental factors including a western style diet, hormonal changes are postulated to up- or downregulate adiposity. Recent evidence indicates that hypogonadism is a predictor of obesity, insulin resistance, diabetes, and coronary artery disease in men (12). Testosterone replacement therapy improves insulin resistance and glycemic control in hypogonadal men with type 2 diabetes (13). Male hypogonadism is a distinctly defined clinical entity associated with sexual dysfunction, inactivity, depression, decreased muscle mass, bone loss, etc. Hence, testosterone replacement also improves these abnormalities (14). On the other hand, although circulating DHEA and testosterone concentrations are known to decline during the aging process (15) in men, the relationship between low plasma DHEA level and cardiovascular disease remains controversial. Barrett-Connor and colleagues reported negative correlation between DHEA sulfate (DHEA-S) level and death from any case and death from cardiovascular disease in men more than 50 years of age (16). The same authors concluded that DHEA-S did not predict cardiovascular death in women (17). Analyses of the relationship of plasma DHEA or DHEA-S levels with obesity or body fat distribution have revealed inconsistent results. Plasma DHEA levels are negatively correlated with total body mass index and abdominal fat accumulation; however, contradictory is true for the relationship between DHEA-S and adiposity. Several studies supported the association of high plasma DHEA level with favorable insulin sensitivity (18). Meanwhile, administration of DHEA has been reported to improve obesity (19), diabetes (20), and cancer (21) in animal studies. However, discrepancies have been reported in the benefit of DHEA administration in human studies. Both positive (22) and negative (23) effects of DHEA replacement in elderly people or in patients with adrenal insufficiency have been reported. A major cause of these discrepancies might be the varied study designs including the selection of subjects, dose, drug administration, and definitions of endpoint in these numerous studies.

Although the specific receptor of DHEA has not been identified, one recently proposed mechanism is that DHEA is a precursor of androgen and estrogen that is converted to active form in peripheral tissues. DHEA is metabolized into androstenedione with 3β-hydroxysteroid dehydrogenase, and then transformed to testosterone with 17β-hydroxysteroid dehydrogenase (intracrine process) (24). The fact that androgen receptor (AR)-deficient mice are obese (25) indicates that AR acts as a mediator to prevent fat accumulation in whole body. Accordingly, several effects of DHEA may be mediated via AR. In this regard, it is possible that DHEA and testosterone have common mechanisms to reduce adiposity. However, few comparative studies between these hormones have been reported (26).

We demonstrated that administration of DHEA reduced adiposity in Otsuka Long-Evans Tokushima Fatty (OLETF) rats. Moreover, we found that DHEA directly downregulated the PPARγ mRNA level in cultured adipocytes, which may explain the anti-obesity effect of DHEA (11). However, contradictory data have been reported lately (27). To understand the weight-reducing effect of DHEA comprehensively, we performed a microarray study. Analysis of approximately 30,000 genes in epididymal fat isolated from mice after treatment with or without DHEA demonstrated that although a few genes involved in energy metabolism (e.g., malonyl-CoA decarboxylase) were affected, genes regulating cell growth (e.g., foxa1, nuclear factor I/X, eukaryotic translation elongation factor 1α, and aurora kinase) and genes regulating apoptosis (e.g., caspase 3, tumor necrosis factor receptor superfamily, and Bcl2) were markedly up- and downregulated, respectively. These results indicate that DHEA regulates cell growth or death, possibly resulting in decreased adiposity. However, we failed to find evidence of increased apoptosis in adipose tissue and cultured adipocytes after DHEA treatment.

2. Materials and methods

Materials. [γ-^{32}P]ATP was purchased from Amersham (Aylesbury, Buckinghamshire, UK). [1,2-^{3}H]2-deoxyglucose ([^{3}H]2-DOG) was purchased from DuPont-NEN (Boston, MA). Anti-phosphotyrosine (PY) antibody was purchased from Transduction Laboratory (Lexington, KY). Anti-PKCζ, anti-Akt and anti-PDK1 antibodies were purchased from Santa Cruz Biotechnology (Santa Cruz, CA). DHEA was purchased from Sigma (St. Louis, MO). All other chemicals were of reagent grade.

Adipocyte experiments. Males Wistar rats weighing 150-200 g were fed ad libitum and killed by decapitation. Isolated adipocytes were obtained by collagenase digestion of rat epididymal fat pads in Krebs-Ringer phosphate (KRP) buffer (pH 7.4) containing 127 mM NaCl, 12.3 mM NaH_2PO_4, 5.1 mM KCl, 1.3 mM $MgSO_4$, 1.4 mM $CaCl_2$, 3% bovine serum albumin (BSA), and 2.5 mM glucose (28). Animal care and use were approved by the Committee for Animal Care and Use in Gifu University Graduate School of Medicine.

Transfection study. Plasmids for expression of wt-PKCζ (M246)/ΔPKCζ (K281W mutant) (kindly supplied by Dr. Shigeo Ohno, Yokohama City University School of Medicine, Japan), wt-PDK1/ΔPDK1 (K110N) and wt-Akt/ΔAkt (T308A) (kindly supplied by Dr. Robert V. Farese, University of South Florida College of Medicine, USA) were constructed in vector SRD, pCDNA3 and pCIS, respectively. Adipocytes (50% vol/vol) were transfected by the electroporation method (5 μg DNA/cuvette) as described by Quon et al in the presence of SRD, pCDNA3 or pCIS eukariocytic expression vector clone, or SRD-, pCDNA3- or pCIS-containing cDNA encoding wtPKCζ/ΔPKCζ, wtPDK-1/ΔPDK-1 or wtAkt/ΔAkt (29). Transfected adipocytes were incubated at 37°C overnight (5% CO2) in Dulbecco's Phosphate-Buffered Saline containing 20 μg/ml ampicilin. After overnight incubation, each protein content was identified by an enhanced chemiluminescence Western blotting detection system according to the manufacturer's protocol. To ensure equal loading of proteins, membrane were stripped and restained with antibodies against β-actin.

PI 3-kinase activity. Isolated rat adipocytes were preincubated with KRP buffer for 30 min. The samples were treated with 1 μM DHEA at 1 min and 10 min, and were lyzed immediately in lysis buffer [20 mM Tris/HCl, pH 7.5, 140 mM NaCl, 20 μM phenylmethylsulfonyl fluoride (PMSF), 0.5 mM Na_3VO_4, 1 mM ethylene glycol bis (β-aminoethylether)-N,N,N',N'-tetraacetic acid (EGTA), 10% Glycerol, 1% Nonidet P-40, and 10 μg/ml aprotinin]. The lysates were centrifuged at 15,000 × g for 10 min at 4°C. Five μg of anti-PY antibody was added to 500 μg of the above resultant supernatant and incubated at 4°C overnight. After addition of protein A sepharose for 2 h, the immunoprecipitates were washed twice with washing buffer A [20 mM Tris/HCl, pH 7.5, 140 mM NaCl, 1 mM dithiothreitol (DTT), and 1% Nonidet P-40], once with LiCl solution (100 mM Tris/HCl, pH 7.5, 0.5 M LiCl, and 1 mM DTT), and twice with buffer B (10 mM Tris/HCl, pH 7.5, 100 mM NaCl, and 1 mM DTT). The PI 3-kinase reaction was started by the addition of a 40 μl solution containing 20 mM Tris/HCl, pH 7.4, 10 μCi [γ-^{32}P]ATP, 250 μM ATP, 10 mM $MgCl_2$, 5 mM EGTA, and 20 μl (1 mg/ml) of sonicated phosphatidylinositol. After a 10 min incubation at 30°C, the reaction was terminated by the addition of 500 μl 1 N HCl. Then, in succession, 500 μl of $CHCl_3$/methanol (2:1, vol/vol) was added to the samples, which were then centrifuged. The extracts were washed with 500 μl of $CHCl_3$/methanol/1 N HCl (4:2:3, vol/vol), then dried and resuspended in $CHCl_3$. The samples were spotted onto silica gel 60 thin-layer chromatography (TLC) plates (Merck, Darmstadt, Germany), and visualized by autoradiography (X-OMAT film, Eastman Kodak, Rochester, NY) (30). These results were then scanned and analyzed with a laser densitometer (UltroScan XL, Pharmacia LKB Biotechnology, Tokyo).

Glucose uptake study Isolated rat adipocytes were incubated with KRP buffer for 30 min, followed by treatment with 1 μM DHEA or 10 nM insulin for 30 min. Uptake of [^{3}H]2-DOG was measured over a 1 min period after treatment with 1 μM DHEA or 10 nM insulin. When overexpressed rat adipocytes were treated with 1 μM DHEA for 30 min, uptake of [^{3}H]2-DOG was measured over a 1 min period after treatment with 1 μM DHEA for 30 min. In another experiment when overexpressed rat adipocytes were incubated with or without 1 μM wortmannin for 10 min, followed by treatment with 1 μM DHEA for 30 min, uptake of [^{3}H]2-DOG was measured over a 1 min period after treatment with 1 μM DHEA for 30 min.

PKC studies Wt-PKCζ-transfected adipocytes were treated with 1 μM DHEA for 10 min, respectively, following pretreatment with or without 1 μM wortmannin, and were terminated by the addition of ice-cold buffer C (20 mM Tris/HCl, pH 7.5, 0.25 M sucrose, 1.2 mM EGTA, 0.1 mM PMSF, 20 μg/ml leupeptin, 20 mM 2-mercaptoethanol, and 10 μg/ml aprotinin). Each sample was sonicated in buffer C. The homogenates were centrifuged for 60 min at 105,000 × g to separate the cytosol and membrane fractions. After the membranes were resuspended in lysis buffer (20 mM Tris/HCl, pH 7.5, 0.25 M sucrose, 20 μg/ml leupeptin, 20 mM 2-mercaptoethanol, 5 mM EGTA, 0.1 mM PMSF, 2 mM ethylenediaminetetraacetic acid, and 1% Triton X-100) for 30 min at 4°C, they were sonicated, and then centrifuged for 60 min at 105,000 × g to obtain solubilized membrane fractions. They were then resuspended in Laemmli sample buffer and boiled for 2 min at 100°C. Thirty μg of each sample was subjected to sodium dodecyl sulfate-polyacrylamide gel electrophoresis, transferred to a nitrocellulose membrane, and subjected to Western analysis with anti-PKCζ antibody as described above. These results were then scanned and analyzed with a laser densitometer.

Animal study

Male Long-Evans Tokushima Otsula (LETO) rats and Otsuka Long-Evans Tokushima Fatty (OLETF) rats were obtained from Otsuka Pharmaceutical Co., Ltd. Animals were fed CE2 powder ad libitum, and treated with (DHEA group) or without (control group) 0.4% DHEA for 52 weeks. They were housed in a specific pathogen-free facility with a 12-h light/12-h dark cycle. All procedures for animal care were carried out in accordance with protocols approved by the University of Gifu's Institutional Animal Care Committee. To compare the effects of DHEA and testosterone on adiposity, male Wistar rats were fed with (control) or without 0.4% DHEA- or 0.4% testosterone-containing food for 4 weeks. Body weight, fat weight, and serum levels of glucose, IRI, DHEA-S, and testosterone were measured.

Statistics

Experimental results were calculated as means ± standard errors. Statistical comparisons were performed by ANOVA. Significance was defined as $P < 0.05$.

3. Results

Overexpression of wild type- and kinase inactive type-PKCζ/PDK1/Akt.

DHEA stimulated both PI 3-kinase activation and DG production as previously described (5). We examined whether DHEA activates PKCζ, which is thought to be a downstream of PI 3-kinase. When isolated adipocytes of LETO rats (control) were treated with or without (control: 0 min) 1 μM DHEA for 5 , 10 and 20 min, cytosolic PKCζ immunoreactivities gradually decreased and membrane-*associated* PKCζ immunoreactivity were inversely increased as previously described (10). Moreover we examined precise mechanism of DHEA action in adipocytes. Although each DNA was transfected to rat adipocytes transiently, these protein contents were significantly overexpressed in rat adipocytes after overnight incubation. Each protein content was identified by an enhanced chemiluminescence Western blotting detection system. Each wild type- and kinase inactive type-PKCζ/PDK1/Akt-transfected cells exhibited a 2 to 3 fold increase in immunoreactive signal of 2-3 fold, compared with nontransfected cells (Fig. 1).

DHEA-induced 2-DOG uptake.

First, we examined DHEA-induced 2-DOG uptake in rat adipocytes. DNA, using the electroporation system was transfected into adipocytes. DHEA-induced 2-DOG uptake in wt-PDK1- and wt-PKCζ-transfected adipocytes significantly increased to 250±30% and 280±50%, respectively, compared with the control cells and vector alone-transfected cells (Fig. 2). However, wt-Akt-transfected adipocytes had no significant influence on DHEA-induced 2-DOG uptake in this system, when compared with the control cells and vector alone-transfected cells (Fig. 2).
Second, we also examined the effect of wortmannin pretreatment on DHEA-induced 2-DOG uptake. DHEA-induced 2-DOG uptake after pretreatment with 1 μM wortmannin for 30 min was significantly reduced in wt-PDK1-transfected adipocytes. Similarly, DHEA-induced 2-DOG uptake after pretreatment with wortmannin for 30 min was significantly reduced in wt-PKCζ-transfected adipocytes (Fig. 2).

DHEA-stimulated PKCζ translocation with or without wortmannin pretreatment.

DHEA-induced membrane-associated PKCζ immunoreactivity for 20 min in PKCζ-transfected cells was greater than that of control cells and tranfected cell without DHEA stimualtion. (Fig. 3, lanes 1 and 2). The DHEA-stimulated PKCζ translocation in PKCζ-transfected cells significantly increased to 3-fold greater than the control (Fig. 3, lane 3). Pretreatment with wortmannin for 15 min completely suppressed DHEA-stimulated PKCζ translocation from the cytosol to the membrane in PKCζ-transfected cells (Fig. 3, lane 4). These results indicate that DHEA-induced PKCζ translocation is provoked via a PI 3-kinase dependent pathway.

Effect of DHEA treatment in vivo on insulin-induced glucose uptake in adipocytes of OLETF/LETO rats

We selected a type 2 diabetes animal model, the OLETF rat, and examined the effect of "in vivo" DHEA treatment on insulin-, TPA- or DHEA-induced [^{3}H]2-DOG uptake. At 10 wk of age, 10 nM insulin-induced [^{3}H]2-DOG uptake in adipocytes of OLETF rat decreased by 45% when compared to LETO rat (control). In the 2 weeks treatment with 0.4% DHEA in vivo, there were no significant differences in body weight or plasma insulin level but there was a

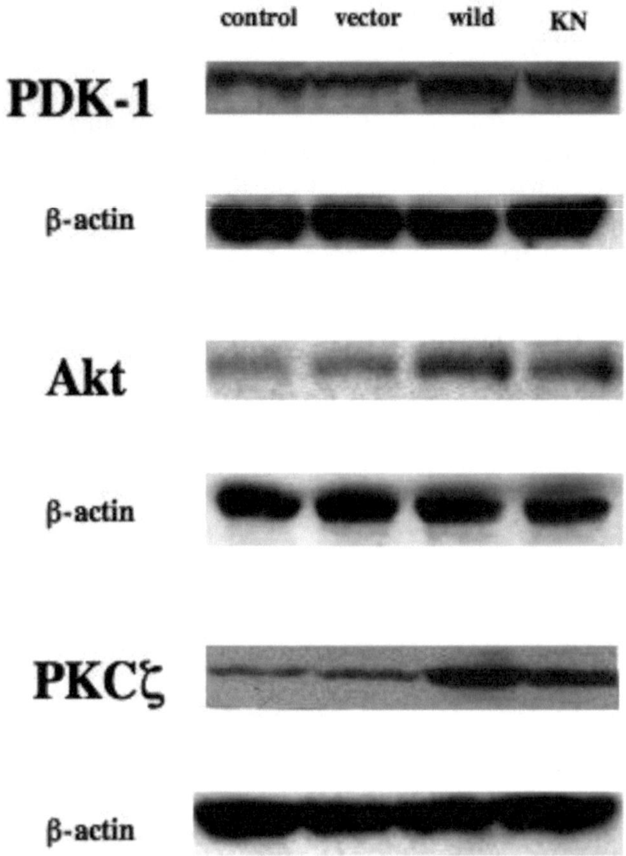

Fig. 1. Overexpression of PDK1, PKCζ and Akt in rat adipocytes. Isolated rat adipocytes were prepared as described in "Materials and Methods". Adipocytes (50%) were transfected by the electroporation method (5 μg/cuvette) in the presence or absence (control) of eucariocytes expression vector-containing wild and kinase-inactive (KN) cDNA encoding PDK-1, Akt and PKCζ. Transfected adipocytes were incubated at 37°C overnight in Dulbeco's modified buffer. Each protein was identified by ECL western blotting system as shown in "Materials and Methods". Equal loading of protein was confirmed by stripping the membrane and staining with anti-β-actin antibody. Transfection with wild type and kinase-negative type (KN) PDK1/PKCζ/Akt significantly increased immunoreactive PDK1/PKCζ/Akt 2-3 fold compared with nontransfected cells, respectively. Statistical significance was determined by Fisher's PLSD test.

significant difference in plasma glucose of OLETF rats as shown in Table 1. After "in vivo" treatment with DHEA, insulin-induced glucose uptakes were significantly increased by 50-100% when compared to untreated OLETF and LETO rats, but not in DHEA- induced glucose uptake. TPA-induced glucose uptake was also significantly increased compared to untreated OLETF and LETO rats as previously described (5). These results suggested that DHEA markedly increased glucose transport activity in not only LETO rats, but also in OLETF rats.

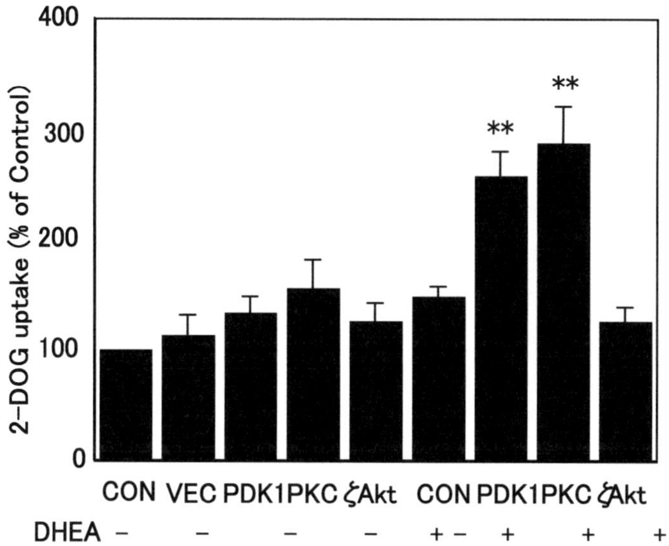

a)

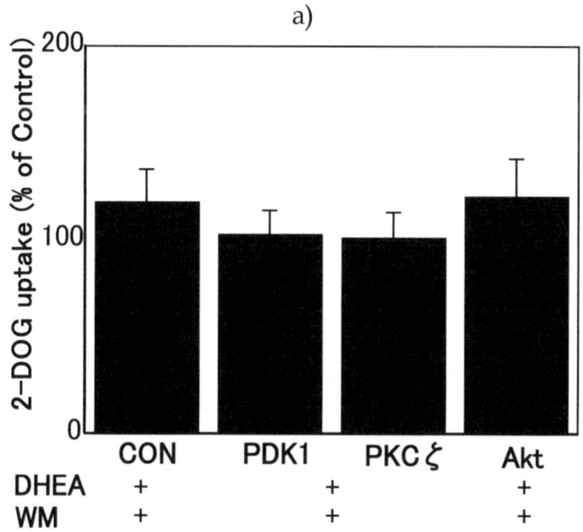

b)

Fig. 2. DHEA-induced 2-DOG uptake in transfected adipocytes. a) Isolated adipocytes obtained by the electroporation system were stimulated with 1 μM DHEA for 30 min. Uptake of [^{3}H]2-DOG was measured as shown in "Materials and Methods". DHEA-induced 2-DOG uptake in wt-PDK1- and wt-PKCζ-transfected adipocytes significantly increased to 250±30% and 280±50%, respectively, compared with the control cells and vector alone-transfected cells. b) Isolated adipocytes obtained by above procedure were pretreated with 1 μM wortmannin for 30 min, and then stimulated with 1 μM DHEA. DHEA-induced 2-DOG uptake after pretreatment with wortmannin for 30 min was significantly reduced in wt-PDK1-transfected and wt-PKCζ-transfected adipocytes. The data are plotted as mean ± SE of three separate experiments. **, $P < 0.01$, vs. control by Fisher's PLSD test.

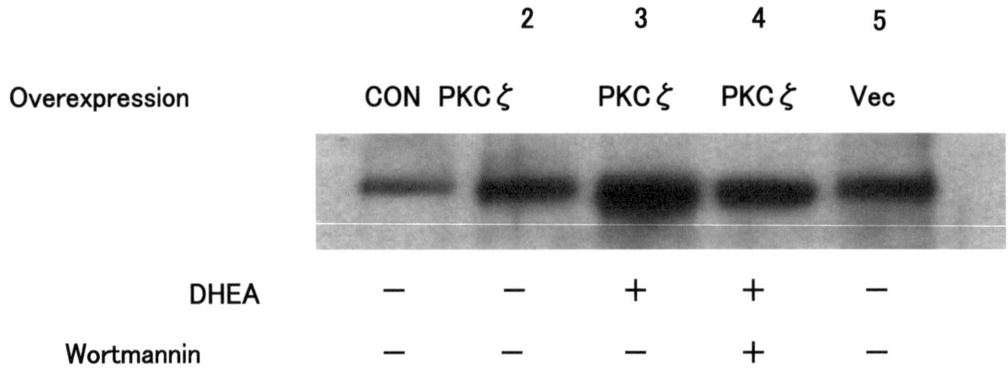

Fig. 3. DHEA-stimulated membrane-associated PKCζ immunoreactivity with or without wortmannin pretreatment. Adipocytes were transfected wt-PKCζ DNA using an electroporation system. Membrane-associated PKCζ immunoreactivity was examined by Western blotting as shown in "Materials and methods". DHEA-induced membrane-associated PKCζ immunoreactivity in PKCζ-transfected cells significantly increased to about 3-fold over the control (lane 3). Pretreatment with wortmannin for 30 min completely suppressed DHEA-stimulated PKCζ immunoreactivity in PKCζ-transfected cells (lane 4). The result is representative one of three separate experiments.

Specimen	LETO		OLETF	
	Control	DHEA	Control	DHEA
Epididymal fat (g)	10.9 ± 1.4	5.5 ± 1.7**	16.6 ± 1.2	11.2 ± 2.1**
Glucose (mg/mL)	140 ± 1	132 ± 2	184 ± 4	168 ± 3 *
TG (mg/mL)	101 ± 14	53 ± 2 *	544 ± 42	171 ± 54 **
T.Chol (mg/mL)	121 ± 5	139 ± 2	226 ± 7	191 ± 7
FFA (mEq/L)	645 ± 115	490 ± 16	1225 ± 96	854 ± 214 *
AST (IU/L)	207 ± 10	331 ± 35 *	202 ± 49	150 ± 21 *
ALT (IU/L)	75 ± 11	118 ± 9	141 ± 4	101 ± 34 *
IRI (ng/mL)	1.8 ± 0.4	2.4 ± 0.3	2.4 ± 1	2.7 ± 0.4

Data are expressed as mean ± SE (N = 6).
$^*P < 0.05$, $^{**}P < 0.01$ vs control.

Table 1. Effect of DHEA Administration on Epididymal Fat Weight and Laboratory Data in LETO and OLETF Rats

Effect of DHEA treatment in vivo on insulin-induced phosphatidylinositol (PI) 3-kinase and PKCz activations in OLETF/LETO rats

Moreover, in order to clarify the effect of DHEA treatment in vivo on PI 3-kinase, which binds to tyrosine phosphorylated insulin receptor substrate-1 (IRS-1) via SH2 domain of PI 3-kinase, downstream of the insulin signaling pathway, we examined whether DHEA treatment improves PI 3-kinase activity in adipocytes of OLETF/LETO rats. When

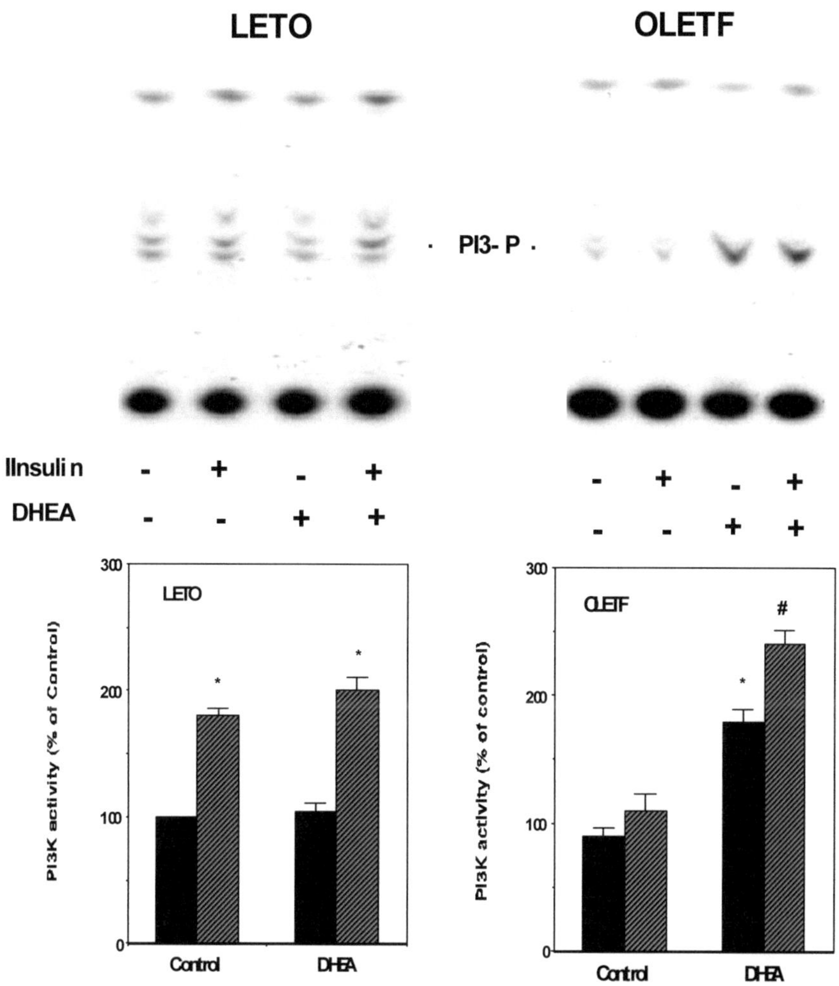

Fig. 4. Effect of in vivo treatment with DHEA on insulin-induced PI 3-kinase activation in adipocytes of OLETF/LETO rats. After treatment with 0.4% DHEA in vivo for 2 wk, isolated adipocytes were obtained from epididymal fat pads in OLETF rats. Isolated adipocytes were incubated with or without (control: 0 min) 10 nM insulin for 10 min, homogenized, and immunoprecipitated with phosphotyrosine antibody. Each PI 3-kinase activity was measured as shown in "Materials and methods". Densitometric data are plotted as the mean ± SE of four separate experiments. *$P < 0.01$ by ANOVA with Fisher's PLSD.

adipocytes were incubated with 10 nM insulin, enzyme activity after immunoprecipitation with antiphosphotyrosine antibody apparently increased for 5 and 10 min in control LETO rats. PI-3kinase activity of OLETF rat was decreased and insulin-stimulated PI-3kinase activity also decreased, compared with those in LETO rats (Fig. 4). In vivo treatment with DHEA increased membrane-associated PKCζ immunoreactivities, especially in OLETF rat as shown in Fig. 5. These results suggest that in vivo treatment with DHEA for 2 weeks increases PI 3-kinase/atypicalPKC signaling and finally ameliorate blood glucose level as shown in Table 1.

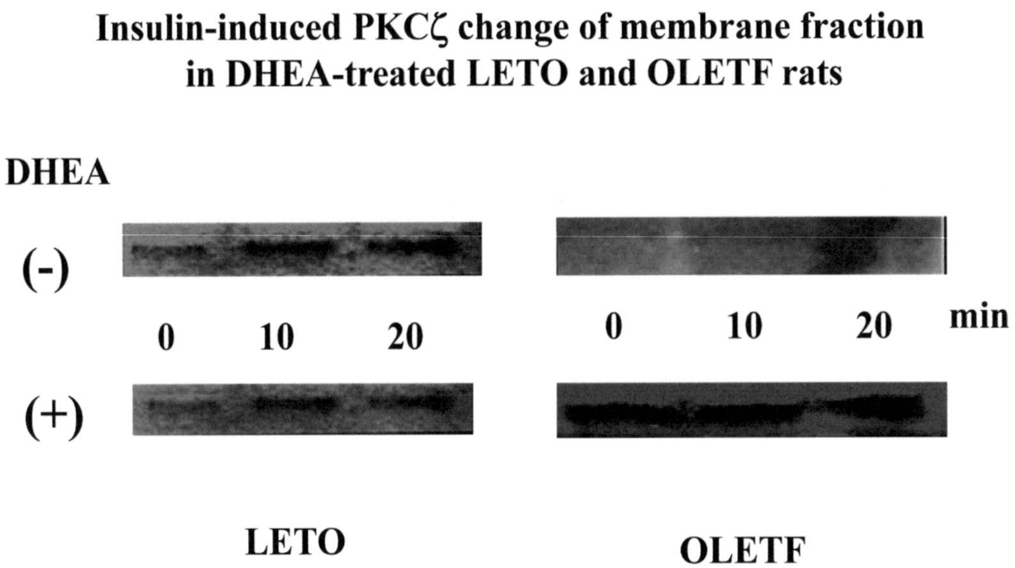

Fig. 5. Effect of in vivo treatment with DHEA on insulin-induced PKCζ translocations in adipocytes of OLETF/LETO rats. After treatment with 0.4% DHEA in vivo for 2 wk, isolated adipocytes were obtained from epididymal fat pads in OLETF rats. Isolated adipocytes were stimulated with or without (control) 10 nM insulin for 10, 20 min. Cells were homogenized and centrifuged to obtain cytosol and membrane fraction. Membrane-associated protein (40 μg) was subjected to SDS-PAGE, transferred to the nitrocellulose membrane, and immunoblotted with PKCζ antibodies using ECL system. The result is representative one of three separate experiments.

Effect of DHEA administration on body weight, food consumption, and laboratory Data in LETO and OLETF rats

DHEA administration reduced body weight of both LETO and OLETF rats over a period of 44 weeks; however, a significant decrease in food consumption was observed only in the first 2 weeks. This indicated that DHEA-induced reduction of body weight could not be attributed to the change in food intake (Fig. 6). As shown in Table 1, DHEA administration significantly reduced epididymal fat weight in LETO and OLETF and plasma glucose level in OLETF rats. Serum triglyceride and free fatty acid levels were also diminished by DHEA administration.

Effects of DHEA and testosterone on body weight and fat weight

Treatment with both 0.4% DHEA and 0.4% testosterone resulted in reduction of body weight and epididymal fat, intestinal fat, and perirenal fat weights (Fig. 7A, B). Animals were treated for 4 weeks to avoid the effect of decreased food intake. Because rodents lack 17α-hydroxylase (CYP17A1) in their adrenal glands, they produce little or no DHEA. Hence, DHEA-S was not detected in control serum, whereas elevated DHEA-S levels were observed in both DHEA-treated and testosterone-treated rats (Fig. 7C). Treatment with DHEA resulted in less elevated testosterone levels than treatment with testosterone (Fig. 7D). No differences were observed in serum levels of glucose, triglyceride, free fatty acid, AST, ALT, and IRI levels among these animals (data not shown).

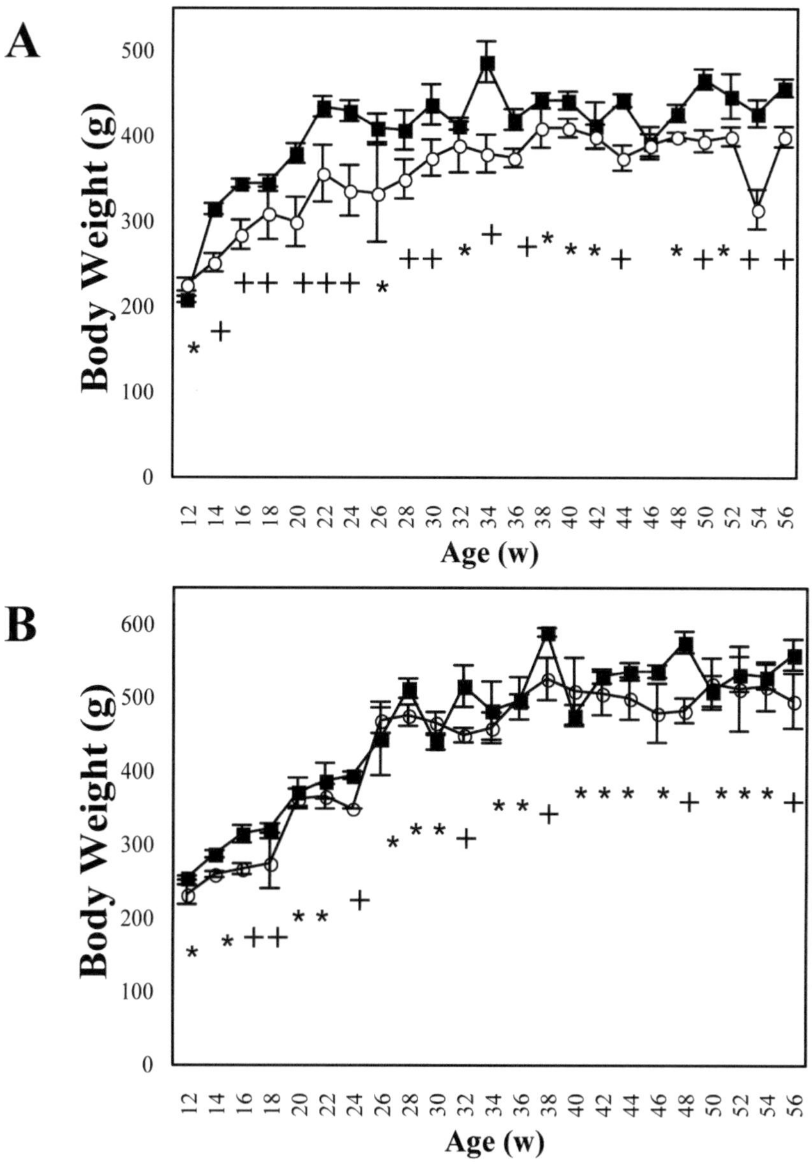

Fig. 6. Effects of DHEA administration on body weight in LETO and OLETF rats
Both LETO and OLETF rats were treated with or without (Control) 0.4% DHEA-containing food. Effects of this treatment on body weight in LETO (A) and OLETF (B) are shown. Closed square: Control, Open circle: DHEA, *: $P < 0.05$, vs Control, +: $P < 0.01$, vs Control, N = 10.

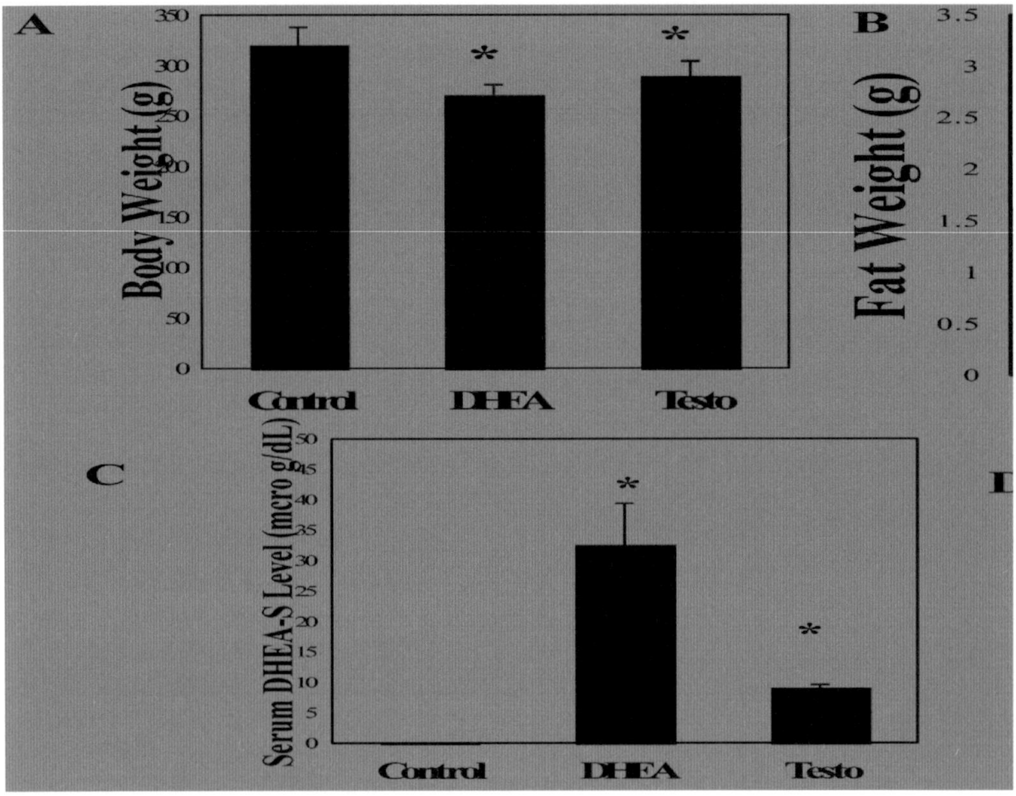

Fig. 7. Effects of DHEA and testosterone administration on body weight, fat weight, and serum concentration of DHEA-S and testosterone
Wistar rats were housed with or without 0.4% DHEA- or 0.4% testosterone-containing food for 4 weeks. DHEA and testosterone administration produced equal and significant decrease in body weight (A), epididymal (black bar), intestinal (white), and perirenal (gray) fat weight. *: $P < 0.05$ vs each control, N = 8. Testosterone (Testo) administration raised serum DHEA-S level (C), while DHEA administration significantly elevated serum testosterone level (D). *: $P < 0.05$ vs control, N = 6.

4. Discussion

We have previously reported that DHEA improves insulin resistance via activation of PI 3-kinase/atypical PKC signaling (5). However, more precise mechanism still remains unclear concerning about downstream signaling of PI 3-kinase and in vivo effect of DHEA on human male adults. Therefore, we have shown in vivo administration of DHEA stimulates glucose uptake via activation of PI3-kinase/atypiacal in OLETF rats and improves insulin resistance in human male adults. It has been reported that insulin receptor-mediated tyrosine phosphorylation of insulin receptor substrate 1 stimulates PI 3-kinase (31). It is believed that PI 3-kinase plays an important role in the insulin-stimulated glucose transport system (32). It has been reported that PI 3-kinase mediated aPKC activation is essential in insulin-induced glucose transporter 4 translocation and glucose uptake (33). The current results demonstrate that PDK1 is necessary for phosphorylation and activation of aPKC (34), and aPKC may provoke glucose transporter translocation to the membrane of insulin sensitive tissues (35). Our previous studies show that DHEA may directly or indirectly activate PI 3-kinase without an increase in tyrosine phosphorylation of IRS-1 (36) and subsequent activation of PKCζ (13). Although DOG uptake by DHEA stimulation significantly increased, it appears to be more than the 150% increases in cultured adipocytes from an unstimulated level, as shown in Fig. 2. In this study, we hypothesize that overexpressions of PKCζ and PDK1 may markedly cause DOG uptake. As a result, DHEA-induced DOG uptake increased 250 and 280% in wt-PDK1- and wt-PKCζ-transfected adipocytes, respectively, when compared with the control and vector-transfected cells, as shown in Fig. 2. DHEA-induce glucose uptake was stimulated by activation of PI-3 kinase and subsequent stimulation of PDK1/atypical PKC by PIP_2/PIP_3 production as already shown (5), and partially mimics insulin-induced activation of glucose uptake.

Although we acknowledge that PDK1 can phosphorylate Akt kinase (known as protein kinase B), DHEA-induced DOG uptake did not increase in wt-Akt-transfected adipocytes (Fig. 2). Moreover, Kotani et al stated that Akt kinase was not associated with insulin-induced glucose uptake in 3T3-L1 adipocytes (37). Further work will be needed to focus on the elucidation of the function of Akt kinase.

In addition, we investigated the effect of wortmannin, a PI 3-kinase inhibitor, on glucose uptake in wt-PKCζ-transfected adipocytes. When treated with DHEA, PKCζ significantly increased in the membrane fractions as indicated in Fig. 3. (lane 3). However, pretreatment with wortmannin for 30 min significantly suppressed DHEA-induced PKCζ translocation to the membrane (Fig. 3, lane 4). We also investigated the effect of wortmannin on DHEA-induced PI 3-kinase and PKCζ activity. After pretreatment with wortmannin, DHEA-induced PI 3-kinase and PKCζ activations were inhibited completely as previously described (10). These results indicate that acute DHEA stimulation may potentiate DOG uptake via a PI 3-kinase-PDK1-PKCζ pathway and subsequent glucose transporter translocation.

Nakashima et al. reported that insulin-stimulated DOG uptake increased by incubating cells with DHEA (38). We also revealed that DHEA could enhance insulin-induced DOG uptake via activation of PI 3-kinase-PKCζ signaling in DHEA-treated (for 2 weeks) OLETF (Otsuka Long-Evans Tokushima Fatty) rat in vivo, when compared with untreated control rats (5). Although the precise mechanism is unknown, the preferential activation of PI 3-kinase and redistribution of PKCζ by chronic DHEA treatment may appear to result in enhancement of insulin sensitivity in OLETF rats and human male adults. On the other hand, DHEA converts into estrogenic and androgenic metabolites, such as 17β-estradiol, 5-androstene-3β,17β-diol, testosterone and 4-androstene-3,17-dione (39). Investigators need to examine whether DHEA-metabolites affect DOG uptake, although in vitro examinations indicated androstenedione and estradiol did not stimulate DOG uptake in native rat adipocytes as previously reported (5). Finally, 4-hydroxy-androstenedione, an aromatase inhibitor, may be useful in evaluating the effect of DHEA.

In this study, DHEA treatment for 2 wk in genetically obese OLETF rats reduced the weight of subcutaneous and visceral adipose tissues, but not total body weight. Although a small effect could also be observed also in control rats, DHEA decreased a broad range of adipose in fatty ones. We also revealed that DHEA treatment significantly reduced plasma leptin level as previously reported (11). Leptin is thought to correlate with the amount of stored body. Therefore, DHEA-induced reduction in adipose tissue mass might contribute to the decrease in plasma leptin concentration. Moreover, we found that DHEA treatment prevented the elevation of PPARγ expression in adipose tissue from OLETF rats (11). The present study could not ascertain whether the expression of PPARγ in adipose tissue is genetically determined or not. However, considering the fact that an increased amount of PPARγ expression in obese human adipose tissue, which is proportional to BMI, can be reduced by a low calorie diet (40), our result seems to suggest an acquired origin. We questioned whether these effects of DHEA on adipose tissue are direct or not. Interestingly, DHEA-S cannot stimulate peroxisomal gene induction in the liver of PPARγ knockout mice, suggesting that some of the DHEA or DHEA-S actions are mediated via the PPAR family (41). These results are supposed to be biologically significant, because Pro 12 Ala substitution in the human PPARγ gene, which exhibits 30-45% less transactivation capacity, leads to prevention of obesity and insulin resistance (24). Our recent preliminary study revealed that the effect of DHEA on PPARγ was enhanced in adipocytes with overexpression of PKCζ (11). We previously reported that DHEA activates phosphatidylinositol 3-kinase (PI 3-kinase) and atypical PKC (10). In addition, TNF-α, another PPARγ reducing agonist, also activated atypical PKC (42).

Based on the above results, DHEA may improve insulin resistance via activation of glucose transport and downregulations of adiposity through the activation of PI 3-kinase/PKCζ signaling and the reduction of PPARγ and, finally, DHEA may contribute to the amelioration of insulin sensitivity in diabetic model animals. These results suggest that DHEA may be useful for clinical application for insulin resistant state such as diabetes, obesity, hyperlipidmia and hypertension, recently called as metabolic syndrome in the future time.

Since the presentation by Coleman and colleagues suggested that DHEA administration prevented diabetes in db/db mice, numerous studies have been published (20). Our previous study revealed that although treatment with DHEA fails to decrease blood glucose in Goto-Kakizaki rats, an animal model of lean type 2 diabetes, it significantly reduces blood glucose in OLETF rats (5). Therefore, we speculated that DHEA administration might improve obesity-associated diabetes in association with preventing obesity-induced insulin resistance. We found that treatment with DHEA for 2 weeks reduced fat mass and that DHEA directly suppressed mRNA levels of PPARγ in isolated adipocytes (11). Since suppression of PPARγ activity leads to reduced adiposity in PPARγ-deficient mice (43) and Pro12Ala polymorphism in humans (44), our result could explain the weight-reducing effect of DHEA. On the other hand, our microarray experiment revealed that genes regulating cell proliferation were more profoundly influenced by DHEA administration than those regulating energy homeostasis in adipose tissue. Hence, we examined the effect of DHEA on cell proliferation in adipose tissue.

In this study, we demonstrated that we compared the effects of DHEA and testosterone administration. Long-term DHEA administration decreased body weight of both LETO and OLETF rats (Fig. 6). Although several studies indicated that the anti-obesity effect of DHEA was associated with decreased food intake, no difference was observed in food consumption except for that in the first 2 weeks. It was suggested that DHEA-induced central neurotransmitter changes suppress the appetite; however, these changes may not persist longer than 3 weeks (45).

Epidemiological studies suggest that high plasma DHEA-S level is associated with longevity (46, 47), whereas, to our knowledge, our study is the first to provide evidence of the anti-aging effect of DHEA. Both DHEA and testosterone led to decreased visceral fat weight when administered for 4 weeks. These results imply that treatment with these hormones acts similarly on adipose tissue. Moreover, dot blot analysis revealed that both testosterone and DHEA administration yielded identical results. In addition, our results suggest that DHEA administration could substitute for testosterone replacement; however, because DHEA is known to act as a neurosteroid and other unique actions of DHEA are known, further study is necessary to understand the difference between these hormones.

5. References

[1] Melby, J.C. (1970)Assessment of adrenocortical function. N. Engl. J. Med. 285, 735- 739

[2] Gordon, G.B., Bush, D.E., Weisman, H.F. (1988) Reduction of atherosclerosis by administration of dehydroepiandrosterone. J. Clin. Invest. 82 712-720

[3] Yen., T.T., Allan, J.A., Pearson, D.V., Acton, J.M., and Greenberg, M.M. (1977) Prevention of obesity in A^{vy}/a mice by dehydroepiandrosterone. Lipid 12, 409-413

[4] Coleman, D.L, Leiter, E.H., and Schwizer, R.W. (1982) Effect of genetic background on the therapeutic effects of dehydroepiandrosterone (DHEA) in diabetes-obesity mutants and aged normal mice. Diabetes 33, 26-32

[5] Ishizuka, T., Kajita, K., Miura, A., Ishizawa, M., Kanoh, Y., Itaya. S., Kimura, M., Muto, N., Mune, T., Morita, H., and Yasuda, K. (1999) Dehydroepiandrosterone improves glucose uptake via activations of protein kinase C and phosphatidylinositol 3-kinase. Am. J. Physiol. 276, E196-E204

[6] Standaert, M.L., Galloway, L., Karnam, P., Bandyopadhyay, G., Moscat, J., and Farese R.V. (1997)Protein kinase C-zeta as a downstream effector of phosphatidylinositol 3-kinase during insulin stimulation in rat adipocytes. Potential role in glucose transport. J Biol. Chem. 272, 30075-30082

[7] Le Good, J A., Ziegler, W.H., Parekh, D.B., Alessi, D.R., Cohen, P., and Parker, P.J. (1998) Protein kinase C isotypes controlled by phosphoinositide 3-kinase through the protein kinase PDK1. Science 281. 2042-2045

[8] Han, D-H., Hansen, P.A., Chen, M.M., and Holloszy, J.O. (1998) DHEAtreatment reduces fat accumulation and protects against insulin resistance in male rats. J. Gerontol. 53, 19-24

[9] Ishizuka, T., Miura, A., Kajita, K., Yamada, K., Wada, H., S. Itaya, S., Kanoh Y., Ishizawa, M., Kimura, M., and Yasuda, K. (1998) Alterations in insulin-induced postreceptor signaling in adipocytes of the Otsuka Long-Evans Tokushima fatty rat strain. J. Endocrinol. 156, 1-13

[10] Kajita, K., Ishizuka, T., Miura, A., Ishizawa, M., Kanoh, Y., Yasuda, K. (2000)The role of atypical and conventional PKC in dehydroepiandrosterone-induced glucose uptake and dexamethasone-induced insulin resistance. Biochem. Biophys. Res. Commun. 277, 361-367.

[11] Kajita, K., Ishizuka, T,, Mune, T,, Miura, A,, Ishizawa, M,, Kanoh, Y,, Kawai, Y., Natsume,Y., Yasuda, K. (2003) Dehydroepiandrosterone down-regulates the expression of peroxisome proliferator-activated receptor γ in adipocytes. Endocrinology 144, 253-259

[12] Kapoor D, Channer KS, Aldred H, Jones TH, Clark S 2007 Clinical and biological assessment of hypogonadism in men with type 2 diabetes. Diabetic Care 30:911-917

[13] Kapoor D, Goodwin E, Channer KS, Jones TH 2006 Testosterone replacement therapy improves insulin resistance, glycaemic control, visceral adiposity and

hypercholesterolaemia in hypogonadal men with type 2 diabetes. Eur J Endocrinol 154:899-906

[14] Wang C, Eyre DR, Clark R, Kleinberg D, Newman C. Iranmanesh A, Veldhuis J, Dudley RE, Berman N, Davidson T, Barstow TJ, Sinow R, Alexander G, Swerdloff RS 1996 Sublingual testosterone replacement improves muscle mass and bone formation markers in hypogonadal men-a clinical research center study. J Clin Endocrinol Metab 81:3654-3662

[15] Orentreich N, Brind JL, Rizer RL, Vogelman JH 1984 Age changes and sex differences in serum dehydroepiandrosterone sulfate concentrations throughout adulthood. J Clin Endocrinol Metab 59:551-555

[16] Barrett-Connor E, Khaw KT, Yen SS 1986 A prospective study of dehydroepiandrosterone sulfate, mortality, and cardiovascular disease. N Engl J Med 315:1519-1524

[17] Barrett-Connor E, Goodman-Gruen D 1995 Dehydroepiandrsterone sulfate does not predict cardiovascular death in postmenopausal women. Circulation 91:1757-1760

[18] Tchernof A, Despres JP, Dupont A, Belanger A, Nadeau A, Prud'homme D, Moorjani S, Lupien PJ, Labrie F 1995 Relation of steroid hormones to glucose tolerance and plasma insulin levels in men. Importance of visceral adipose tissue. Diabetes Care 18:292-299

[19] Berdanier CD, Parente Jr JA, Mcintosh MK 1993 Is dehydroepiandrosterone an antiobesity agent? FASEB J 7:414-419

[20] Coleman DL, Leiter EH, Schwizer RW 1982 Therapeutic effects of dehydroepiandrosterone (DHEA) in diabetic mice. Diabetes 31:830-833

[21] Shilkaitis A, Green A, Punj V, Steele V, Lubet R, Christov K 2005 Dehydroepiandrosterone inhibits the progression phase of mammary carcinogenesis by inducing cellular senescence via a p16-dependent but p-53-independent mechanism. Breast Cancer Research 7:R1132-R1140

[22] Villareal DT, Holloszy JO, Kohrt WM 2000 Effect of DHEA replacement on bone mineral density and body composition in elderly women and men. Clin Endocrinol 53:561-568

[23] Callies F, Fassnacht M, Christoph van Vlijmen J, Koehler I, Huebler D, Seibel MJ, Arlt W, Allolio B 2001 Dehydroepiandrosterone replacement in women with adrenal insufficiency: Effects on body composition, serum leptin, bone turnover, and exercise capacity. J Clin Endocrinol Metab 86:1968-1972

[24] Labrie F 1991 Intracrinology. Mol Cell Endocrinol 78:C113-C118

[25] Sato T, Matsumoto T, Yamada T, Watanabe T, Kawano H, Kato S 2003 Late onset of obesity in male androgen receptor–deficient (AR KO) mice. Biochem Biophys Res Commun 300:167-171

[26] Sato K, Iemitsu M, Aizawa K, Ajisaka R 2008 Testosterone and DHEA activate the glucose metabolism-related signaling pathway in skeletal muscle. Am J Physiol Endocrinol Metab 294:E961-E968.

[27] Karbowska J, Kochan Z 2005 Effect of DHEA on endocrine functions of adipose tissue, the involvement of PPARγ. Biochemical Pharmacology 70:249-257

[28] Rodbell,M. (1964) Metabolism of isolated fat cells. J. Biol. Chem. 239, 375-380

[29] Quon, M.J., Butte, A.J., Zarnowski, L., Sesti, G., Cushman, S.W., and Taylor, S.I. (1994) Insulin receptor substrate 1 mediates the stimulatory effect of insulin on GLUT4 translocation in transfected rat adipose cells. J. Biol. Chem. 1994; 269 27920-27924.

[30] Ruderman, N.B., Kapeller, R., White, M.F., and Cantley, L.C. (1990) Activation of phosphatidylinositol 3-kinase by insulin. Proc. Natl. Acad. Sci. USA. 87, 1411-1415

[31] Endemann, G., Yonezawa, K., and Roth, R. A. (1990) Phosphatidylinositol kinase or an associated protein is a substrate for the insulin receptor tyrosine kinase. J. Biol. Chem. 265, 396-400

[32] Myers, M.G., and White, M.F. (1993) The new elements of insulin signaling. Insulin receptor substrate-1 and proteins with SH2 domains. Diabetes 42, 643-650.

[33] Standaert, M. L, Bandyopadhyay, G,, Pert, L., Price, D., Galloway, L., Poklepovic, A., Sajan, M.P,, Cenni., V., Sirri, A., Moscat, J., Toker, A., and Farese, R.V. (1999) Insulin activates protein kinase C-ζ and C-λ be an autophosphorylation-dependent mechanism and stimulates their translocation to GLUT4 vesicles and other membrane fraction in rat adipocytes. J. Biol. Chem. 274, 25308-25316

[34] Balendran, A., Hare,G.R., Kiekoch, A., Williams, M.R., and Alessi, D.R. (2000) Further evidence that 3-phosphoinositide-dependent protein kinase-1 (PDK-1) is required for the stability and phosphorylation of protein kinase C (PKC) isoforms. FEBS. lett. 484, 217-223

[35] Balendran, A., Biondi, R.M., Cheung, P.C., Casamayor, A., Deak, M., and Alessi, D.R. (2000) A 3-phosphoinositide-dependent protein kinase-1 (PDK1) docking site is required for the phosphorylation of protein kinase C zeta (PKC zeta) and PKC-related kinase 2 by PDK1. J Biol Chem 2000; 275 20806-20813

[36] Kajita, K, Ishizuka, T,, Miura, A., Kanoh, Y., Ishizawa, M., Kimura, M., Muto, N. and Yasuda, K. (2001) Glucocorticoid-induced insulin resistance associates with activation of protein kinase C isoforms. Cellular Signalling 13, 169-175

[37] Kotani, K., Ogawa, W., Matsumoto, M., Kitamura, T., Sakaue, H., Hino, Y., Miyake, K., Sano, W., Akimoto, K., Ohno,S., and Kasuga, M. (1998) Requirement of atypical protein kinase C lambda for insulin stimulation of glucose uptake but not for Akt activation in 3T3-L1 adipocytes. Mol. Cell. Biol. 18 6971-6982.

[38] Nakashima, N., Haji, M., Sakai,Y., Ono, Y., Umeda, F., Nawata, H. (1995) Effect of dehydroepiandrosterone on glucose uptake in cultured human fibroblasts. Metabolism 44, 543-548

[39] Kaufman, F.R., Stanczyk, F.Z., Matteri, R.K., Gentzschein, E., Delgado, C., and Lobo, R.A. (1990) Dehydroepiandrosterone and dehydroepiandrosterone sulfate metabolism in human genital skin. Fertil. Steril. 54 251-254

[40] Vidal-Puig, A.J., Considine, R.V., Linan, M.J., Werman, A., Pories, W..J., Caro, J.F., and Flier, J.S. (1997) Peroxisome proliferator-activated receptor γ gene expression in human tissues: Effect of obesity, weight loss, and regulation by insulin and glucocorticoids. J. Clin. Invest. 99, 2416-2422

[41] Peters, J.M., Zhou, Y.C., Ram, P.A., Lee, S.S., Gonzalez, F.J. and Waxman, D.J. (1996) Peroxisome proliferator-activated receptor alpha required for gene induction by dehydroepiandrosterone-3 beta-sulfate. Mol. Pharmacol. 50, 67-74

[42] Bourbon, N.A. (2002) Sandirasegarane L & Kester M. Ceramide-induced inhibition of Akt is mediated through protein kinase ζ. J. Biol. Chem. 277, 3286-3292

[43] Kubota N, Terauchi Y, Miki H, Tamemoto H, Yamauchi T, Komeda K, Satoh S, Nakano R, Ishii C, Sugiyama T, Eto K, Tsubamoto Y, Okuno A, Murakami K, Sekihara H, Hasegawa G, Naito M, Toyoshima Y, Tanaka S, Shiota K, Kitamura T, Fujita T, Ezaki O, Aizawa S, Kadowaki T 1999 PPARgamma mediates high-fat diet-induced adipocyte hypertrophy and insulin resistance. Mol Cell 4:597-609

[44] Deeb SS, Fajas L, Nemoto M, Pihlajamaki J, Mykkanen L, Kuusisto J, Laakso M, Fujimoto W, Auwerx J 1998 A Pro12Ala substitution in PPARgamma2 associated with decreased receptor activity, lower body mass index and improved insulin sensitivity. Nat Genet 20:284-287

[45] Wright BE, Svec F, Porter JR 1995 Central effects of dehydroepiandrosterone in Zucker rats. Int J Obes Relat Metab Disord 19:887-892

[46] Matsumoto M, Ishizuka T, Kajita K, Sugiyama C, Morita H, Uno Y, Ikeda T, Mori I, Matsubara K, Takeda N, Yamakita N, Yasuda K 2007 Dehydroepiandrosterone-sulfate concentration in men from a Japanese longevity district. Geriatr Gerontol Int 7:352-356

[47] Roth GS, Lane MA, Ingram DK, Mattison JA, Elahi D, Tobin JD, Muller D, Metter EJ 2002 Biomarkers of caloric restriction may predict longevity in humans. Science 297:811

7

A Review of Clinical Trials in Emerging Botanical Interventions for Type 2 Diabetes Mellitus

Cheow Peng Ooi, Seng Cheong Loke and Tengku-Aizan Hamid
Institute of Gerontology, Universiti Putra Malaysia
Malaysia

1. Introduction

Although type 2 diabetes mellitus (T2DM) is pandemic globally, Asia-Pacific has the largest diabetes burden in the world (International Diabetes Federation, 2009). This region is home to more than half of the world's population with some of the richest and most developed countries alongside many developing as well as a significant number of poorest and least developed ones. Despite existing knowledge and recent progress in therapy, the majority of diabetic patients do not achieve an optimal blood glucose control. With a predisposition to disproportionate effect on the lower socioeconomic groups, the combination with the resulting poor health consequences, disability, and dependency is of concern (L.E. Egede, 2004). Taken together with the confluence of the recent upsurge of obesity and an ageing population, this will have far-reaching implications in terms of income security, social welfare and medical services (J.C. Chan et al., 2009; C. Pan et al., 2010). The consequent enormous health, social and economic burden will overwhelm the social and health care systems, particularly of the low and middle-income developing countries in the Asia-Pacific (D.O. Abegunde et al., 2007).

Controlling this disease is important for reducing complications, improving quality of life, and reducing the economic burden associated with disability and dependency (UKPDS 37, 1999). Strategies for the effective treatment of this devastating disease are of great interest to the general public, government organisations, and the healthcare industry. Besides nutritional intervention as an essential component of diabetes management, botanicals and associated products are also remedies for T2DM in traditional medicine practices. In the past decade, enhanced global research into botanicals has identified more than 600 plants as potential contributors to the management of T2DM (M. Modak et al., 2007; L.W. Qi et al., 2010).

Use of plant-based complementary and alternative medicine is common in many communities (H.Y. Chang et al., 2007; A. Metcalfe et al., 2010; H.T. Nguyen et al., 2010). In the past, the traditional 'observation' as remedies in complimentary alternative medicines, preliminary preclinical studies, and anecdotal evidence, have endorsed the use of these plants. However, their safety and efficacy in humans are of concern. Adding to the complexity of such issues are the challenges in the management of T2DM. Specifically, these are the use of pluralistic medical practices and the relevant roles of these botanicals in the management of T2DM in mainstream medicine (C.C. Shih et al., 2010). In addition, there are also issues of adequate regulatory standards and patients' disclosures to their mainstream medical practitioners (S. Tyreman, 2010). Thus, rigorous research in translating these botanicals to the clinical arena is warranted (M. Kantor, 2009).

There has been no evaluation of the clinical trials for the use of these emerging botanicals for type 2 diabetes mellitus. The aim of this review is to assess the effects of botanicals on type 2 diabetes mellitus. Existing opportunity for these botanicals in the management of diabetes and the state of the evidence for their anti-diabetic usefulness will be discussed. This includes issues pertaining to these clinical trials, the quality of antihyperglycemic efficacy data and related complementary metabolic effects. The adverse effects of interventions, a critical aspect of diabetic care, will also be emphasised. Finally, important limitations, which may affect the interpretation of data from these clinical studies and the implications for future research; in the context of T2DM in developing Asia-Pacific countries, will also be addressed.

2. Research methodology

2.1 Methods

Search was carried out in the following databases: MEDLINE, CINHAL, Proquest Health & Medical Complete, ProQuest Dissertations & Theses, CAM-PubMed, and the Cochrane Library Database from April 2006 to March 2011 using the MeSH terms *CAM, alternative therapies, hypoglycemic plants or botanicals, anti-diabetic plants or botanicals* and individual botanicals and supplement names from popular sources, each crossed with the term *diabetes mellitus*. Databases of ongoing trials (http://www.controlled-trials.com/ with links to several databases and https://www.clinicaltrialsregister.eu/) were also searched.

Only emerging botanical derived products or drugs not in the established armamentarium of modalities used in the current management of T2DM were included. Supplements in which animal products were major components were excluded. We also did not include soluble or dietary fibre supplements that were already established in conventional diabetes nutrition advice.

Specific filters for retrieving controlled clinical trial, double-blind, placebo-controlled, phase II, or III randomised controlled trials of any duration; published systematic reviews and meta-analyses of randomised controlled trials; and randomised controlled trials (RCT) in human adults (aged ≥18), were incorporated. Hand searching was not performed, but reference lists of identified systematic reviews, meta-analyses, and pooled analyses were reviewed to identify further studies. Unpublished studies were also not sought. References in any articles that met the inclusion criteria were included. There were no language restrictions.

2.1.1 Studies selection

The results of the search from the various databases were entered in a bibliographic manager software, Endnote X4 (Thomson Reuters). Duplicates were automatically discarded. We screened the identified articles to ensure they met pre-determined inclusion criteria. To ensure uniformity of appraisal for each study a checklist of specified inclusion criteria was used. The initial review for all identified citations included titles or abstracts, or both. Following, a second review stage of full text publications for citations remaining after the first pass was carried out. We used a positive exclusion method to exclude only those publications that did not meet one or more of the inclusion criteria. In ambiguous cases, inclusion of studies was based on expert opinion.

2.1.2 Data extraction

A structured table was developed for data extraction to ensure uniformity of appraisal for each study as well as capturing all relevant data. Extracted data consisted of study characteristics (such as treatments and doses, status of T2DM and associated conditions, duration, and study location) and relevant outcomes (glycaemic control, adverse effects, morbidity, blood lipids level, body weight or body mass index).

2.1.3 Outcome measures

There were two primary outcomes: glycaemic control and adverse effects. These were considered as measures of efficacy and measures of tolerability respectively. Secondary outcomes were included when present. These included serum insulin, body weight or body mass index, blood lipids level and morbidity. Morbidity included both type 2 diabetes mellitus as well as cardiovascular-related comorbidity and all cause morbidity. The above data were only extracted and analysed when reported.

Data for glycaemic control, FBG and 2HPBG, was collected for trials of at least 6 weeks and over. For HbAic, trials over three months were considered. Data of all other outcomes will be collected from studies of any duration.

2.1.4 Statistical analysis

Analyses were performed on data that were explicitly reported in the individual papers, with no imputations for data that were not reported. When available, we analysed the intention-to-treat population; when this was not possible, we used data from the last observation carried forward. The analyses were conducted using RevMan 5.0 meta-analytic software (The Cochrane Collaboration, 2008).

2.2 Results

The search returned a total of 45 publications and abstracts (Figure 1). After review of titles and abstracts, we identified and included 22 relevant papers. All were clinical trials (1 clinical trial, 1 controlled clinical trial, and 20 randomised controlled trials) (Table 1). Six were excluded because duration of these studies were less than 6 weeks. Another was excluded because the primary outcome was not glycaemic control or adverse effects. Of the 15 remaining studies, all were randomised controlled trials. All the trials consisted of different plant-based interventions.

2.2.1 Characteristics of included studies

There were fifteen studies that met all the inclusion criteria. Table 1 shows the characteristics of the trials. The study participants for each trial range from 24 to 109. All studies included both genders. The participants were middle-age and older adults. Study length ranged from 12 weeks to 4 months.

Four papers provided information on different forms of cinnamon extracts (S.M. Blevins et al., 2007; P. Crawford, 2009; B. Mang et al., 2006; S. Suppapitiporn& N. Kanpaksi, 2006). Two papers provided information on different forms of *Silybum marianum* preparations (H.F. Huseini et al., 2006; S.A. Hussain, 2007) and another two papers provided findings of

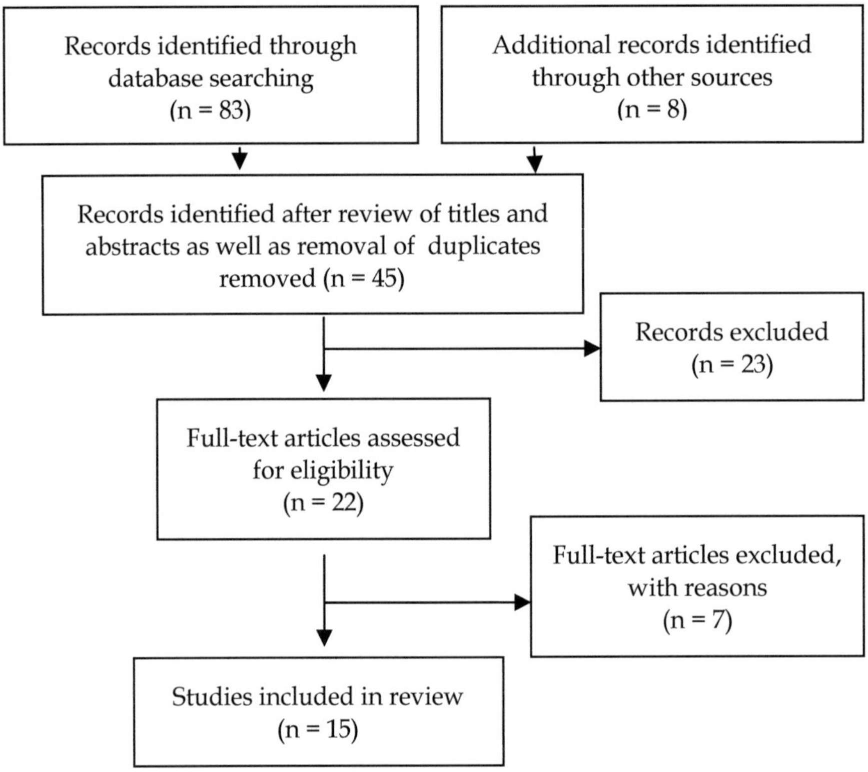

Fig. 1. Modified PRISMA (Preferred Reporting Items for Systematic Reviews and Meta-Analyses) flow-chart of study selection (D. Moher et al., 2009)

catechin-containing tea preparations (T. Mackenzie et al., 2007; T. Nagao et al., 2009). The rest of the seven papers were focussed on 7 diffent plant-based preparations for T2DM (A.M. Dans et al., 2007; H.F. Huseini et al., 2009; V.T. Huyen et al., 2010; R. Kuriyan et al., 2008; F.R. Lu et al., 2008; V. Vuksan et al., 2008; S. Zibadi et al., 2008).

2.2.2 Risks of bias

Risk of bias assessments included assessments of minimisation of selection, performance, attrition, reporting biases as well as other sources of biases (A.R. Jadad et al., 1996; L.L. Kjaergard et al., 2001; K.F. Schulz et al., 1995).

One trial was a crossover randomised trial (V. Vuksan et al., 2008), while the rest was parallel-group design. Recruitment of patients was limited to the centres of the studies. Of the 15 included randomised trials, five trials described the methods of randomisation (P. Crawford, 2009; A.M. Dans et al., 2007; H.F. Huseini et al., 2006; T. Mackenzie et al., 2007; V. Vuksan et al., 2008). Among them, three used simple randomisation methods (random number generator, table and computer generated sequence) (A.M. Dans et al., 2007; T. Mackenzie et al., 2007; V. Vuksan et al., 2008), one used block randomisation technique (P. Crawford, 2009) and another used a balanced randomisation technique (H.F. Huseini et al., 2006). Only three trials reported generation of allocation concealment (P. Crawford, 2009; A.M. Dans et al., 2007; H.F. Huseini et al., 2006). The rest of the trials did not document adequate methods of randomisation.

Ref	Study design	Subjects	Intervention	Control
(S.M. Blevins et al., 2007)	DBRPCT	58 with T2DM	Cinnamon powder capsule (*C. cassia)*	Wheat flour placebo capsule
(B. Mang et al., 2006)	DBRPCT	65 with T2DM	Aqueous cinnamon extract (*C. cassia)* capsule	Microcrystalline cellulose placebo capsule
(S. Suppapitiporn& N. Kanpaksi, 2006)	SBRPCT	60 with T2DM	Cinnamon powder capsule (*C. Cassia)*	Placebo
(P. Crawford, 2009)	RCT	109 with T2DM	Cinnamon capsule (*C. Cassia)*	No placebo intervention
(A.M. Dans et al., 2007)	DBRPCT	40 with T2DM	*Momordica charantia* leaf capsules	Placebo
(H.F. Huseini et al., 2009)	DBRPCT	50 with T2DM	*Citrullus. colocynthis* dried fruit powder capsules	Placebo
(H.F. Huseini et al., 2006)	DBRPCT	51 with T2DM	*Silybum marianum* seed extract tablets	Placebo
(S.A. Hussain, 2007)	DBRPCT	59 with T2DM	*Silybum marianum* extract tablets	Placebo
(V.T. Huyen et al., 2010)	DBRPCT	24 with T2DM	*Gynostemma pentaphyllum* tea	Placebo tea
(R. Kuriyan et al., 2008)	DBRPCT	60 with T2DM	*Coccinia cordifolia* leaves and fruit extract capsules	Maltosedextrin capsule placebo
(F.R. Lu et al., 2008)	RCT	69 with T2DM	*Trigonella foenum-graecum* powder capsules	*Chinese yam* powder placebo
(T. Mackenzie et al., 2007)	DBRPCT	49 with T2DM	Green and black tea extract capsules	Cellulose capsule placebo
(T. Nagao et al., 2009)	RCT	43 with T2DM	Green tea extract (catechin-rich 528 mg) beverage	Low dose catechin (96.3 mg) placebo tea
(V. Vuksan et al., 2008)	DBRPCT, crossover	19 with T2DM	*Panax ginseng* extract capsules	Vanilla flavoured cornstarch capsule placebo
(S. Zibadi et al., 2008)	RCT	48 with T2DM	*Pinus maritima* bark extract pill	Placebo

Table 1. Clinical trials of botanical interventions for type 2 diabetes mellitus.

Blinding of all patients, trials investigators and assessors were reported in five trials (A.M. Dans et al., 2007; H.F. Huseini et al., 2009; H.F. Huseini et al., 2006; S.A. Hussain, 2007; T. Mackenzie et al., 2007). Eight trials did not report any aspects of blinding at all (V.T. Huyen et al., 2010; A, Khan et al., 2003; R. Kuriyan et al., 2008; F.R. Lu et al., 2008; B. Mang et al., 2006; T. Nagao et al., 2009; S. Suppapitiporn& N. Kanpaksi, 2006; V. Vuksan et al., 2008). While the rest documented blinding of patients and trial investigators (S.M. Blevins et al., 2007) or assessors only (P. Crawford, 2009; S. Zibadi et al., 2008). Both dropouts of patients and intention-to-treat analysis were reported in five trials (S.M. Blevins et al., 2007; P. Crawford, 2009; A.M. Dans et al., 2007; F.R. Lu et al., 2008; S. Zibadi et al., 2008). One trial reported only dropouts of patients but not intention-to-treat analysis (H.F. Huseini et al., 2006).

Four papers did not mention appropriate inclusion, exclusion criteria or both (P. Crawford, 2009; R. Kuriyan et al., 2008; B. Mang et al., 2006; V. Vuksan et al., 2008). A statement of power calculation had been undertaken or give any justification for the numbers of participants needed to detect an effect of differences with intervention was documented in five papers (S.M. Blevins et al., 2007; P. Crawford, 2009; A.M. Dans et al., 2007; T. Mackenzie et al., 2007; V. Vuksan et al., 2008). Potential confounding factors were not elaborated in four papers (S.M. Blevins et al., 2007; P. Crawford, 2009; H.F. Huseini et al., 2009; B. Mang et al., 2006). There was also no uniform tool to assess adjunct dietary management in all these trials.

2.2.3 Effects of interventions

In view of the quality of data and variability of treatment, meta-analysis was not performed. One trial compared single botanical preparation without adjunct oral hypoglycaemics with placebo. The rest of the trials compared the botanical preparation with adjunct oral hypoglycaemicis with placebo. These tested botanicals included preparations of *Cinnamon cassia, Momordica charantia, Citrullus Colocynthis, Silybum marianum, Gynostemma pentaphyllum, Coccinia cordifolia, trigonella foenum-graecum L, Camelia sinesis* (tea) and *Pinus maritima.* Among them, *Cinnamon cassia* was tested in 4 trials, while *Silybum marianum* and *Camelia sinesis* (tea) were each tested in two trials. The reported outcomes included fasting blood glucose, postprandial blood glucose, HbA1c, fasting serum insulin levels, serum lipids level, symptoms, and adverse effects.

Single botanical preparations versus placebo

Compared with placebo (maltodextrin capsules), *Coccinia cordifolia* showed significantly better effect on normalisation of fasting blood glucose. There was a mean decrease of 15.6% in the intervention group compared to mean increase of 6% in the placebo group. Similarly, with the 2 hour postprandial blood glucose, there was a significant mean decrease of 18.5% in the intervention group. No significant change was noted in the placebo control group. There was also significant decrease in the glycosylated haemoglobin level in the intervention group.

Mild hypoglycaemic symptoms, perspiration, excessive hunger and slight dizziness, was noted post-prandially in 59% of the participants in the intervention group. However, there was no significant difference in minor gastrointestinal adverse effects between the two groups.

Single botanical preparations with oral hypoglycaemic agent (OHA) adjuncts versus placebo

The effect of *Cinnamon cassia* preparations and OHA in reducing fasting blood glucose level was not consistent. One trial showed a significant reduction in fasting blood glucose levels (B. Mang et al., 2006). However, two others reported no significant change with trials of 3 to 4 months (S.M. Blevins et al., 2007; S. Suppapitiporn& N. Kanpaksi, 2006). There was no overall effect on HbA1c changes. Only one trial reported significant improvement in HbA1c level after 3 months (Standard mean difference (SMD) 0.12 g%; 95%CI -0.26 to 0.50) (P. Crawford, 2009). However, this change did not translate into an overall significant effect size. Further, three trials of 3 and 4 month durations reported no significance improvement in the HbA1c with this botanical intervention (S.M. Blevins et al., 2007; B. Mang et al., 2006; S. Suppapitiporn& N. Kanpaksi, 2006). Three trials of 3 and 4 months duration did not find any significant effect on the lipid levels (S.M. Blevins et al., 2007; B. Mang et al., 2006; S. Suppapitiporn& N. Kanpaksi, 2006).

Adverse effect of hypersensitivity rash was reported in only one trial (P. Crawford, 2009). Comparison of these studies was difficult in view of different baseline biochemical characteristics (blood glucose, HbA1c, insulin, lipid level), weight, diet and concurent medications.

There was no significant difference between *Camelia sinesis* extracts (catechin and theaflavin) with OHA and placebo in HbA1c (T. Mackenzie et al., 2007; T. Nagao et al., 2009) and fasting blood glucose levels (T. Nagao et al., 2009). Although there was a significant increase in the insulin level in the catechin-rich beverage group, the number of participants was too small (n=23) for further interpretation (T. Nagao et al., 2009). Adverse effects reported were profuse sweating and rash, which led to withdrawal from the study.

Compared with placebo, combination *Silybum marianum* and OHA significantly reduced both the FBG and HbA1c levels in two trials of four month durations (H.F. Huseini et al., 2006; S.A. Hussain, 2007). Even so, results of other parameters such as 2HPBG, BMI and lipid levels, were not consistent. No side-effects were reported.

Compared with placebo, the fruits and seeds capsules preparation of *Momordica charantia* and OHA showed no statistically significant effect on reduction of fasting blood glucose and HbA1c levels (A.M. Dans et al., 2007). Similarly, when compared with placebo, the treatment also showed no statistically significant reduction in secondary outcome measures, total cholesterol levels or body mass index when compared to placebo. However, the minor adverse effects of gastrointestinal discomfort led to discontinuation of treatment.

Ingestion of tea prepared from *Gynostemma pentaphyllum* and OHA for 12 weeks showed a significant reduction in FBG, HbA1c and insulin resistance, compared with placebo and OHA (V.T. Huyen et al., 2010). There were no adverse effects reported.

Intervention with *Citrullus colocynthis* and OHA in 25 patients for 2 months demonstrated significant reduction in both FBG and HbA1c levels , compared with patients taking placebo and OHA (H.F. Huseini et al., 2009). There were no significant changes in secondary outcome measures of lipid levels. However, three patients reported mild diarrhoea at the beginning of the study.

Patients on *Trigonella foenum-graecum* capsules and OHA for 12 weeks showed significant improvement glycaemic profile, FBG, 2HPBG and HbA1c, as well as symptoms, compared with placebo (F.R. Lu et al., 2008). However, there were no significant secondary outcomes change of BMI, hepatic and renal functions. Adverse effects of abdominal discomforts and diarrhoea led to withdrawal from intervention.

Compared with placebo, intervention with *Panax ginseng* extract capsules and OHA, significantly improved glucose tolerance and insulin sensitivity in a double-blind, placebo-controlled crossover randomised clinical trial (V. Vuksan et al., 2008). There were no significant changes in HbA1c as well as safety biochemical parameters of liver and kidneys. Adverse effects of hypoglycaemia was reported. In addition, there was a high number of dropouts (50%). This was attributed to conflicting approaches used in the management of T2DM in mainstream medical practice and traditional herbal practice in the country of the trial.

Finally, *Pinus maritima* bark extract pill and OHA demonstrated significant reduction in FBG, HbA1c and LDL-cholesterol, compared with placebo and OHA (S. Zibadi et al., 2008). This was over a relatively short duration of 3 months. However, there was no documentation of adverse effects.

2.3 Discussions

2.3.1 Summary of main results

Fifteen randomised trials were included in this review. The exclusion of 7 trials was due to treatment duration of less than six weeks or reported outcomes not relevant to this review. The included trials compared different botanical preparation with or without combinations with hypoglycaemic agents versus placebo. Not all the trials provided data on dietary and lifestyle modification in patients with type 2 diabetes mellitus. Majority of the trials measured surrogate primary outcomes, some evaluated symptoms or adverse events. Two trials failed to demonstrate any improvements in the blood glucose control in terms of normalisation, reduction of fasting blood glucose, reduction of 2HPBG responses and reduction of HbA1c. This is in contrast with the majority that demonstrated improvements in the surrogate primary outcomes.

Only some trials examined secondary outcomes such as lipid levels or BMI. Safety biochemical parameters of the kidney and liver were examined in a limited number of trials. The low methodological quality and the general small sample size in these trials contributing to the low power of all the studies. Taken together with the limited number of the trials identified for individual botanical preparations, caution is needed in interpreting the findings of these trials. In all these studies, there were no statements on the health-related quality of life, well-being, socioeconomic status or costs.

Compared with placebo, six botanical preparations with oral hypoglycaemics, *Cinnamon cassia, Citrullus Colocynthis, Silybum marianum, Gynostemma pentaphyllum, trigonella foenum-graecum L* and *Pinus maritima* seemed to have varying effects on blood glucose control. The hypoglycaemic agents used are sulphonylureas, metformin, thiazoledinediones, glinides, glitazones, acarbose or combination therapies. In addition to the conflicting findings of the four trials using preparations of *Cinnamon cassia,* the botanical preparations above with potential effects on glucose, warrant further trials.

2.3.2 Applicability of evidence

The fifteen trials available for this review were only a small fraction (less than 3%) of the vast resources of potential botanicals for T2DM. For the four trials using *Cinnamon cassia* intervention, the extracts were of derived from different techniques, dosages and sources. Moreover, the placebos used as control of three of these trials also varied. One trial did not elaborate on the contents (S. Suppapitiporn& N. Kanpaksi, 2006), while two others used

wheat flour and microcrystalline cellulose (S.M. Blevins et al., 2007; B. Mang et al., 2006). Another trial did not use any placebo as control (P. Crawford, 2009). In addition, the time point for assessment of the effect of intervention for the four trials was not uniform. This time point was 3 months for two trials (S.M. Blevins et al., 2007; S. Suppapitiporn& N. Kanpaksi, 2006)and 4 months for the other two(T. Mackenzie et al., 2007; B. Mang et al., 2006). Thus, these methodological issues may affect the results.
Even though there were two trials for each of the botanical, *Camillia sinensis* and *Silybum marianum,* different preparations were used. This means that none of the preparations of trials in this review were tested at least twice. Furthermore, many trials used the 'double-blind'design but few reported blinding of outcome assessors. This may predisposed to the possibility of performance and reporting bias (D. Moher et al., 1998; K.F. Schulz et al., 1995).

2.3.3 Quality of evidence

Since all the trials in this review did not meet one or more essential risk of bias criteria, these trials were assessed having high risk of bias. There was no trial with moderate or low risk of bias. When quality criteria in terms of minimisation of selection, performance, attrition, and detection biases are met, trial of low risk of bias is indicated. Similarly, categorization into moderate risk of bias required the quality criteria to be partially fulfilled.

2.3.4 Safety of botanical preparations

The botanical preparations evaluated in this review generally did not report severe adverse effects. Thus, the conclusion on the safety of using these botanicals in the management of diabetic patients cannot be made. Further, many of the adverse effects were not sufficiently reported. None of the reviews looked for the effects of 'botanical-drug' interaction. It is important that both the beneficial and harmful effects in clinical trials of human given equal attention.
Previous reviews examined the use the different modalities of complementary and alternative medicine (R. Nahas& M. Moher, 2009) or the use herbs and dietary supplements (G.Y. Yeh et al., 2003). This review differs in the respect that we are focussed on the update of the clinical trials of botanical preparations for type 2 diabetes mellitus of the last five years. This included randomised controlled clinical trials comparing botanical preparation with placebo or hypoglycaemic drugs in type 2 diabetes mellitus of duration exceeding six weeks. Previous reviews included both randomised and non-randomised controlled trials with interventions consisting of herbs, dietary supplements as well as minerals (vanadium and chromium) in both types of diabetics and healthy individuals. However, we limited our focus to potential botanicals for T2DM. Furthermore, our search strategy has no restriction to language. This is important as many of the trials with botanicals may appear in the languages in the regions where the use of botanicals is common, particularly in Asia. Finally, stringent criteria for quality assessment were used in this review based on recommendations by several authors (A.R. Jadad et al., 1996; L.L. Kjaergard et al., 2001; K.F. Schulz et al., 1995).
Current approaches to the use of botanical preparations differ with the type of medical practices. The expectation of mainstream medical practice is standardisation of extracts of botanicals extracts of predominantly specific parts of single plant (P. Talalay, 2001). This preparation is further investigated based on a set of criteria, which include preparation consistent with the description in the pharmacopoeia, chemical standardisation, biological assays, animal models, and clinical testing for the particular condition. In comparison,

traditional medical practices may include non-herbal or herbal modalities or combination (H.T. Debas et al., 2006). The focus may be on symptoms, well-being and customising for each individual patient based on the differentiation of the patients' 'syndrome' based on the particular traditional medicine practice philosophy. However, in many communities in Asia, the use of plural practices for management of type 2 diabetes is common (K.L. Tackett& M.C. Jones, 2009). Since there is evidence of the potential of botanicals contributing to management of T2DM, it is important to further understand their uses. The pleiotropic properties may have other benefits for these diabetics. Further insight may allow the use as possible expanding armamentarium of the glucose lowering therapeutic agents or complementing other aspects of treatment such as medical nutritional therapy. Improving the morale of the patients rather than creating conflict with the patient's use of other approaches, is important to ensure continuity of treatment and ultimately control of disease.
In summary, the selected studies in this review showed variability of treatment interventions, control interventions and generally small effect sizes. None of the preparations were tested twice. As a result, there is insufficient evidence for any reliable conclusion of the potential benefits or harmful effects of these botanicals for type 2 diabetes mellitus.

2.3.5 Limitations

This systematic review has several limitations. First, there are limited trials available for selection. This may be due to the fact that research of these botanicals is still in the early days or publication bias. With the included trials, methodological issues were predominant. The poor quality of randomisation and blinding may exaggerate effects of the interventions due to systematic errors (bias). Potential bias may also occur during selection of patients, administration of treatment, and assessment of outcomes. Therefore, these methodologically less rigorous trials may show inappropriately skewed larger significant intervention effects than trials with more rigors (M. Egger et al., 2003; L.L. Kjaergard et al., 2001).
Small sample size of the trials leads to diminished power of the results. This may explain the absence of a statistically significant difference between botanical preparations used for interventions (E. Christensen, 2007; G. Piaggio& A.P. Pinol, 2001). In other words, the analyses from the size of these trials may not establish with confidence that two interventions have equivalent effects.
All the selected trials reported end-of treatment responses, ranging from six weeks to four months. Important long-term responses beyond this period are not known. Finally, not all the trials provide information on ethnicity of the participants. The recruitment of patients was limited to the respective centre of study. In addition, all the preparations used in the intervention arms were tested only once, which made it impossible to pool data. Thus, the applicability of the results to other ethnic groups or populations is not known.

3. Conclusion

Some of the botanical preparations in this review may have beneficial effects on glycaemic glucose control in people with T2DM. However, at this point of time, we cannot recommend any for routine clinical use. All the trials had low methodological quality. The beneficial effects need to be confirmed by large rigorous randomised controlled trials of high-quality. In addition, the adverse effects also need to be further elucidated. Nevertheless, results from ongoing studies may provide more information on the potential clinical use of *Cinnamon cassia, Momordica charantia* and *Camellia sinesis* (Table 2).

3.1 Implications for future research

Although preclinical and early clinical trials suggest that the botanicals in this review may contribute to the management of T2DM, a potential methodological problem is the issue of the quality of these botanical preparations. An example is the varying effect of *C. cassia* preparations from different sources on glycaemic control. Some of the differences may arise with the varying climates, conditions for growing, harvesting and processing (U. Solimene et al., 2007). Different parts of the plant may have a different proportion of bioactive compounds present. This may add to the complexity of characterisation, production of reliable and consistently effective products. Therefore, there is a need to address the standardisation and the quality of the products used in clinic trials.

Ref	Study design	Country	Intervention	Control
(P. Crawford, 2011)	DBRCT	USA	*Cinnamon* bark and Cinnulin PF dietary supplements	metformin
(A. Tsiami, 2009)	DBRPCT	UK	*Cinnamon* capsules	Starch capsule placebo
(R. Ridout et al., 2007)	DBRPCT	Canada	Cinnamonforce capsule	Placebo
(K. Khawaja, 2009)	DBRPCT	Pakistan	Momordica charantia capsule	Wheat flour placebo capsule
(C.H. Hsu, 2007)	DBRPCT	Taiwan	*epigallocatechin gallate* predominant green tea extract	Green tea extract placebo

Table 2. Ongoing clinical trials of botanical interventions for type 2 diabetes mellitus.

The trials in this review did not examine the effect of the botanical interventions over a prolonged period (over 4 months). Thus, the effects on the micro and macro-complications well as other benefits in the patients with T2DM are not known. Moreover, with the different methodologies used, the presence of confounders, the varieties in the diet and the difficulty in recording dietary intake make it difficult to interpret the results. Furthermore, there is also the practicality of maintaining a 'stable' oral hypoglycaemic agents regime over a long period. Introduction of relevant clinically important outcome measures for long-term follow up may improve the quality of the trial.

Design of future trials comparing such botanical interventions with established hypoglycaemic drugs should be based on 'equivalence principle'. In view of the findings of preclinical studies suggesting benefits beyond glycaemic control, when comparing these botanical interventions combined with one or more established oral hypoglycaemic agents, verifying these potential benefits is suggested. Particularly, for the middle-aged and older patients with T2DM, relevant outcome measures should include functional outcomes, quality of life, well-being, socioeconomic status and costs.

The quality of assessment of adverse events may be improved with a standardised format. Several components of selection bias that affect the quality of randomised controlled trials of this review required attention. This is the detailed reporting of the methods used to generate allocation sequence and allocation concealment. Adequate descriptions of withdrawal or drop-out during the trial and use of intention-to-treat analysis will also contribute to the quality of the trial.

4. Acknowledgment

The authors would like to acknowledge the kind support given by Institute of Gerontology, Universiti Putra Malaysia.

5. Abbreviations

MeSH, Medical Subject Headings; CAM, Complementary and Alternative Medicine; CCT, controlled clinical trial; DBRPCT, double-blind randomised placebo-controlled trial; DBRCT, double-blind randomised controlled trial; SBRPCT, single-blind randomised placebo-controlled trial; RCT, randomised controlled trial; T2DM, type 2 diabetes mellitus; UK, United Kingdom; USA, United States of America

6. References

Abegunde, D.O.; Mathers, C.D.; Adam, T.; Ortegon, M. & Strong, K. (2007). The burden and costs of chronic diseases in low-income and middle-income countries. *Lancet*, Vol. 370, No. 9603 (Dec 8 2007), pp. 1929-38, ISSN 1474-547X (Electronic) 0140-6736 (Linking)

Blevins, S.M.; Leyva, M.J.; Brown, J.; Wright, J.; Scofield, R.H. & Aston, C.E. (2007). Effect of cinnamon on glucose and lipid levels in non insulin-dependent type 2 diabetes. *Diabetes Care*, Vol. 30, No. 9 (Sep 2007), pp. 2236-7, ISSN 1935-5548 (Electronic) 0149-5992 (Linking)

Chan, J.C.; Malik, V.; Jia, W.; Kadowaki, T.; Yajnik, C.S.; Yoon, K.H. & Hu, F.B. (2009). Diabetes in Asia: epidemiology, risk factors, and pathophysiology. *JAMA*, Vol. 301, No. 20 (May 27 2009), pp. 2129-40, ISSN 1538-3598 (Electronic) 0098-7484 (Linking)

Chang, H.Y.; Wallis, M. & Tiralongo, E. (2007). Use of complementary and alternative medicine among people living with diabetes: literature review. *J Adv Nurs*, Vol. 58, No. 4 (May 2007), pp. 307-19, ISSN 0309-2402 (Print) 0309-2402 (Linking)

Christensen, E. (2007). Methodology of superiority vs. equivalence trials and non-inferiority trials. *J Hepatol*, Vol. 46, No. 5 (May 2007), pp. 947-54, ISSN 0168-8278 (Print) 0168-8278 (Linking)

Crawford, P. (2009). Effectiveness of cinnamon for lowering hemoglobin A1C in patients with type 2 diabetes: a randomized, controlled trial. *J Am Board Fam Med*, Vol. 22, No. 5 (Sep-Oct 2009), pp. 507-12, ISSN 1557-2625 (Print) 1557-2625 (Linking)

Crawford, P. (2011). *Cinnamon Bark, Water-Soluble Cinnamon Extract, and Metformin as Initial Treatment for Type 2 Diabetes Mellitus: A Randomized, Controlled Trial, ClinicalTrials.gov identifier: NCT01302743* In: ClinicalTrials.gov, US National Institute of Health, Date of access: 12/04/2011, Available from:

http://clinicaltrials.gov/ct2/show/NCT01302743?term=cinnamon+diabetes&rank=1.

Dans, A.M.; Villarruz, M.V.; Jimeno, C.A.; Javelosa, M.A.; Chua, J.; Bautista, R. & Velez, G.G. (2007). The effect of Momordica charantia capsule preparation on glycemic control in type 2 diabetes mellitus needs further studies. *J Clin Epidemiol,* Vol. 60, No. 6 (Jun 2007), pp. 554-9, ISSN 0895-4356 (Print) 0895-4356 (Linking)

Debas, H.T.; Laxminarayan, R. & Straus, S.E. (2006). Complementary and Alternative Medicine, *Disease Control Priorities in Developing Countries.* In: Jamison, D.T.; Breman, J.G.; Measham, A.R.; Alleyne, G.; Claeson, M.; Evans, D.B.; Jha, P.; Mills, A. &Musgrove, P., pp. 1281-1291, The International Bank for Reconstruction and Development/The World Bank Group, ISSN Washington, D. C.

Egede, L.E. (2004). Diabetes, major depression, and functional disability among U.S. adults. *Diabetes Care,* Vol. 27, No. 2 (Feb 2004), pp. 421-8, ISSN 0149-5992 (Print) 0149-5992 (Linking)

Egger, M.; Juni, P.; Bartlett, C.; Holenstein, F. & Sterne, J. (2003). How important are comprehensive literature searches and the assessment of trial quality in systematic reviews? Empirical study. *Health Technol Assess,* Vol. 7, No. 1 (February 2003), pp. 1-76, ISSN 1366-5278 (Print) 1366-5278 (Linking)

Hsu, C.H. (2007). *Effect of Green Tea Extract on Type 2 Diabetes (GTT-DM), ClinicalTrials.gov Identifier: NCT00567905* In: ClinicalTrials.gov, US National Intitutes of Health, Date of access: 04/12/2011, Available from: http://clinicaltrials.gov/ct2/show/NCT00567905?term=tea+diabetes&rank=3.

Huseini, H.F.; Darvishzadeh, F.; Heshmat, R.; Jafariazar, Z.; Raza, M. & Larijani, B. (2009). The clinical investigation of Citrullus colocynthis (L.) schrad fruit in treatment of Type II diabetic patients: a randomized, double blind, placebo-controlled clinical trial. *Phytother Res,* Vol. 23, No. 8 (Aug 2009), pp. 1186-9, ISSN 1099-1573 (Electronic) 0951-418X (Linking)

Huseini, H.F.; Larijani, B.; Heshmat, R.; Fakhrzadeh, H.; Radjabipour, B.; Toliat, T. & Raza, M. (2006). The efficacy of Silybum marianum (L.) Gaertn. (silymarin) in the treatment of type II diabetes: a randomized, double-blind, placebo-controlled, clinical trial. *Phytother Res,* Vol. 20, No. 12 (Dec 2006), pp. 1036-9, ISSN 0951-418X (Print) 0951-418X (Linking)

Hussain, S.A. (2007). Silymarin as an adjunct to glibenclamide therapy improves long-term and postprandial glycemic control and body mass index in type 2 diabetes. *J Med Food,* Vol. 10, No. 3 (Sep 2007), pp. 543-7, ISSN 1096-620X (Print) 1096-620X (Linking)

Huyen, V.T.; Phan, D.V.; Thang, P.; Hoa, N.K. & Ostenson, C.G. (2010). Antidiabetic effect of Gynostemma pentaphyllum tea in randomly assigned type 2 diabetic patients. *Horm Metab Res,* Vol. 42, No. 5 (May 2010), pp. 353-7, ISSN 1439-4286 (Electronic) 0018-5043 (Linking)

International Diabetes Federation. (2009). *IDF Diabetes Atlas,* (4th), International Diabetes Federation, ISBN -13: 978-2-930229-71-3, Brussels, Belgium

Jadad, A.R.; Moore, R.A.; Carroll, D.; Jenkinson, C.; Reynolds, D.J.; Gavaghan, D.J. & McQuay, H.J. (1996). Assessing the quality of reports of randomized clinical trials: is blinding necessary? *Control Clin Trials,* Vol. 17, No. 1 (Feb 1996), pp. 1-12, ISSN 0197-2456 (Print) 0197-2456 (Linking)

Kantor, M. (2009). The role of rigorous scientific evaluation in the use and practice of complementary and alternative medicine. *J Am Coll Radiol*, Vol. 6, No. 4 (Apr 2009), pp. 254-62, ISSN 1558-349X (Electronic) 1546-1440 (Linking)

Khan, A.; Safdar, M.; Ali Khan, M.M.; Khattak, K.N. & Anderson, R.A. (2003). Cinnamon improves glucose and lipids of people with type 2 diabetes. *Diabetes Care*, Vol. 26, No. 12 (Dec 2003), pp. 3215-8, ISSN 0149-5992 (Print) 0149-5992 (Linking)

Khawaja, K. (2009). *Glycemic Response to Momordica Charantia in Type 2 Diabetes, ClinicalTrials.gov Identifier: NCT00823953*. In: ClinicalTrials.gov, US National Institutes of Health Date of access: 04/12/2011, Available from: http://clinicaltrials.gov/ct2/show/NCT00823953?term=Momordica+charantia+diabetes&rank=1.

Kjaergard, L.L.; Villumsen, J. & Gluud, C. (2001). Reported methodologic quality and discrepancies between large and small randomized trials in meta-analyses. *Ann Intern Med*, Vol. 135, No. 11 (Dec 4 2001), pp. 982-9, ISSN 0003-4819 (Print) 0003-4819 (Linking)

Kuriyan, R.; Rajendran, R.; Bantwal, G. & Kurpad, A.V. (2008). Effect of supplementation of Coccinia cordifolia extract on newly detected diabetic patients. *Diabetes Care*, Vol. 31, No. 2 (Feb 2008), pp. 216-20, ISSN 1935-5548 (Electronic) 1935-5548 (Linking)

Lu, F.R.; Shen, L.; Qin, Y.; Gao, L.; Li, H. & Dai, Y. (2008). Clinical observation on trigonella foenum-graecum L. total saponins in combination with sulfonylureas in the treatment of type 2 diabetes mellitus. *Chin J Integr Med*, Vol. 14, No. 1 (Mar 2008), pp. 56-60, ISSN 1672-0415 (Print) 1672-0415 (Linking)

Mackenzie, T.; Leary, L. & Brooks, W.B. (2007). The effect of an extract of green and black tea on glucose control in adults with type 2 diabetes mellitus: double-blind randomized study. *Metabolism*, Vol. 56, No. 10 (Oct 2007), pp. 1340-4, ISSN 0026-0495 (Print) 0026-0495 (Linking)

Mang, B.; Wolters, M.; Schmitt, B.; Kelb, K.; Lichtinghagen, R.; Stichtenoth, D.O. & Hahn, A. (2006). Effects of a cinnamon extract on plasma glucose, HbA, and serum lipids in diabetes mellitus type 2. *Eur J Clin Invest*, Vol. 36, No. 5 (May 2006), pp. 340-4, ISSN 0014-2972 (Print) 0014-2972 (Linking)

Metcalfe, A.; Williams, J.; McChesney, J.; Patten, S.B. & Jette, N. (2010). Use of complementary and alternative medicine by those with a chronic disease and the general population--results of a national population based survey. *BMC Complement Altern Med*, Vol. 10, No. (Oct 2010), pp. 58, ISSN 1472-6882 (Electronic) 1472-6882 (Linking)

Modak, M.; Dixit, P.; Londhe, J.; Ghaskadbi, S. & Paul, A.D.T. (2007). Indian herbs and herbal drugs used for the treatment of diabetes. *J Clin Biochem Nutr*, Vol. 40, No. 3 (May 2007), pp. 163-73, ISSN 0912-0009 (Print) 0912-0009 (Linking)

Moher, D.; Liberati, A.; Tetzlaff, J. & Altman, D.G. (2009). Preferred reporting items for systematic reviews and meta-analyses: the PRISMA statement. *PLoS Med*, Vol. 6, No. 7 (Jul 2009), pp. e1000097, ISSN 1549-1676 (Electronic) 1549-1277 (Linking)

Moher, D.; Pham, B.; Jones, A.; Cook, D.J.; Jadad, A.R.; Moher, M.; Tugwell, P. & Klassen, T.P. (1998). Does quality of reports of randomised trials affect estimates of intervention efficacy reported in meta-analyses? *Lancet*, Vol. 352, No. 9128 (Aug 22 1998), pp. 609-13, ISSN 0140-6736 (Print) 0140-6736 (Linking)

Nagao, T.; Meguro, S.; Hase, T.; Otsuka, K.; Komikado, M.; Tokimitsu, I.; Yamamoto, T. & Yamamoto, K. (2009). A catechin-rich beverage improves obesity and blood glucose control in patients with type 2 diabetes. *Obesity (Silver Spring)*, Vol. 17, No. 2 (Feb 2009), pp. 310-7, ISSN 1930-7381 (Print) 1930-7381 (Linking)

Nahas, R. & Moher, M. (2009). Complementary and alternative medicine for the treatment of type 2 diabetes. *Can Fam Physician*, Vol. 55, No. 6 (Jun 2009), pp. 591-6, ISSN 1715-5258 (Electronic) 0008-350X (Linking)

Nguyen, H.T.; Grzywacz, J.G.; Lang, W.; Walkup, M. & Arcury, T.A. (2010). Effects of complementary therapy on health in a national U.S. sample of older adults. *J Altern Complement Med*, Vol. 16, No. 7 (Jul 2010), pp. 701-6, ISSN 1557-7708 (Electronic) 1075-5535 (Linking)

Pan, C.; Shang, S.; Kirch, W. & Thoenes, M. (2010). Burden of diabetes in the adult Chinese population: A systematic literature review and future projections. *Int J Gen Med*, Vol. 3, No. (Aug 2010), pp. 173-9, ISSN 1178-7074 (Electronic) 1178-7074 (Linking)

Piaggio, G. & Pinol, A.P. (2001). Use of the equivalence approach in reproductive health clinical trials. *Stat Med*, Vol. 20, No. 23 (Dec 2001), pp. 3571-7, ISSN 0277-6715 (Print) 0277-6715 (Linking)

Qi, L.W.; Liu, E.H.; Chu, C.; Peng, Y.B.; Cai, H.X. & Li, P. (2010). Anti-diabetic agents from natural products--an update from 2004 to 2009. *Curr Top Med Chem*, Vol. 10, No. 4 (Feb 2010), pp. 434-57, ISSN 1873-4294 (Electronic) 1568-0266 (Linking)

Ridout, R.; Dugoua, J.; Koren, G. & Einarson, T. (2007). *The Anti-Diabetic and Cholesterol-Lowering Effects of Cinnamon and Cassia Bark, ClinicalTrials.gov Identifier: NCT00479973.* In: ClinicalTrials.gov, US National Institutes of Health Date of access: 04/12/2011, Available from: http://clinicaltrials.gov/ct2/show/NCT00479973?term=cinnamon+diabetes&rank=6.

Schulz, K.F.; Chalmers, I.; Hayes, R.J. & Altman, D.G. (1995). Empirical evidence of bias. Dimensions of methodological quality associated with estimates of treatment effects in controlled trials. *JAMA*, Vol. 273, No. 5 (Feb 1995), pp. 408-12, ISSN 0098-7484 (Print) 0098-7484 (Linking)

Shih, C.C.; Su, Y.C.; Liao, C.C. & Lin, J.G. (2010). Patterns of medical pluralism among adults: results from the 2001 National Health Interview Survey in Taiwan. *BMC Health Serv Res*, Vol. 10, No. (Jul 2010), pp. 191, ISSN 1472-6963 (Electronic) 1472-6963 (Linking)

Solimene, U.; Alkofahi, A.; Allemann, C.; Amigoni, M.; Aspan, R.; Azimova, S.; Bloodworth, B.C.; Caccialanza, G.; Caizzi, A.; Cheraghali, M.; Discalzi, A.; Eagles, P.; Fong, H.; Giachetti, D.; Goda, Y.; Harris, S.; Keller, K.; Law, R.; Ruichao, L.; Minelli, E.; Oh, M.; Rizzo, I.; Roll, D.B.; Serrano, S.; Scrabbi, L.; Sulaikah, M.; Tsang, R.; Guorong, W.; Wongsinkongman, P. & Yusufu, H.U. (2007). *WHO guidelines for assessing quality of herbal medicines with reference to contaminants and residues.* WHO, Report 978 92 4 159444 8, Geneva.

Suppapitiporn, S. & Kanpaksi, N. (2006). The effect of cinnamon cassia powder in type 2 diabetes mellitus. *J Med Assoc Thai*, Vol. 89 No. Suppl 3 (Sep 2006), pp. S200-5, ISSN 0125-2208 (Print) 0125-2208 (Linking)

Tackett, K.L. & Jones, M.C. (2009). Complementary and Alternative Medicines for the Treatment of Diabetes. *Journal of Pharmacy Practice*, Vol. 22, No. 6 (Dec 2009), pp. 546-552, ISSN 0897-1900 (Print) 1531-1937 (Linking)

Talalay, P. (2001). The importance of using scientific principles in the development of medicinal agents from plants. *Acad Med*, Vol. 76, No. 3 (Mar 2001), pp. 238-47, ISSN 1040-2446 (Print) 1040-2446 (Linking)

The Cochrane Collaboration. (2008). *Review Manager (RevMan)* 5.0, The Nordic Cochrane Centre, Copenhagen.

Tsiami, A. (2009). *Is There a Metabolic Effect of Cinnamon on HbA1c, Blood Pressure and Serum Lipids in Type 2 Diabetes Mellitus? ClinicalTrials.gov Identifier: NCT00846898* In: ClinicalTrials.gov, US National Institutes of Health, Date of access: 04/12/2011, Available from: http://clinicaltrials.gov/ct2/show/NCT00846898?term=cinnamon+diabetes&rank=4.

Tyreman, S. (2010). Values in complementary and alternative medicine. *Med Health Care Philos*, Vol. 13, No. 4 (Nov 2010), pp. Online First™, 23 November 2010, ISSN 1572-8633 (Electronic) 1386-7423 (Linking)

UKPDS 37. (1999). Quality of life in type 2 diabetic patients is affected by complications but not by intensive policies to improve blood glucose or blood pressure control (UKPDS 37). U.K. Prospective Diabetes Study Group. *Diabetes Care*, Vol. 22, No. 7 (Jul 1999), pp. 1125-36, ISSN 0149-5992 (Print) 0149-5992 (Linking)

Vuksan, V.; Sung, M.K.; Sievenpiper, J.L.; Stavro, P.M.; Jenkins, A.L.; Di Buono, M.; Lee, K.S.; Leiter, L.A.; Nam, K.Y.; Arnason, J.T.; Choi, M. & Naeem, A. (2008). Korean red ginseng (Panax ginseng) improves glucose and insulin regulation in well-controlled, type 2 diabetes: results of a randomized, double-blind, placebo-controlled study of efficacy and safety. *Nutrition Metabolism & Cardiovascular Diseases*, Vol. 18, No. 1 (Jan 2008), pp. 46-56, ISSN

Yeh, G.Y.; Eisenberg, D.M.; Kaptchuk, T.J. & Phillips, R.S. (2003). Systematic review of herbs and dietary supplements for glycemic control in diabetes. *Diabetes Care*, Vol. 26, No. 4 (Apr 2003), pp. 1277-94, ISSN 0149-5992 (Print) 0149-5992 (Linking)

Zibadi, S.; Rohdewald, P.J.; Park, D. & Watson, R.R. (2008). Reduction of cardiovascular risk factors in subjects with type 2 diabetes by Pycnogenol supplementation. *Nutr Res*, Vol. 28, No. 5 (May 2008), pp. 315-20, ISSN 1879-0739 (Electronic) 0271-5317 (Linking)

Part 3

Prevention

8

Prevention of Diabetes: Effects of a Lifestyle Intervention

Kátia Cristina Portero McLellan[1], Antonio Carlos Lerário[2] and Roberto Carlos Burini[1]
[1]*Sao Paulo State University/ UNESP - School of Medicine, Botucatu/SP*
[2]*University of Sao Paulo/USP - School of Medicine, São Paulo/SP*
Brazil

1. Introduction

Lifestyle is directly related to the incidence of type 2 diabetes mellitus (DM2), a risk dramatically elevated by obesity and inactivity. Sedentary lifestyle, inadequate eating habits, aging, educational backgrounds and the increased life expectancy observed in Brazil suggested to be the main culprits for the increased prevalence of DM2 seen in this country. Therefore, many epidemiologists have been emphasizing the importance of primary prevention for obesity and DM in Brazil (Sartorelli & Franco, 2003).

Some studies have shown that people consuming a diet rich in whole grains (Salmeron et al. 1997a; Salmeron et al. 1997b) and polyunsaturated fatty acids (Salmeron et al. 2001), combined with low intake of trans fatty acids and foods with low glycemic index (Salmeron et al. 1997a; Salmeron et al. 1997b; Salmeron et al. 2001; Burani &Longo, 2006), present lower risk for the development of DM2. Several studies have verified the benefit of educational interventions on the progression of impaired glucose tolerance (IGT) to DM2. Some of the interventions strategies utilized medication and diet, diet and/or physical exercise or the combination of diet and exercise, generally referred to a change in lifestyle (Pan et al. 1997; Tuomilehto et al. 2001; Knowler et al. 2002). The Finnish Diabetes Prevention Study showed that lifestyle counseling can be effective and feasible in routine health care (Tuomilehto et al. 2001; Lindstron et al. 2003; Absetz et al. 2009).

Brazilian studies evaluating the impact of DM2 on primary care or "at risk" populations are still scarce. Preliminary data from an intervention study for DM2 prevention among adults suggests that these programs are not only viable in Primary Public Health Care (Sartorelli et al. 2004) but also help to improve the health of the population. Since DM2 is one of the biggest problems in public health worldwide, it should receive special attention from health-related government entities.

In order to identify the effects of a 12-month nutritional education and lifestyle intervention program in a Brazilian urban community, on metabolic improvement, body composition and eating behavior, we evaluated subjects recruited primarily through 2 Diabetes Prevention Campaigns, carried out in November 2002 and November 2003 in a small urban Brazilian community. A total of 2043 individuals were screened for capillary glucose levels and among them 142 people presented fasting plasma glucose above 100mg/dL and also 2 risk factors for developing DM2 and cardiovascular disease (CVD). Fasting plasma glucose and an oral glucose tolerance test were repeated in these subjects to confirm the diagnosis of impaired glucose tolerance and/or fasting glucose levels. A total of 67 subjects aged from 30 to 85 years were included in the study and were divided in two groups: compared (n=43) and intervention (n=24) group (CG and IG respectively). Availability to attend the group session was considered for including individuals in the IG. All individuals in both groups had their clinical, metabolic and dietetic profiles examined. The subjects in the IG were given detailed advice about diet, exercise and lifestyle modification through monthly individual visits and group meetings every two weeks for 12 months. An individual visit was offered to the GC at the beginning of the study and after 12 months. Dropout rates were 8.3% (n=2) in the IG and 31% (n=13) in the CG. Principles of the Declaration of Helsinki were followed. Subjects gave their informed consent for the study, which was reviewed and approved by the Medical Ethics Committee of the University of São Paulo. A paired *t* test was used to examine differences in the outcomes between baseline and 12 months. Statistical analyses were performed using the Bioestat program.

Baseline characteristics of the participants are given in Table 1. The IG patients achieved a weight loss of 5.10% ($p<0.001$) while the CG had an increase of 0.54% from their initial weight. IG patients reduced 3.3% ($p<0.05$), and 6.8% ($p<0.01$) of their waist circumference (WC) and body fat %, respectively. Fasting and postprandial glucose levels were reduced 13.5% ($p<0.05$) and 20.9% ($p<0.05$), respectively, in the IG. The assessment of dietary composition at the beginning and at the end of the study showed that cholesterol and caloric intake significantly decreased inside the IG patients (49.5% and 4.7%, respectively).

The individuals in the IG showed a 5% weight loss at the end of the study and this was attributed to their participation in the nutrition intervention program. In parallel to weight loss, the IG also presented a significant decrease in body fat. Interventions to reduce the incidence of diabetes should aim at weight loss as the primary determinant of success (Hamman et al. 2006). The Finnish Diabetes Prevention Study (Tuomilehto et al. 2001) showed that a weight reduction of 5% or more can promote better metabolic control, prevent DM2 and improve quality of life. Interventions to reduce diabetes risk should primarily target weight reduction. The identification of abdominal obesity has become important due to its association with the risk for obesity-associated diseases, regardless of overall obesity.

After a 12-months follow-up, the IG presented a reduced intake of calories, saturated fatty acids and cholesterol. Qualitative assessment showed that eating habits of the individuals in both groups were within the dietary recommendations intake at the beginning and at the end of the study. The main objective of the nutritional counseling supplied by this study was not to encourage the individuals to adhere to a specific diet, but to encourage them to gradually change their diets as follows: eat smaller meals at more frequently intervals, select complex and whole carbohydrates; increase fiber, fruit and vegetable consumption; and increase unsaturated fatty acid intake by consuming olive oil and fish. Modifying the eating behavior of an individual is a complicated process since guidance needs to be on a personal level and individuals need to be encouraged to adhere to the process since people eat foods and not nutrients alone.

This study showed that a lifestyle modification program can reduce known risk factors for DM2 and CVD in a Brazilian urban community. This suggests that carrying out primary prevention of DM2 and CVD through lifestyle education, especially by emphasizing nutrition and physical activity, is very important in terms of public health and should be part of the routine of Health Care System. Further research is necessary to understand better how to facilitate effective and efficient programs for the primary prevention of DM2 in developing countries.

	IG					CG				
	Baseline		12 months		P value	Baseline		12 months		P value
	Value	SD	Value	SD		value	SD	value	SD	
Weight (kg)	67.61	14.8	64.18	13.5	<0.001	75.78	15.2	76.20	16.3	0.43
BMI (kg/m^2)	26.59	5.3	25.00	4.5	<0.001	28.46	4.5	28.60	5.2	0.98
WC (cm)	88.53	10.6	85.57	9.9	<0.05	91.19	17.0	92.50	18.1	0.34
Body fat (%)	33.36	9.61	31.10	9.51	<0.01	35.98	7.4	36.21	8.03	0.88
FPG (mg/dl)	105.0	21.6	90.83	14.2	<0.05	91.79	18.3	90.20	28.9	0.72
2-h PG (mg/dl)	138.0	40.8	109.17	27.4	<0.05	117.80	31.5	109.57	38.9	0.36
TC (mg/dl)	213.42	85.5	164.50	49.9	<0.05	170.43	62.7	163.73	45.1	0.60
Calories (kcal)	1 668.75	616.7	1 589.57	289.3	<0.05	1 445.16	686.7	1 785.75	552.5	0.04
Carbohydrates (g)	241.47	91.3	214.20	41.0	0.29	191.25	25.0	260.87	69.9	0.07
Proteins (g)	85.54	37.7	68.87	12.8	0.14	65.67	34.0	74.41	30.5	0.40
Lipids (g)	54.43	18.4	48.90	14.0	0.20	40.52	23.1	53.83	30.6	0.10
SFA (g)	18.32	10.2	8.51	1.4	0.18	9.91	6.5	10.98	8.3	0.71
Cholesterol (mg)	183.69	55.4	92.72	44.7	<0.001	155.01	81.0	118.25	81.7	0.15
Fibers (g)	12.23	5.7	12.13	5.5	0.94	7.72	10.7	7.93	7.8	0.93

IG = Intervention Group; CG = Compared Group; Values in Mean; SD = Standard Deviation; FPG = Fasting Plasma Glucose; 2-h PG = 2-hour Plasma Glucose; TC = Total Cholesterol; SFA = Saturated fatty acids.

Table 1. Changes in clinical, metabolic and dietetic characteristics from baseline and 12 months of the participants.

2. Diet

In the last twenty years, Brazil and many other Latin American countries have experienced an accelerated demographic, epidemiological and nutritional transition. The so-called "nutritional transition," which refers to changes in secular nutritional patterns, that is, to structural dietary changes, is directly correlated to economic and demographic changes and health conditions (Kac, 2003; Ferreira et al., 2005).

As the nutritional transition advanced, the consumption of high-fat products increased, especially from animal fat and sugars. Additionally, the consumption of complex carbohydrates and dietary fiber is decreasing. This reduction has been pointed out as a critical factor for the increasing prevalence of obesity and its comorbidities.

The Diabetes Prevention Program (Tuomilehto et al. 2001) showed that it is possible to achieve primary prevention of type 2 diabetes by changing lifestyle (diet and exercise) in subjects with impaired glucose tolerance. The reduction in weight, in total intake of fat to less than 30 percent of energy, and in intake of saturated fat to less than 10 percent of energy, along with an increase in fiber intake to at least 15 g per 1000 kcal and physical activity, resulted in lost at least 5 percent of the initial weight, and reveals a cumulative incidence of diabetes 58 percent lower compared to individuals in the control group. The

Diabetes Prevention Program (Knowler et al. 2002) showed that lifestyle changes and treatment with metformin both reduced the incidence of diabetes in persons at high risk. The intensive lifestyle intervention aimed achieving and maintaining a weight reduction of at least 7 percent of initial body weight through a healthy low-calorie, low-fat diet, along with physical activity of moderate intensity. The lifestyle intervention reduced the incidence by 58 percent and metformin by 31 percent, as compared with placebo.

2.1 Carbohydrates, glycemic index and glycemic load

Diet is one of the main modifiable lifestyle factors and relates to the prevention of diabetes mellitus and/or its complications (Portero & Cattalini, 2005, Mclellan et al., 2007, Mclellan et al., 2009). Carbohydrates are responsible for postprandial hyperglycemia and insulin secretion (Bao et al. 2011), and are related to the etiology of many chronic diseases.

Epidemiological evidences show that a better choice of carbohydrates is promising for the nutritional therapy and metabolic control of people with DM (Willett et al., 2002; Sartorelli & Cardoso, 2006; AMB, 2005; Jenkins et al., 2008). Diets with low Glicemic Index (GI) and Glicemic Load (GL) are independently associated with a reduced risk of developing chronic diseases (Barclay et al., 2008). Increased consumption of fruits and vegetables, whole foods and products that have undergone less processing, as well as limited consumption of potatoes, white rice and white bread are measures that help to reduce dietary GI (Silva & Mello, 2006).

In the prospective epidemiological study called Nurses' Health Study (1997), which included 65173 American women aged 40 to 65 years, a positive association was found between the habitual consumption of a high-GI diet and incidence of DM after six years of follow-up (Salmeron et al., 1997a). Furthermore, the Nurses' Health Study II (2004), which included 91249 women aged 20 to 44 years, found that high GI values were associated with risk of DM after 8 years of follow-up (Schulze et al., 2004). Another prospective American study, the Health Professionals Follow-Up Study (1997), which included 42759 men aged 40 to 75 years, also observed a positive association between high dietary GI and incidence of DM after six years of follow-up (Salmeron et al., 1997b).

It is suggested that diets with low GI increase satiety, delay hunger and reduce the consumption of calories in subsequent meals. One of the main means of preventing DM and controlling metabolism is controlling the glycemic load. Blood glucose is modulated mainly by the speed in which carbohydrates enter the blood after meals, by its removal time determined by insulin synthesis and by the sensitivity of peripheral tissue to insulin. Thus, quantity and quality of carbohydrates have long been considered an important dietary factor involved in glycemic homeostasis (Ludwig, 2000; Sartorelli et al., 2006; Brand-Miller et al., 2003). According to the results of many studies, diets with low GI can in fact aid glycemic control and probably reduce the risks of DM complications.

GI is defined as the relationship between the area under the glycemic response curve two hours after the consumption of a test food containing 25 or 50 grams of carbohydrates, and the area under the glycemic response curve corresponding to the consumption of the same amount of carbohydrates from a reference food, that is, glucose or white bread (refined flour) (Jenkins et al., 1981; Jenkins et al., 2002; Sartorelli e Cardoso, 2006; Foster-Powell et al., 2002; Silva e Mello, 2006; Willett et al., 2002).

The GL is a mathematical calculation based on the GI of a food and its carbohydrate content. It represents a global indicator of the glycemic response and insulin demand induced by a serving of a food (Salmeron et al., 1997a; Salmeron et al., 1997b). The glycemic load of a food is calculated by multiplying the glycemic index by the amount of carbohydrates in grams provided by a food and dividing the total by 100 (Liu & Willett, 2002) When GI and GL are used together, they provide more tangible information about how the food affects blood glucose (Silva e Mello, 2006).

Glycemic index and glycemic load can be classified as low, medium or intermediate and high (Sampaio et al. 2007; Foster-Powell et al. 2002) as shown in Table 2.

	Glycemic index	Glycemic load
Low	≤55	≤10
Medium / Intermediate	56 to 69	11 to 19
High	≥70	≥20

Table 2. Classification of glycemic index and glycemic load

2.2 Dietary fiber

Fibers are classified as soluble and insoluble. Soluble fibers are represented by oat bran, pectin (fruits) and gums (oat, barley and legumes: beans, chickpeas, peas and lentils). Insoluble fibers are represented by cellulose (wheat), hemicellulose (cereals) and lignin (non-starchy vegetables). The recommended total fiber intake for adults is 20 to 30g/day, where 5 to 10g should be soluble (SBD, 2006).

Many studies have shown that diets rich in fibers, especially from whole grains, are associated with a significantly reduced risk of developing DM2 (Salmeron et al. 1997a; Salmeron et al. 1997b; Stevens et al. 2002; Montonen et al. 2003; Schulze et al 2004; Schulze et al. 2007). This is due to the production of short-chain fatty acids in the colon which increases hepatic insulin sensitivity (Schuze et al. 2007). Increased fiber intake may also improve insulin sensitivity (Behall et al. 2006; Weickert et al. 2006) and reduce systemic inflammation (Qi et al. 2006).

The soluble fibers found in fruits and legumes improve satiety by providing bulk and increasing digestion time (Institute of Medicine, 2002; Liu et al. 2000). The mechanisms that explain this action are related to the fact that dietary fibers are capable of reducing the speed in which glucose is absorbed, which in turn prevents glycemic and insulin peaks (Slavin, 2008). Studies show that a diet rich in fibers (>30g/day) can change biochemical parameters, reduce the likelihood of developing DM2 and reduce the risk factors associated with the development of cardiovascular diseases (ADA, 2002; Weickert et al. 2006; Qi et al. 2006).

Intervention studies done by Tuomilehto et al. (2001) and Knowler et al (2002) combined lifestyle changes with increased fiber consumption, which resulted in adults having a reduced risk of developing DM2 and IGT.

There are many factors related to the development of DM2, such as obesity, physical inactivity and genetic factors. Data from observational and intervention studies indicate that high-fiber diets improve glucose metabolism and reduce the risk of developing DM2, especially among high-risk individuals (Meyer et al. 2000; Liu & Willett, 2002; Liu, 2002; Priebe et al. 2008). A multi-ethnic study done in Hawaii with 75,512 individuals found that fiber intake was associated with reduced development of DM in men and women. High fiber intake reduced the risk of developing DM by 10% in the study individuals. High intake of fibers from non-starchy vegetables and fruits reduced the risk of DM by 22% in men (Hopping et al. 2010).

The prospective epidemiological study Nurses' Health Study followed 7822 American women with diabetes and investigated whether fiber intake affected mortality and cardiovascular risk. The study found a positive association between fiber intake and reduced mortality and cardiovascular diseases in diabetic women. This study shows the potential effect of fibers in the prevention of mortality and risk of cardiovascular disease in diabetic patients (He et al. 2010).

2.3 Dietary fat intake

The dietary pattern of the Brazilian population has been changing (Levy-Costa et al. 2005; Molina et al. 2007). Data from household budget surveys from 1974 to 2003 that showed time-trends in metropolitan areas indicating a decline in the consumption of traditional food (rice and beans); noticeable increases in the consumption of processed items such as cookies and soft drinks (Mondini & Monteiro, 1994; Monteiro et al. 2000); a continued excessive consumption of sugar; and a continued increase in total fat and saturated fat content in the diet (Levy-Costa et al. 2005).

The type and amount of dietary fat intake has been associated with insulin sensitivity (Storlien et al. 1991), monounsaturated or polyunsaturated fats appear to have beneficial effects on insulin action, whereas saturated fats and diets with high total-fat content appear to decrease insulin sensitivity in studies with animal (Storlien et al. 1991; Lardinois & Starich, 1991) and human (Vessby et al. 2001). Changes in dietary fatty acids may influence insulin action in the body through many mechanisms such as by affecting membrane lipid composition, metabolism, signal-transduction pathways, and by the direct control of gene expression (Vessby 2003).

Prospective studies such as the Nurses' Health Study suggest the role of specific types of fat in the development of DM2 mellitus (Salmeron et al 2001) and weight gain (Field et al 2007). There was an inverse association between development of diabetes and intake of vegetable fat and polyunsaturated fat, and a positive association for *trans*-fatty acids. The investigators found no association for total fat in the diet and development of diabetes (Salmeron et al 2001). Field et al (2007) investigate the association of dietary fat and weight gain among 41,518 adult women in the Nurses' Health Study. The results showed that the percent of calories from fat had a weak positive association with weight gain, and the percentage of calories from animal, saturated fat, and *trans*-fatty acids had stronger associations.

The Finnish prospective cohort study, with a 4 years follow-up, assessed the association of serum fatty acid composition and the development of impaired fasting glycemia (IFG) or DM2 in a cohort of middle-aged normoglycaemic men (n = 895). The results showed that a high proportion of linoleic acid in plasma fatty acids, indicating a high intake of dietary linoleic acid, had a lower risk of developing DM2 and showed lower increases in serum insulin and blood glucose over the follow-up period (Laaksonen et al. 2002). These findings are compatible with other studies (Vessby et al. 1994; Feskens, 2001), which indicated that individuals with a low proportion of linoleic acid or vegetable fat in the diet have an increased risk of developing DM2.

3. Medication

Although long term studies demonstrated that changes in lifestyle could prevent or retard the development of IFG or IGT to clinical diabetes, in practice, the achievement of changes in lifestyle for most of individuals are not easily observed indicating that the early intervention with pharmacological in addition to diet and exercise, could improve the success of preventing or delaying the incidence of the disease. To solve this difficulty, several randomized placebo-controlled clinical trials specifically designed to demonstrate the efficacy and potential disadvantages of precocious pharmacological intervention to prevent the progression of prediabetes to diabetes were performed using different anti-diabetic drugs, specially agents that improve insulin sensitivity.

3.1 Metformin

The two major studies that had included metformin were the DPP study performed in United States and the IDPP-1 study in India. In the DPP trial 1073 participants with IGT were allocated to 850 mg of metformin twice a day and 1082 to placebo that were followed-up for a median period of 2.8 years. At the end of the study metformin reduced the incidence of DM2 by 31% compared to placebo being metformin more effective in individuals who had baseline Body Mass Index (BMI) of 35 kg/m^2 or more in whom incidence of diabetes was reduced in 50% and in individuals younger than 60 years (Knowler et al, 2002). The weight loss was 1.7 kg in metformin group compared with a weight gain of 0.3 kg in placebo group. However, in comparison to the study arm that changed only lifestyle (LSC), the reduction of incidence of diabetes at the end of the study in individuals using metformin (Met) was significantly less pronounced (LSC: 59% vs. Met: 31%). After the end of the original study a 10 years follow-up was offered to the active participants that continued to follow the original study protocol. A total of 88% of the participants (n= 2766) enrolled for and additional median follow up of 5.7 years. Diabetes incidence in 10 years since DPP randomization was reduced by 37% in the LMC group and 18% metformin group in comparison to placebo. The study confirmed that prevention or delay of diabetes with LSC or metformin can be maintained for at least 10 years (Diabetes Prevention Program Reasearch Group, 2009). The IDPP-1 study showed a 25% relative reduction in 120 patients who used metformin 250 mg twice a day. The beneficial changes were similar to those observed with LSC and also showed that the combination of LSC with metformin did not have an additional benefit (Ramachandran et al, 2006). A Chinese study randomizing 70 participants with IGT to receive placebo and metformin at a dosage of 250 mg 3 times a day for a period of 12 months and observed a beneficial effect of metformin in reducing diabetes incidence in comparison to placebo (Met: 16.2% vs. Pbo: 3%) (Li et al, 1999). A meta-analysis of 31 randomized studies including 4570 participants of at least 8 weeks of metformin use showed that the incidence of DM2 was reduced by 40% with an absolute risk reduction of 6% (Sally, 2008).

3.2 Thiazolidenidione

Since experimental and clinical evidences indicated that TZDs could improve insulin sensitivity and restore pancreatic B cell function, this class of agent have been used in several clinical trials to evaluate the prevention of DM2. Troglitazone was the first of this drug class tested in the Trogliazone in Prevention of Diabetes Study (TRIPOD) in women with story of gestational diabetes. In a medium follow up of 30 months it was observed a risk reduction of 55% and the effect of treatment was found to persist months after the drug withdrawal (Buchanan et al, 2002). An open labeled 3 years follow up study for pioglitazone entitled Pioglitazone in Prevention of Diabetes (PIPOD) showed similar results to those observed with troglitazone (Xiang, 2006). In the DPP trial troglitazone was prescribed in 585 participants with IGT for 9 months before its withdrawal due to hepatotoxicity, being observed a remarkable reduction of 75% of clinical DM2 in a relatively short period (Knowler et al, 2002). Rosiglitazone was tested alone in 2 randomized studies: the Diabetes REduction Assessment with Ramipril and Rosiglitazone Medication (DREAM trial) and the Canadian Normoglycemia Outcomes Evaluation (CANOE). The Dream Trial, one of the largest multicentric study demonstrated in 5269 patients recruited with IFG, IGT or both that rosiglitazone was highly effective in reducing the incidence of DM2 by 60% in comparison to placebo (Gerstein et al 2006). The CANOE Study randomly assigned in 207 patients with IGT to receive either a combination of rosiglitazone (2mg) and metformin (500 mg) twice daily for a median period of 3.9 years matched for placebo showed a effective reduction of incidence of DM2 (Zinman et al, 2010). Pioglitazone use to prevent progression of diabetes was observed for a average off 3.75 years in the randomized-placebo controlled study ACT NOW in which 602 patients with IGT received either 45 mg/day pioglitazone or placebo. Patients randomized to pioglitazone treatment showed a reduction 82% reduction in progression in comparison to those treated with placebo (DeFronzo et al, 2009). Despite there are no evidences of association of pioglitazone to cardiovascular risk and hepatotoxicity related respectively to rosiglitazone and troglitazone (that caused their withdrawal of the market), one must also consider the drug´s long term adverse effects like edema, weight gain, increased risk to heart failure and osteoporosis could be a limitation for the drug for diabetes prevention (Nissen et al, 2007).

3.3 Acarbose

Acarbose, a α-glicosidase inhibitor, was tested for its potential to prevent diabetes in persons with IGT in the Study to Prevent Non-insulin dependent Diabetes (STOP-NIDDM) in 1429 participants randomized either to 100 mg of acarbose or placebo, 3 times a day for a mean period of 3.3 years. A relative reduction of 35.8% was seen with acarbose group when compared to placebo. However one third of those in the acarbose group could not complete the study because of gastrointestinal side effects. The study also showed a 49% relative risk reduction in cardiovascular events (Chiasson et al, 2002).

3.4 Other antidiabetic drugs

Meteglinide a rapid acting insulin secretor and valsartan, a angiotensin receptor blocker, were tested to their potential to prevent the development of diabetes and cardiovascular in 9306 participants with IGT in the Nateglinide and Valsartan Improved Glucose Tolerance Outcomes Research (NAVIGATOR) study in a median follow up period of 4 years. Neither the drug or the combination reduced the incidence of diabetes progression or cardiovascular disease (Navigator Study Group, 2010).

Although intestinal hormone GLP-1 and incretin-mimetics drugs have been showed to preserve β cell function in animal models, the role in human β cell preservation remains to be established. Clinical studies using for exanatide and liraglutide have presented significant reduction in body weight and in glucagon secretion reduction and insulin secretion and improvement of insulin secretion in short and median term studies but no specific long term randomized studies designed to demonstrate the efficacy of preventing the progression of diabetes was already published (Blonde et al, 2006; Buse et al, 2009). In a similar way DPP-4 inhibitors, despite being demonstrated to improve glucose control with minimal side effects need to be tested in specific studies to demonstrate the advantage of its use precociously in DM2 to prevent β cell deterioration.

3.5 Other drugs

Besides anti-diabetic drugs, other pharmacologic agents as angiotensin converting enzyme inhibitors, calcium channel blockers, thiazides diuretics, beta-blockers, angiotensin receptor blockers were tested in several randomized studies for their potential benefits in reducing diabetes incidence, but evidences were insufficient to demonstrate their efficacy in reducing diabetes (Yussuf et al 2000, Fonseca, 2006; Padwal & Laupacis, 2004). In one study named Xenical in the Prevention of Diabetes in Obese Subjects (Xendos Study) an antiobesity agent, orlistat (Xenical), in comparison to placebo was tested for prevention of Diabetes and CVD (Torgerson et al 2004). Although it was observed in comparison to placebo a reduction in incidence of diabetes from 9 to 6% and a mean weight reduction of 2.8 kg, the results were not conclusive because the high attrition rate (57%).

Despite that experimental and clinical data based in long term randomized studies have demonstrated that the precocious pharmacological intervention of insulin sensitizing drugs metformin and TZD can reduce diabetes progression of IGF to clinical diabetes, their clinical systematic recommendation is still debated considering their superior efficacy and safety observed with lifestyle modifications, the coexistence with possible long term effect side effects associated to the drug use and difficultly to determine which kind of subjects will have real future benefits from the precocious drug intervention. Based on this concerns, organizations involved to diabetes study and care as the American Diabetes Association (ADA) and the Brazilian Diabetes Society (SBD) have not, until now, endorsed any recommendations to introduction of pharmacologic intervention in patients with prediabetes.

4. Future research / perspective

Despite the significant increase in DM2 prevalence and in the risk factors for metabolic syndrome, preventive intervention is still limited, as much in primary as in secondary care. Nutritional intervention programs and lifestyle changes can benefit the population at risk for developing chronic diseases such as DM2 and CVD (Ratner et al. 2005; Jörgensen et al. 2006), becoming therefore these programs strongly noteworthy.

Structuralized programs that emphasize lifestyle changes, including nutritional counseling, reducing fat intake (less than 30% of the total energy intake) increasing whole grain, fruit and vegetable intake, together with regular physical activity, are important for a better quality of life and prevention of DM2.

5. References

[ADA] American Diabetes Association. Evidence-based nutrition principles and recommendations for the treatment and prevention of diabetes and related complications. *Diabetes Care* 2002; 25:50-60.

[AMB] Associação Médica Brasileira [AMB]. Diabetes Mellitus: *Recomendações Nutricionais.* Projeto Diretrizes, 2005. [In portuguese].

Absetz P, Oldenburg B, Hankonen N, Valve R, Heinonen H, Nissinen A, Fogelhom M, Talja M, Uutela A. Type 2 Diabetes Prevention in Real World: Three-year results of the GOAL Lifestyle Implementation Trial. *Diabetes Care* 2009; 8: 1418-1420.

Bao J, Atkinson F, Petocz P, Willett W, Brand-Miller JC. Prediction of postprandial glycemia and insulinemia in lean, young, healthy adults: glycemic load compared with carbohydrate content alone. *Am J Clin Nutr* 2011; 93:984-996.

Barclay AW, Petocz P, Mcmillan-Price J, Flood VM, Prvan T, Mitchel PL, Brand-Miller JC. Glycemic index, glycemic load, and chronic disease risk - a meta analysis of observational studies. *Am J Clin Nutr* 2008; 87:627–637.

Behall KM, Scholfield DJ, Hallfrisch JG, Liljeberg-Elmstãhl HGM. Consumption of both resistant starch and β-glucan improves postprandial plasma glucose and insulin in women. *Diabetes Care* 2006; 29:976-981.

L. Blonde L, Klein EJ, Han J, Zhang B, Mac SM, Poon TH, Taylor KL, Trautmann ME, Kim DD, Kendall DM. Interim analysis of of the effects of exanatide treatment on A1c, weight and cardiovascular risk factors over 82 weeks in 314 overweight patients with type 2 diabetes. *Diab Obes Metab* 2006; 8:436-447.

Brand-Miller JC, Hayne S, Petocz P, Colagiuri S. Low glycemic index diets in the management of diabetes: a meta-analysis of randomized controlled trials. *Diabetes Care* 2003; 26: 2261-2267.

Buchanan TA, Xiang AH, Peters RK, Kjos SL, Marroquin A, Goico J, Ochoa C, Tan S, Berkowitz K, Hodis HN, Azen SP. Preservation of beta-cell function and diabetes by pharmacologic treatment of insulin resistance in high risk Hispanic women. *Diabetes* 2002; 51:2769-2803.

Burani J & Longo PJ. Low–Glycemic Index Carbohydrates: An Effective Behavioral Change for Glycemic Control and Weight Management in Patients With Type 1 and 2 Diabetes. The *Diabetes Educator* 2006; 32, 78-88.

Buse JB, Rosenstock J, Sesti G, Schmidt WE, Montanya E, Brett JH, Zychma M, Blonde L. Liraglutide once a day versus exenatide twice a day for type 2 diabetes: a 26-week randomized, parallel-group, multinational, open-label trial (LEAD-6). *Lancet* 2009; 374 (9683): 39-47

Chiasson JL, Josse RG, Gomis R, Hanefeld M, Karasik A, Laakso M. Acarbose for prevention of type 2 diabetes mellitus: the Stop-NIDDM randomized trial. *Lancet* 2002; 359:2072-2077.

Defronzo RA, Banerji M, Bray GA, Buchanan TA, Clement S, Henry RR, Kitabchi AE, Mudaliar S, Musi N, Ratner R, Reaven PD, Schwenke D, Stentz FB, Tripathy D. Actos Now for the prevention of diabetes (ACT NOW) study. *BMC Endocr Disord* 2009; 29; 9:17.

Diabetes Prevention Program Research Group. 10-year follow-up of diabetes incidence and weight loss in the Diabetes Prevention Program Outcomes Study. *Lancet* 2009; 374:1677 - 1686.

Ferreira HS, Florêncio TMTM, Fragoso MAC, Melo FP, Silva TG. Hypertension, abdominal obesity and short stature: aspects of nutritional transition within a shantytown in the city of Maceió (Northeastern Brazil). *Rev Nutr* 2005;18:209-18.

Field AE, Willett WC, Lissner L, Colditz GA. Dietary fat and weight gain among women in the Nurses' Health Study. *Obesity* 2007; 15:967–976

Fonseca VA Insulin resistance, diabetes, hypertension, and renin-angiotensin-converting-enzyme inhibitor reducing risk of cardiovascular disease. *J Clin Hypertens* 2006; 8:713-720.

Foster-Powell K, Holt SHA, Brand-Miller JC. International table of glycemic index and glycemic load value: 2002. *Am J Clin Nutr* 2002; 76: 5-56.

Gerstein HC, Yusuf S, Bosch J, Pogue J, Sheridan P, Dinccag N, Hanefeld M, Hoogwerf B, Laakso M, Mohan V, Shaw J, Zinman B, Holman RR. Effect of rosiglitazone on the frequency of diabetes in patients with impaired glucose: a randomized controlled trial. *Lancet* 2006; 368: 1096-1105.

Hamman RF, Wing RR, Edelstein SL, Lachin JM, Bray GA & Delahanty L. Effect of Weight Loss With Lifestyle Intervention on Risk of Diabetes. *Diabetes Care* 2006; 29, 2102-2107.

He M, van Dam RM, Rimm E, Hu FB, Qi L. Whole-Grain, Cereal Fiber, Bran, and Germ Intake and the Risks of All-Cause and Cardiovascular Disease-Specific Mortality Among Women With Type 2 Diabetes Mellitus. *Circulation* 2010; 121:2162-2168.

Hopping BN, Erber E, Grandinetti A, Verheus M, Kolonel LN, Maskarinec G. Dietary Fiber, Magnesium, and Glycemic Load Alter Risk of Type 2 Diabetes in a Multiethnic Cohort in Hawaii. *J Nutr* 2010; 140: 68–74.

Institute of Medicine. Dietary reference intakes for energy, carbohydrate, fiber, fat, fatty acids, cholesterol, protein, and amino acids (macronutrients). Washington, DC: The National Academies Press; 2002.

Jenkins DJ, Wolever TM, Taylor RH, Barker H, Fielden H, Baldwin JM, Bowling AC, Newman HC, Jenkins AL, Goff DV. Glycemic index of foods: a physiological basis for carbohydrate exchange. *Am J Clin Nutr* 1981; 34: 362-366.

Jenkins DJA, Kendall CWC, Augustin LSA, Franceschi S, Hamidi M, Marchie A, Jenkins AL, Axelsen M. Glycemic index: overview of implications in health and disease. *Am J Clin Nutr* 2002; 76:266S–273S.

Jenkins DJA, Kendall CWC, Mckeown-Eyssen G, Josse RG, Silverberg J, Booth GL. Effect of a Low-Glycemic Index or a High-Cereal Fiber Diet on Type 2 Diabetes. A Randomized Trial. *JAMA* 2008; 300: 2742-2753.

Jörgensen ME, Borch-Johnsen K & Bjerregaard P. Lifestyle modifies obesity-associated risk of cardiovascular disease in a genetically homogeneous population. *Am J Clin Nutr* 2006; 84: 29-36.

Kac G, Velásquez-Meléndez G. A transição nutricional e a epidemiologia da obesidade na América Latina. *Cad Saude Publica* 2003; 19:S4-S5. [In portuguese].

Knowler WC, Barret-Connor E, Fowler SF, Hamman RF, Lachin JM & Walker EA. Reduction in the incidence of type 2 diabetes with lifestyle intervention or metformin. *N Eng J Med* 2002; 346, 393-403.

Lardinois CK, Starich GH: Polyunsaturated fats enhance peripheral glucose utilization in rats. *J Am Coll Nutr* 1991; 10: 340–345.

Levy-Costa RB, Sichieri R, Pontes NS, Monteiro CA. Disponibilidade domiciliar de alimentos no Brasil: distribuição e evolução (1974-2003). *Rev Saúde Pública* 2005; 39:530-540 [In portuguese].

C. L. Li CL, Pan CY, Lu JM, Zhu Y, Wang JH, Deng XX, Xia FC, Wang HZ, Wang HY. Effect of metformin on patients with impaired glucose tolerance *Diabet Med* 1999; 16:477-461.

Lindstrom J, Louheranta A, Mannelin M, Rastas M, Salminen V, Eriksson J, Uusitupa M, Tuomilehto J. The Finnish Diabetes Prevention Study (DPS): lifestyle intervention and 3-year result on diet and physical activity. *Diabetes Care* 2003; 26: 3230-3236.

Liu S, Manson JE, Stampfer MJ, Hu FB, Giovannucci E, Colditz GA, Hennekens CH, Willett WC. A prospective study of whole-grain intake and risk of type 2 diabetes mellitus in US women. *Am J Public Health* 2000; 90:1409–1415.

Liu S, Willett WC. Dietary glycemic load and atherothrombotic risk. *Curr Atheroscler Rep.* 2002; 4:454-461.

Liu S. Intake of refined carbohydrates and whole grain foods in relation to risk of type 2 diabetes mellitus and coronary heart disease. *J Am Coll Nutr* 2002; 21:298-306.

Ludwig DS. The Glycemic Index: Physiological Mechanisms Relating to Obesity, Diabetes and Cardiovascular Disease. *JAMA* 2002; 287:2414 - 2423.

Mclellan KCP, Barbalho SM, Cattalini M, Lerario AC. Diabetes *mellitus* do tipo 2, sindrome metabólica e modificação no estilo de vida. *Rev Nutr* 2007; 20: 515-524 [In portuguese].

Mclellan KCP, Cattalini M, Barbalho SM, Souza MC, Oshiiwa M, Lerario AC. Benefícios de um programa de educação nutricional e mudança no estilo de vida em pessoas que apresentam fatores de risco para o desenvolvimento de diabetes mellitus tipo 2. *Ciência, Pesquisa e Consciência* 2009; 1: 56-62 [In portuguese].

Meyer KA, Kushi LH, Jacobs DR, Jr., Slavin J, Sellers TA, Folsom AR. Carbohydrates, dietary fiber, and incident type 2 diabetes in older women. *Am J Clin Nutr* 2000; 71:921-930.

Molina MC, Bettiol H, Barbieri MA, Silva AAM, Conceição SIO, Dos-Santos JE. Food consumption by young adults living in Ribeirao Preto, SP, 2002/2004. *Braz J Med Biol Res* 2007; 40:1257-1266.

Mondini L, Monteiro CA. Changes in the diet pattern of the Brazilian urban population (1962-1988). *Rev Saúde Pública* 1994; 28:433-439.

Monteiro CA, Mondini L, Costa RB. Changes in composition and appropriate nutrition of family diet in the metropolitan areas of Brazil (1988-1996). *Rev Saúde Pública* 2000; 34: 251-258.

Montonen J, Knekt P, Jarvinen R, Aromaa A, Reunanen A. Whole-grain and fiber intake and the incidence of type 2 diabetes. *Am J Clin Nutr* 2003; 77:622-629.

Navigator Study Group Hollman RR, Haffner SM et al. Effect of nateglinide on incidence of diabetes and cardiovascular events. *N Engl J Med* 2010; 262:1463-1490.

Nissen SE, Wolski K. Effect of rosiglitazone on the myocardial infarction and death from cardiovascular causes. *N Engl J Med* 2007; 356:2457-2471.

Padwal R, Laupacis A. Antihipertensive therapy and incidence of type 2 diabetes: a systematic review. *Diabetes Care* 2004; 24:247-255.

Pan XR, Li GW, Wang WY, An ZX, Hu ZX & Lin J. Effect of diet and exercise in preventing NIDDM in people with impaired glucose tolerance. The Da Qing IGT and Diabetes Study. *Diabetes Care* 1997; 20, 537-544.

Portero KCC, Cattalini M. Mudança no estilo de vida para prevenção e tratamento do Diabetes Mellitus tipo 2. *Saúde em Revista* 2005; 7: p.63-69 [In portuguese].

Priebe MG, van Binsbergen JJ, de Vos R, Vonk RJ. Whole grain foods for the prevention of type 2 diabetes mellitus. *Cochrane Database Syst Rev* 2008;(1):CD006061.

Qi L, Van Dam RM, Liu S, Franz M, Mantzoros C, Hu FB. Whole-Grain, bran, and cereal fiber intakes and markers of systemic inflammation in diabetic womem. *Diabetes Care* 2006; 29:207-211.

Ramachandran A, Snehalatha C, Mary S, Mukesh B, Bhaskar AD, Vijay V. The Indian-Diabetes Prevention Programe shows that lifestyle and metformin prevent type 2 diabetes in Asian Indian subjects with impared glutose tolerance (IDPP-1). *Diabetologia* 2006; 49:289-297.

Ratner R, Goldberg R, Haffner S, Marcovina S, Orchard T & Fowler S. Impact of intensive lifestyle and metformim therapy on cardivascular disease risk factors in Diabetes Prevention Program. *Diabetes Care* 2005; 28, 888-894.

Sally S. Meta-analysis: metformin treatment in patients at risk for diabetes mellitus. *Am J Med* 2008; 121:149-157.

Salmeron J, Ascherio A, Rimm EB, Colditz GA, Spiegelman D, Jenkins DJ, Stampfer MJ, Wing AL, Willett WC. Dietary fiber, glycemic load and risk of NIDDM in men. *Diabetes Care.* 1997b; 20(4):545-50.

Salmeron J, Hu FB, Manson JE, Stampfer MJ, Colditz GA, Rimm EB & Willett WC. Dietary fat intake and risk of type 2 diabetes in women. *Am J Clin Nutr* 2001; 73,1019-1026.

Salmeron J, Manson JE, Stampfer MJ, Colditz GA, Wing AL & Willet WC. Dietary fiber, glycemic load, and risk of non-insulin-dependent-diabetes mellitus in women. *JAMA* 1997a; 277, 472-477.

Sampaio HAC, Silva BYC, Sabry MOD, Almeida PC. Índices Glicêmicos e Cargas Glicêmicas de dietas consumidas por indivíduos obesos. *Rev Nutr* 2007; 20: 615-624 [In portuguese].

Sartorelli D S, Franco LJ, Cardoso MA. Intervenção nutricional e prevenção primária do diabetes mellitus tipo 2: uma revisão sistemática. *Cad Saúde Pública* 2006; 22:7-18 [In portuguese].

Sartorelli DS & Franco LJ. Tendências do diabetes mellitus no Brasil: o papel da transição nutricional. *Cad Saúde Pública* 2003; 19, 29-36.

Sartorelli DS, Cardoso MA. Associação entre carboidratos da dieta habitual e Diabetes Mellitus Tipo 2: Evidências epidemiológicas. *Arq Bras Endocrinol Metab* 2006; 50: 415-426 [In portuguese].

Sartorelli DS, Sciarra EC, Franco LJ & Cardoso MA. Primary prevention of type 2 diabetes through nutritional counseling. *Diabetes Care* 2004; 27, 3091.

Schulze MB, Liu S, Rimm EB, Manson JE, Willett WC, Hu FB. Glycemic index, glycemic load, and dietary fiber intake and incidence of type 2 diabetes in younger and middle-aged women. *Am J Clin Nutr* 2004; 80: 348-356.

Schulze MB, Schulz M, Heidemann C, Schienkiewitz A, Hoffmann K, Boeing H. Fiber and magnesium intake and incidence of type 2 diabetes: a prospective study and meta-analysis. *Arch Intern Med* 2007; 167:956-965.

Silva FM, Mello VDF. Índice glicêmico e carga glicêmica no manejo do diabetes melito. *Revista do Hospital das Clinicas de Porto Alegre* 2006; 26: 73-81 [In portuguese].

Slavin JL. Position of the American Dietetic Association: health implications of dietary fiber. J Am Diet Assoc. 2008;108:1716–31.

[SBD] Sociedade Brasileira de Diabetes. *Tratamento e acompanhamento do Diabetes Mellitus: Diretrizes da Sociedade Brasileira de Diabetes.* Diagraphic Editora: Rio de Janeiro, 2006, 153p. [In portuguese].

Stevens J, Ahn K, Juhaeri, Houston D, Steffan L, Couper D. Dietary fiber intake and glycemic index and incidence of diabetes in African-American and white adults: the ARIC study. *Diabetes Care* 2002; 25:1715–1721.

Storlien LH, Jenkins AB, Chisholm DJ, Pascoe WS, Khouri S, Kraegen EW: Influence of dietary fat composition on development of insulin resistance in rats. Relationship to muscle triglyceride and omega-3 fatty acids in muscle phospholipid. *Diabetes* 1991; 40: 280–289

Torgerson JS, Hauptman J, Boldrin MN, Sjöström L. Xenical in the prevention of diabetes in obese subjects (XENDOS) study: a randomized study of orlistat as an adjunct to lifestyle changes for prevention of type 2 diabetes in obese patients. *Diabetes Care* 2004; 27:155-161.

Tuomilehto J, Lindström J, Eriksson JG, Valle TT, Hämäläinen H & Ilanne-Parikka P. Prevention of type 2 diabetes mellitus by changes in lifestyle among subjects with impaired glucose tolerance. *N Eng J Med* 2001; 344, 1343-1350.

Vessby B, Unsitupa M, Hermansen K, Riccardi G, Rivellese AA, Tapsell LC, Nalsen C, Berglund L, Louheranta A, Rasmussen BM, Calvert GD, Maffetone A, Pedersen E, Gustafsson IB, Storlien LH: Substituting dietary saturated for monounsaturated fat impairs insulin sensitivity in healthy men and women: The KANWU Study. *Diabetologia* 2001; 44: 312–319.

Vessby B. Dietary fat, fatty acid composition in plasma and the metabolic syndrome. *Current Opinion in Lipidology* 2003, 14: 15-19

Xiang AH, Peters RK, Kjos SL, Marroquin A, Goico J, Ochoa C, Tan S, Berkowitz K, Hodis HN. Effect of pioglitazone on pancreatic beta cell function and diabetes in Hispanic women with prior gestational diabetes. *Diabetes* 2006; 55:517-522.

Weickert MO, Mohlig M, Schöel C, Arafat AM, Otto B, Viehoff H, et al. Cereal fiber improves whole-body insulin sensitivity in overweight and obese women. *Diabetes Care* 2006; 29:775-780.

Willett W, Manson J, Liu S. Glycemic index, glycemic load, and risk of type 2 diabetes. *Am J Clin Nutr* 2002; 76:274–280.

Yusuf S, Sleight P, Pogue J, Bosch J, Davies R, Dagenais G. Effects of an angiotensin-converting-enzyme inhibitor, ramipril, on cardiovascular events in high-risk patients. The Heart Outcomes Prevention Evaluation Study Investigators. *N Engl J Med* 2000; 342:145-153.

Zinman B, Harris SB, Neuman J, Gerstein HC, Retnakaran RR, Raboud J, Qi Y, Hanley AJ. Low dose combination therapy of rosiglitazone and metformin to prevent type 2 diabetes mellitus.(CANOE trial): a double-blind randomized controlled study. *Lancet* 2010; 376:103-111.

9

Fiber and Insulin Sensitivity

Kevin C. Maki and Tia M. Rains
Provident Clinical Research, Biofortis North America
United States of America

1. Introduction

The prevalence of type 2 diabetes mellitus (T2DM) continues to increase at an alarming rate. Approximately 18.8 million people in the United States have diagnosed diabetes, whereas 7.0 million people are estimated to be living with the disease undiagnosed (Centers for Disease Control and Prevention [CDC], 2011). Another 79 million adults 20 years and older have pre-diabetes: impaired glucose tolerance (IGT) and/or impaired fasting glucose (IFG) (CDC, 2011). Approximately 20-30% of individuals with pre-diabetes progress to T2DM within 3-4 years (DeFronzo et al., 2011; Knowler et al., 2002).

The progression from normal glucose tolerance to the onset of T2DM is protracted and preceded by metabolic abnormalities that ultimately lead to hyperglycemia. Early in the disease process, individuals typically exhibit resistance to insulin-stimulated glucose uptake at the cellular level (Reaven et al., 2005). Insulin resistance is also associated with a cluster of metabolic disorders including central obesity, dyslipidemia and hypertension that are risk factors for T2DM and atherosclerotic cardiovascular disease (Alexander et al., 2000). The aggregation of these disorders is often referred to as metabolic syndrome or cardiometabolic syndrome (Reaven et al., 2005).

Insulin resistance manifests as decreased insulin-stimulated glucose uptake at adipose and skeletal muscle tissues, as well as impaired suppression of hepatic glucose output by a given circulating level of insulin (DeFronzo, 2009; Goldstein 2003). Normal glucose tolerance is maintained via compensatory hyperinsulinemia, thus preventing hyperglycemia in the earliest stages (Reaven et al., 2005). Over time, the pancreatic beta-cell response becomes inadequate to maintain normoglycemia, and hyperglycemia ensues. It is unclear whether there is an exhaustion of the beta-cells, or if the beta-cells become progressively less responsive to the changes in circulating glucose, or a combination of these defects (Ferannini et al., 2005; Butler et al., 2003; Khan, 2001). Regardless, progressive beta-cell dysfunction ultimately leads to an inability to secrete sufficient insulin to maintain normoglycemia after a carbohydrate load. In frank T2DM, insulin secretion becomes sufficiently impaired to result in hyperglycemia in the fasting state (Stolar, 2010). By the time T2DM is diagnosed, the insulin secretory response is generally 70-80% below that which would be appropriate for the prevailing level of insulin resistance (Ferannini et al., 2005; Maki et al., 2009). The interplay between insulin resistance and beta-cell dysfunction in the development of T2DM (DeFronzo, 2009; Khan 2001) and methods of assessing insulin sensitivity in clinical research (Muniyappa et al., 2008; Singh 2010) have been reviewed in detail elsewhere.

2. Dietary patterns and diabetes risk

Diabetes prevention trials have shown that interventions which increase insulin sensitivity significantly reduce the rate of conversion to diabetes in high risk individuals (Knowler et al., 2002; Tuomilehto et al., 2001; Lindstrom et al., 2003; Pan et al., 1997; Zinman et al., 2010; DeFronzo et al., 2011). In the Diabetes Prevention Program, a lifestyle intervention with targets of 150 minutes per week of moderate intensity physical activity and weight loss of 7% reduced the rate of progression to diabetes by 58% relative to a group that received placebo without lifestyle intervention (Knowler et al., 2002), which was greater than the 31% reduction in new-onset diabetes with metformin treatment. Other lifestyle intervention studies of weight loss and enhanced physical activity have shown reductions in the incidence of new-onset type 2 diabetes of 25-60% over 3-6 year timeframes in individuals with pre-diabetes (Lindstrom et al., 2003; Pan et al., 1997). Both weight loss and increased physical activity enhance insulin sensitivity, which results in a reduced requirement for insulin secretion, thus "unloading" the beta-cells. In turn, this may extend the time during which the available insulin secretory response can maintain normoglycemia. In addition, there is evidence that some interventions that improve insulin sensitivity may arrest, or even partially reverse, the progression of beta-cell dysfunction (Utzschneider et al., 2008; Gastaldelli et al., 2007).

Although weight loss and increased physical activity have received the most attention, particularly in clinical intervention trials, a number of other lifestyle factors may have important influences on the risk for T2DM. Dietary patterns characterized by high intakes of fruits and vegetables, whole grains, low-fat dairy products, and a low glycemic load have been inversely associated with T2DM risk (Figure). In contrast, dietary patterns characterized by high intakes of processed meats, refined grains, and foods containing high

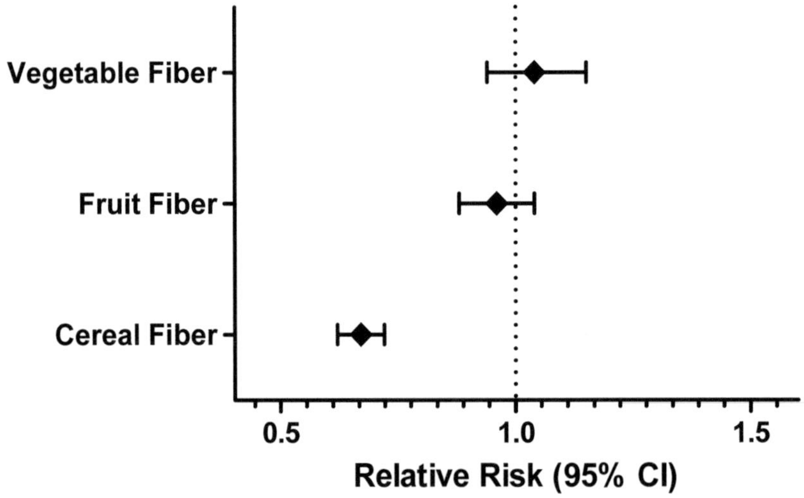

Fig. Relative risks for the associations between cereal fiber, fruit fiber, and vegetable fiber with risk of type 2 diabetes mellitus. Adapted from Schulze et al. 2007. CI = confidence interval.

amounts of added sugars have been associated with increased T2DM risk (Heidemann et al., 2005; Montonen et al., 2005; Fung et al., 2007; Gittelsohn et al., 1998; van Dam et al., 2002; Hodge et al., 2007; Montonen et al., 2005; Brunner et al., 2008; Williams et al., 2000). In particular, an inverse association with T2DM risk has been identified for higher consumption of whole-grain foods (Liu et al., 2000; Murtaugh et al, 2003). Prospective studies have shown that consumption of approximately 3 servings per day of whole grain foods is associated with a reduced risk for T2DM by 20-30% versus consumption of <3 servings of whole grain foods per week (de Munter et al., 2007; Kastorini & Panagiotakos, 2009).

Whole grains contain a number of constituents that may influence T2DM risk, including fibers, vitamins, minerals, lignans, and phytochemicals. The focus of this review is on the potential influences of dietary fibers on risk for T2DM, and the mechanisms that may account for these associations. Nevertheless, the reader should keep in mind that dietary fiber intake correlates with a number of other dietary and lifestyle factors that may influence risk for T2DM, thus fiber intake is likely only one component of the apparent protective effect of a low-risk eating pattern.

3. Intakes of dietary fibers and risk for T2DM

Greater consumption of dietary fiber is associated with lower risk for the development of T2DM, and this may explain, at least in part, the relationship between consumption of whole grains and diabetes risk (Björck& Elmståhl, 2003). Previously, it was thought the reduction in risk might be attributable to the consumption of viscous soluble fibers such as beta-glucan, psyllium, and pectin. Such fibers form viscous solutions when mixed with fluid in the gastrointestinal (GI) tract, creating a physical barrier to digestive enzymes and through which simple sugars must travel to reach the intestinal brush border for absorption (Dikeman & Fahey, 2006; Wolever, 1991; Jenkins et al., 1978). As such, postprandial glucose responses are attenuated when viscous fibers are consumed as part of carbohydrate-rich meals, effectively lowering the glycemic index of such foods (Jenkins et al., 2000, Maki et al., 2007). Prospective epidemiological and observational studies have shown associations between intakes of high-glycemic index foods and high-glycemic load diets and a greater risk of T2DM, consistent with this potential mechanism (Biesalski 2004, Salmeron et al., 1997a, 1997b).

However, results from prospective cohort studies have shown that consumption of insoluble cereal fibers is more strongly inversely associated with risk of T2DM than consumption of soluble fibers (McKeown et al., 2004; Schulze et al., 2007; Weickert & Pfeiffer, 2008). For example, in a cohort of ~25,000 men and women ages 35 to 65 years, greater intake of cereal fibers, but not fruit or vegetable fibers, was inversely associated with developing diabetes over an 11 year period after adjusting for lifestyle and dietary confounders (Schulze et al., 2007). Similarly, a meta-analysis of nine cohort studies on fiber also showed an inverse association for cereal fiber and T2DM risk, but not other fibers (Schulze et al., 2007). Most sources of dietary fiber contain both soluble and insoluble fiber in varying amounts, but whole grain products generally contain a high proportion of insoluble cereal fiber (Weickert & Pfeiffer, 2008; McKee & Latner, 2000). In the U.S. diet, the main sources of soluble fiber are fruits and vegetables, and to a smaller extent, oats and barley (McKee & Latner, 2000).

4. Dietary fiber, colonic fermentation and T2DM risk

Results from several recent studies suggest that fermentability may be a more important factor in the association between dietary fiber intake and T2DM risk than solubility or viscosity. In particular, there is accumulating evidence for a metabolic link between consumption of fibers which are fermented in the lower intestine and insulin sensitivity. This relationship appears likely to be mediated, at least in part, by the inverse association between short chain fatty acid (SCFA) and free fatty acid (FFA) levels in circulation (Robertson et al, 2003, 2005).

Elevated levels of circulating FFA are associated with insulin resistance and it is thought that they contribute to reduced insulin action in the skeletal muscle and liver (Kim et al, 2007). FFA disrupt glucose metabolism by enhancing beta-oxidation in peripheral tissues and by competing with glucose for oxidation, resulting in a reduction of peripheral glucose uptake (Tarini & Wolever, 2010). Sustained elevation of FFA, induced through intravenous infusion of a lipid emulsion, down regulates glycogen storage and leads to a reduction of non-oxidative glucose disposal, thus reducing insulin sensitivity (Ferrannini et al., 1983; Kashyap et al., 2003; Homko et al., 2003). Potential mechanisms by which FFA might affect glycogen regulation include increased expression and activation of glucose-6-phosphatase (Clore et al., 2000; Van de Werve et al., 2000). Conversely, suppression of FFA levels with an infusion of acipimox, a niacin derivative that inhibits hormone sensitive lipase, improves glucose tolerance and peripheral insulin sensitivity (Ferrannini et al., 1983).

The release of FFA shows diurnal variation and is correlated with hepatic glucose output during sleep (Morgan et al., 1999, Kim et al., 2007). In normal weight individuals the fall of hepatic glucose output during sleep is highly synchronized with a decrease in FFA levels (Clore et al., 1989). Conversely, T2DM subjects have an increased rate of FFA appearance at night and elevated plasma FFA levels that are correlated with increased overnight hepatic glucose output (Miles et al., 2003; Taskinen et al., 1989). This increase in FFA levels and release of insulin can be acutely reduced with a pharmacological block of lipoloysis, suggesting that a reduction in FFA release may lead to improved glucose homeostasis (Andreotti et al., 1994). In the canine model of moderate obesity, an increase in nocturnal FFA levels and reduced insulin sensitivity occurred after 6 weeks of high-fat feeding, despite no changes in fasting FFA, fasting glucose or postprandial glucose levels, providing further support that the overnight period may be particularly important (Kim et al., 2007). Given the known diurnal fluctuations of FFA observed in overweight and obese subjects, and in the moderately obese canine model, it is likely that the nocturnal increase in FFA is a key factor in the development of insulin resistance and may play a significant role in the risk for T2DM.

Consumption of indigestible fibers provides available substrate for resident microbiota in the large intestine, which form fermentation products, particularly SCFA (acetate, butyrate, and propionate). Upon absorption into the circulation, SCFA suppress the release of FFA from adipose tissue, thus lowering the concentrations of FFA in circulation, which, in turn, could lead to improved insulin sensitivity and concomitant reduced risk for T2DM (Tarini & Wolever, 1991).

Feeding studies in humans support this proposed relationship between colonic fermentation and peripheral metabolic effects (Table). Nilsson et al. (2008) provided healthy subjects evening meals containing a variety of cereal-based foods with varying levels of resistant starch and fermentable fiber. They demonstrated a relationship between colonic fermentation, as measured by breath hydrogen, and glucose tolerance at the subsequent breakfast meal more than nine hours later (Nilsson et al., 2008). Compared to white bread in the evening, consumption of bread made with barley kernels, high beta-glucan barley, or white bread supplemented with resistant starch and barley fiber all reduced the postprandial curves for glucose and insulin after a subsequent standard breakfast, consistent with improved insulin sensitivity. Additionally, the glucose response was inversely associated with SCFA concentrations (butyrate and acetate) and was positively correlated with FFA during the postprandial period.

Several studies have demonstrated enhanced insulin sensitivity, measured with the euglycemic clamp (the reference standard method) or other methods, after consumption of fermentable fibers or resistant starches over periods ranging from several hours to several weeks (Landin et al., 1988; Robertson et al., 2003, 2005; Maki et al., 2011). Landin et al. (1988) showed improved insulin sensitivity in healthy, nonobese men measured by euglycemic-clamp following intake of 30 g/d guar gum. More recently, Robertson et al (2003) examined the role of resistant starch (RS) on insulin sensitivity in healthy subjects following a 60 g load of RS consumed over the course of one day. Increased insulin sensitivity was positively associated with fasting breath hydrogen levels and lower FFA levels in the late postprandial period (Robertson et al., 2003). In a subsequent study comparing 30 g RS/day for four weeks versus a control starch, insulin sensitivity during a meal tolerance test was 33% higher and glucose clearance adjusted for insulin concentration was 44% higher following RS intake compared with the control condition. Insulin sensitivity, as measured by the euglycemic-hyperinsulinemic clamp, was also higher following RS (Robertson et al., 2005). In a chronic (12-week) study in insulin resistant subjects, 40 g RS/day (supplied in sachets to mix into their daily foods) was associated with improved insulin sensitivity compared to placebo (Johnston et al., 2010). Insulin sensitivity was also correlated with changes in waist circumference, however there was no difference in body mass index, total adipose tissue content or regional distribution between the groups suggesting the observed improvement in insulin sensitivity is not directly attributable to changes in body composition (Johnston et al., 2010). In a study of overweight and obese subjects with normal glucose metabolism, Weikert et al. (2006) reported a 13% improvement in insulin sensitivity in subjects who consumed white bread supplemented with 31.2 g/d insoluble fiber fraction from oat fiber over 72 hours, compared to a white bread control.

Not all studies have shown favorable effects of fermentable fibers on insulin sensitivity. Ebeling et al. (1988) studied the effects of 5 g/d guar gum for 4 weeks in individuals with type 1 diabetes mellitus and showed that guar gum lowered the postprandial glucose response and reduced insulin requirements, suggesting an improvement in hepatic insulin sensitivity. However, there was no measurable effect on peripheral insulin sensitivity, as measured by euglycemic insulin clamp. Given that this study was small (n = 9), a type II error (lack of power) cannot be ruled out. A study in 21 men with metabolic syndrome also failed to show differences in insulin sensitivity measured by euglycemic insulin clamp following a 5-week dietary intervention with 28 g/day of acacia gum and pectin (Pouteau et al., 2010).

Authors	Study Population	Design	Study Products	Results
Andersson et al., 2007	Healthy volunteers (n=30) Age (y): 59±5 BMI (kg/m²): 28.3±2.0	Randomized crossover 6-week study of diet rich in whole grains vs. diet containing equal amount of refined grain	• Whole grain diet contained 112 g/d of whole grain, 18 g fiber • Refined grain diet contained 6 g/d fiber	No effect of whole grains on insulin sensitivity
Ebeling et al., 1988	Type 1 diabetics (n=9) Age (y): 27±2 Body Weight (kg): 71±3	Double-blind crossover with two 4-week study periods	• 5 g/d granulated guar • Control- 0 g/d	No effect on insulin sensitivity
Johnston et al., 2010	Insulin resistant subjects (n=20) Age (y): • Resistant starch- 45.2±3.55 • BMI (kg/m²): • Resistant starch- 31.3±1.70 • Placebo- 30.4±1.15	Single-blind, randomized, parallel 12-week intervention	• Resistant starch supplement -40 g/d • Control- 0 g/d	Improved insulin sensitivity with resistant starch
Landin et al., 1992	Healthy, nonobese middle –aged men (n=25) Age (y): 52.0±5.2 BMI (kg/m²): 24.6±1.6	Double-blind placebo-controlled, cross-over with two 6-week interventions	• 30 g/d granulated guar, given in 3-10 g doses • 30 g/d granulated gelling starch (control), given in 3-10 g doses	Improved insulin sensitivity with guar diet
Maki et al., 2011	Healthy subjects with increased waist circumference (n = 33) Age (y): 49.5 ± 1.6 BMI (kg/m²): 30.6 ± 0.5	Double-blind crossover with two 4-week interventions.	• High-resistant starch diet- 30 g/d • Low-resistant starch diet- 15 g/d • Control- 0 g/d	Improved insulin sensitivity with both resistant starch diets, but effect only reached statistical significance for men.

Authors	Study Population	Design	Study Products	Results
Nilsson et al., 2008	Healthy volunteers (n=15) Age (y): 25.9±3.2 BMI (kg/m^2): 22.5±2.1	Crossover of cereal-based evening test meals with varying GI and amount of resistant starch	Cereal-based meals: • White bread (control) • White bread enriched with barley fiber and 8 g resistant starch • Barley kernel based bread	Improved glucose tolerance with resistant starch
Pouteau et al., 2010	Men with metabolic syndrome (n=21) Age (y): 47±12 BMI (kg/m^2): 33.4±3.0	Double-blind crossover with two 5-week interventions.	Beverages: • 28 g/d acetogenic fibers (acacia gum and pectin) • Control	No effect on insulin sensitivity
Robertson et al., 2003	Healthy subjects (n=10) Age (y): 23-65 BMI: (kg/m^2): 20.3-35.9	Single-blind crossover with two 24-hour interventions	• High-resistant starch diet- 60 g/d • Low-resistant starch diet- 0 g/d	Improved insulin sensitivity with resistant starch.
Robertson et al., 2005	Healthy subjects (n=10) Age (y): 48.5±3.4 BMI (kg/ m^2): 23.4±1.4	Single-blind, crossover with two 4-week interventions	• Resistant starch diet-30 g /d • Control-0 g/d	Improved insulin sensitivity with resistant starch.
Weickert et al., 2006	Overweight and obese subjects with normal glucose metabolism (n=17) Age (y): 52.9±8.7 BMI (kg/ m^2): 30.4±2.0	Single-blind crossover with two 72-hour interventions	Macronutrient-matched breads • Fiber-enriched with 31.2 g insoluble fiber • Control (white bread)	Improved insulin sensitivity with increased insoluble fiber

Table: Clinical trials on the effects of fermentable fibers on insulin sensitivity

5. Conclusion

A dietary pattern characterized by high intakes of whole grains, fruits and vegetables, low-fat dairy products, and a low glycemic load has been associated with lower T2DM risk. Whole grains possess a number of constituents that may influence T2DM risk, including vitamins, minerals, lignans and phytochemicals. Greater dietary fiber intake is also associated with lower risk for the development of T2DM, and this may explain, at least in part, the relationship between consumption of whole grains and reduced diabetes risk. Results from recent intervention studies suggest that fermentability may be the key characteristic of fibers associated with improved insulin sensitivity, providing a metabolic link between dietary fiber intake and reduction in T2DM risk. Future studies on the relationships between dietary fiber, production of SCFAs, circulating FFA release, and physiological mediators such as incretins (glucagon-like peptide-1 and glucose-dependent insulinotropic polypeptide), and inflammatory markers (e.g., interleukin-6, adiponectin), are warranted. There is also a need for longer-term intervention trials to determine the mechanisms by which dietary fibers, particularly fermentable fibers, influence health and T2DM risk.

6. References

Alexander C.M., Landsman P.B., & Teutsch S.M. (2000). Diabetes mellitus, impaired fasting glucose, atherosclerotic risk factors, and prevalence of coronary heart disease. *American Journal of Cardiology,* Vol. 86, No. 9 (November 2000), pp. 897-902. ISSN 0002-9149

Andersson A., Tengblad S., Karlström B., Kamal-Eldin A., Landberg R, Basu S., Åman P., & Vessby B. (2007). Whole-grain foods do not affect insulin sensitivity or markers of lipid peroxidation and inflammation in healthy, moderately overweight subjects, *The Journal of Nutrition,* Vol. 137, No. 6 (June 2007), pp. 1401-1407. ISSN 0022-3166

Andreotti A.C., Lanzi R., Manzoni M.F., Caumo A., Moreschi A., & Pontiroli A.E. (1994). Acute pharmacologic blockade of lipolysis normalizes nocturnal growth hormone levels and pulsatility in obese subjects. *Metabolism,* Vol. 43, No. 10 (October 1994), pp. 1207-1213. ISSN 0026-0495

Bergman R.N., Kim S.P., Hsu I.R., Catalano K.J., Chiu J.D., Kabir M., Richey J. M., & Ader M. (2007). Abdominal obesity role in the pathophysiology of metabolic disease and cardiovascular risk. *The American Journal of Medicine,* Vol. 120, No. 2A (February 2007), pp. S3-S8. ISSN 0002-9343

Biesalski H.K. (2004). Diabetes preventive components in the Mediterranean diet. *European Journal of Nutrition.,* Vol. 43, No. Suppl 1 (March 2004), pp. I/26-30. ISSN 1436-6207

Björck I. & Elmståhl H.L. (2003). The glycaemic index: importance of dietary fibre and other food properties. *Proceedings of the Nutrition Society, Vol. 62, No.* 1 (February 2003), pp. 201-206. ISSN 0029-6651.

Brunner E.J., Mosdøl A., Witte D.R., Martikainen P., Stafford M., Shipley M.J., & Marmot M.G. (2008). Dietary patterns and 15-y risks of major coronary events, diabetes, and mortality. *American Journal of Clinical Nutrition.* Vol. 87, No. 5, (May 2008), pp. 1414-1421. ISSN 0002-9165

Butler A.E., Janson J., Bonner-Weir S., Ritzel R., Rizza R.A., & Butler P.C. (2003). Beta-cell deficit and increased beta-cell apoptosis in humans with type 2 diabetes. *Diabetes.* Vol. 52, No. 1, pp. 102-110. ISSN 0012-1797

Center for Disease Control and Prevention. National diabetes fact sheet: national estimates and general information on diabetes and prediabetes in the United States, 2011.

Atlanta, GA: U.S. Department of Health and Human Services, Centers for Disease Control and Prevention, 2011.

Clore J.N., Nestler J.E., & Blackard W.G. (1989). Sleep-associated fall in glucose disposal and hepatic glucose output in normal humans. Putative signaling mechanism linking peripheral and hepatic events. *Diabetes,* Vol. 38, No. 3 (March 1989), pp. 285-290. ISSN 0012-1797

Clore J.N., Stillman J., & Sugerman H. (2000). Glucose-6-phosphatase flux in vitro is increased in type 2 diabetes. *Diabetes,* Vol. 49, No. 6 (June 2000), pp. 969-974. ISSN 0012-1797

Defronzo R.A. (2009). Banting Lecture. From the triumvirate to the ominous octet: a new paradigm for the treatment of type 2 diabetes mellitus. *Diabetes.* Vol. 58, pp. 773-795. ISSN 0012-1797

DeFronzo R.A., Tripathy D., Schwenke D.C,. Banerji M., Bray G.A., Buchanan T.A., Clement S.C., Henry R.R., Hodis H.N., Kitabchi A.E., Mack W.J., Mudaliar S., Ratner R.E., Williams K., Stentz F.B., Musi N., & Reaven P. (2011). Pioglitazone for diabetes prevention in impaired glucose tolerance. *New England Journal of Medicine,* Vol. 364, No. 12 (March 2011), pp. 1104-1115. ISSN 0028-4793

de Munter J.S., Hu F.B., Spiegelman D., Franz M., & van Dam R.M. (2007). Whole grain, bran, and germ intake and risk of type 2 diabetes: a prospective cohort study and systemic review. *PLoS Medicine,* Vol. 4, No. 8 (August 2007), pp. e261. ISSN 1549-1277

Dikeman C.L. & Fahey G.C. Viscosity as related to dietary fiber: a review. (2006). *Critical Reviews in Food Science and Nutrition,*Vol. 46, No. 8, pp. 649-663. ISSN 1040-8398

Ebeling P., Yki-Järvinen H., Aro A., Helve E., Sinisalo M., & Koivisto V.A. (1988). Glucose and lipid metabolism and insulin sensitivity in type 1 diabetes: the effect of guar gum. *The American Journal of Clinical Nutrition,* Vol. 48, No. 1 (July 1988), pp. 98-103. ISSN 0002-9165

Ferrannini E., Gastaldelli A., Miyazaki Y., Matsuda M., Mari A., & DeFronzo R.A. (2005) beta-Cell function in subjects spanning the range from normal glucose tolerance to overt diabetes: a new analysis. *Journal of Clinical Endocrinology and Metabolism.* Vol. 90, No. 1, pp. 493-500. ISSN 0021-972X

Ferrannini E., Barrett E.J., Bevilacqua S., & DeFronzo R.A. (1983) Effect of fatty acids on glucose production an utilization in man. *Journal of Clinical Investigation,* Vol. 72, No. 5 (November 1983), pp. 1737-1747. ISSN 0021-9738

Fung T.T., McCullough M., van Dam R.M., & Hu F.B. (2008). A prospective study of overall diet quality and risk of type 2 diabetes in women. *Diabetes Care.* Vol. 30, No. 7 (July 2008), pp. 1753-1757. ISSN 0149-5992

Gastaldelli A., Ferrannini E., Miyazaki Y., Matsuda M., Mari A., & DeFronzo R.A. (2007). Thiazolidinediones improve beta-cell function in type 2 diabetic patients. *American Journal of Physiology- Endocrinology and Metabolism,* Vol. 292, No. 3 (March 2007), pp. E871-883. ISSN 0193-1849

Gittelsohn J., Wolever T.M., Harris S.B., Harris-Giraldo R., Hanley A.J., & Zinman B. (1998). Specific patterns of food consumption and preparation are associated with diabetes and obesity in a Native Canadian community. *Journal of Nutrition,* Vol. 128, No.3 (March 1998), pp. 541-547. ISSN 0022-3166

Goldstein B.B. (2003). Insulin resistance: from benign to type 2 diabetes mellitus. *Reviews Cardiovascular Medicine,* Vol. 4, No. Suppl 6, pp. S3-S10. I SSN 1530-6550

Heidemann C., Hoffmann K., Spranger J., Klipstein-Grobusch K., Möhlig M., Pfeiffer A.F., & Boeing H. (2005). A dietary pattern protective against type 2 diabetes in the European Prospective Investigation into Cancer and Nutrition (EPIC)- Potsdam Study cohort. *Diabetologia,* Vol. 48, No. 6 (June 2005), pp. 1126-1134. ISSN 0012-186X

Hodge A.M., English D.R., O'Dea K., & Giles G.G. Dietary patterns and diabetes incidence in the Melbourne Collaborative Cohort Study. (2007). *American Journal of Epidemiology,* Vol. 165, No. 6 (March 2007), pp. 603-610. ISSN 0002-9262

Homko C.J., Cheung P., & Boden G. (2003). Effects of free fatty acids on glucose uptake and utilization in healthy women. *Diabetes,* Vol. 52, No 2 (February 2003), pp. 487-491. ISSN 0012-1797

Jenkins D.J., Wolever T.M., Leeds A.R., Gassull M.A., Haisman P., Dilawari J., Goff D.V., Metz G.L., & Alberti K.G. (1978). Dietary fibres, fibre analogues, and glucose tolerance: importance of viscosity. *British Medical Journal,* Vol. 27, No. 1 (May 1978), pp. 1392-1394. ISSN 0959-8138

Jenkins D.J., Axelsen M., Kendall C.W., Augustin L.S., Vuksan V., Smith U. (2000). Dietary fibre, lente carbohydrates and the insulin-resistant diseases. *British Journal of Nutrition,* Vol. 83, Suppl. 1 (March 2000), pp. S157-163. ISSN 0007-1145

Johnston K.L., Thomas E.L., Bell J.D., Frost G.S., & Robertson M.D. (2010). Resistant starch improves insulin sensitivity in metabolic syndrome, *Diabetic Medicine,* Vol. 27, No. 4 (April 2010), pp. 391-397. ISSN 0742-3071

Kastorini C.M. & Panagiotakos D.B. (2009). Dietary patterns and prevention of type 2 diabetes: from research to clinical practice: a systematic review. *Current Diabetes Reviews,* Vol. 5, No. 4 (November 2009), pp. 221-227. ISSN 1573-3998

Kashyap S., Belfort R., Gastaldelli A., Pratipanawatr T., Berria R., Pratipanawatr W., Bajaj M., Mandarino L., DeFronzo R., & Cusi K. (2003). A sustained increase in plasma free fatty acids impairs insulin secretion in nondiabetic subjects genetically predisposed to develop type 2 diabetes. *Diabetes,* Vol. 52, No. 10 (October 2003), pp. 2461-2474. ISSN 0012-1797

Khan, S.E. (2001). The importance of beta-cell failure in the development and progression of type 2 diabetes. *Journal of Clinical Endocrinology & Metabolism, Vol.* 86, No. 9 , pp. 4047-4058. ISSN0021-972X

Kim S.P., Catalano K.J., Hsu I.R., Chiu J.D., Richey J.M., & Bergman R.N. (2007). Nocturnal free fatty acids are uniquely elevated in the longitudinal development of diet-induced insulin resistance and hyperinsulinemia. *American Journal of Physiology-Endocrinology and Metabolism,* Vol. 292, No. 6 (June 2007), pp. E1590-E1598. ISSN 0193-1849

Knowler W.C., Barrett-Connor E., Fowler S.E., Hamman R.F., Lachin J.M., Walker E.A., & Nathan D.M. (2002). Reduction in the incidence of type 2 diabetes with lifestyle intervention or metformin. *New England Journal of Medicine,* Vol. 346, No. 6 (February 2002), pp. 393-403. ISSN 0028-4793

Landin K., Holm G., Tengborn L., & Smith U. (1992). Guar gum improves insulin sensitivity, blood lipids, blood pressure, and fibrinolysis in healthy men. *The American Journal of Clinical Nutrition*, Vol. 56, No. 6 (December 1992), pp. 1061-1065. ISSN 0002-9165

Lindström J., Eriksson J.G., Valle T.T., Aunola S., Cepaitis Z., Hakumäki M., Hämäläinen H., Ilanne-Parikka P., Keinänen-Kiukaanniemi S., Laakso M., Louheranta A., Mannelin M., Martikkala V., Moltchanov V., Rastas M., Salminen V., Sundvall J., Uusitupa M., & Tuomilehto J. (2003). Prevention of diabetes mellitus in subjects with impaired glucose tolerance in the Finnish Diabetes Prevention Study: results from a randomized clinical trial. *Journal of the American Society of Nephrology*, Vol. 14, No. 7 Suppl 2 (July 2003), pp. S108-113. ISSN 1046-6673

Liu S., Manson J.E., Stampfer M.J., Hu F.B., Giovannucci E., Colditz G.A., Hennekens C.H., & Willett W.C. (2000). A prospective study of whole-grain intake and risk of type 2 diabetes mellitus in US women. *American Journal of Public Health*, Vol. 90, No. 9 (September 2000), pp. 1409-1415. ISSN 1541-0048

Maki K.C., McKenney J.M., Farmer M.V., Reeves M.S., & Dicklin M.R. (2009). Indices of insulin sensitivity and secretion from a standard liquid meal test in subjects with type 2 diabetes, impaired or normal fasting glucose. *Nutrition Journal*. Vol. 28, pp. 8-22. ISSN 1475-2891

Maki K.C. Carson M.L., Miller M.P., Turowski M., Bell M., Wilder D.M., & Reeves M.S. (2007). High-viscosity hydroxypropylmethylcellulose blunts postprandial glucose and insulin responses. *Diabetes Care*, Vol. 30, No. 5 (May 2007), pp. 1039-1043. ISSN 0149-5992

Maki KC, Pelkman CL, Kelley KM, Lawless AL, Schild A, Rains TM. (2011). Effects of type 2 resistant starch consumption on insulin sensitivity in men and women. *Experimental Biology*. Abstract 2914 (April, 2011).

McKee L.H. & Latner T.A. (2000). Underutilized sources of dietary fiber: a review. *Plant Foods for Human Nutrition*, Vol. 55, No 4, pp. 285-304. ISSN 0921-9668

McKeown N.M. (2004) Whole grain intake and insulin sensitivity: evidence from observational studies. Nutrition Reviews, Vol. 62 (7 Pt 1), pp. 286-291. ISSN 0029-6643

Miles J.M., Wooldridge D., Grellner W.J., Windsor S., Isley W.L., Klein S., & Harris W.S. (2003). Nocturnal and postprandial free fatty acid kinetics in normal and type 2 diabetic subjects: effects of insulin sensitization therapy. *Diabetes*, Vol. 52, No. 3 (March 2003), pp. 675-681. ISSN 0012-1797

Montonen J., Knekt P., Härkänen T., Järvinen R., Heliövaara M., Aromaa A., & Reunanen A. (2005). Dietary patterns and the incidence of type 2 diabetes. *American Journal of Epidemiology*, Vol. 161, No. 3 (February 2005), pp. 219-227. ISSN 0002-9262

Morgan L.M., Aspostolakou F., Wright J., & Gama R. (1999). Diurnal variations in peripheral insulin resistance and plasma non-esterified fatty acid concentrations: a possible link? *Annals of Clinical Biochemistry*, Vol. 36, No. 4 (July 1999), pp. 447-450. ISSN 0004-5632

Muniyappa R., Lee S., Chen H., & Quon M.J. (2008). Current approaches for assessing insulin sensitivity and resistance in vivo: advantages, limitations, and appropriate usage. *American Journal of Physiology, Endocrinology, and Metabolism.* Vol. 294, No. 1, (January 2008), pp. E15-26. ISSN 0193-184915

Murtaugh M.A., Jacobs D.R. Jr, Jacob B., Steffen L.M., & Marquart L. (2003) Epidemiological support for the protection of whole grains against diabetes. *Proceedings of the Nutrition Society,* Vol. 62, No. 1 (February 2003), pp. 143-149. ISSN 0029-6651

Nilsson A. C., Östman E.M., Holst J.J., & Björck M.E. (2008). Including indigestible carbohydrates in the evening meal of healthy subjects improves glucose tolerance, lowers inflammatory markers, and increases satiety after a subsequent standardized breakfast. *The Journal of Nutrition,* Vol. 138, No. 4 (April 2008), pp. 732-739. ISSN 0022-3166

Pan X.R., Li G.W., Hu Y.H., Wang J.X., Yang W.Y., An Z.X., Hu Z.X., Lin J., Xiao J.Z., Cao H.B., Liu P.A., Jiang X.G., Jiang Y.Y., Wang J.P., Zheng H., Zhang H., Bennett P.H., & Howard B.V. (1997). Effects of diet and exercise in preventing NIDDM in people with impaired glucose tolerance. The Da Qing IGT and Diabetes Study. *Diabetes Care,* Vol. 20, No. 4 (April 1997), pp. 537-544. ISSN 0149-5992

Pouteau E., Ferchaud-Roucher V., Zair Y., Paintin M., Enslen M., Auriou N., Macé K., Godin J.P., Ballèvre O., & Krempf M. (2010). Acetogenic fibers reduce fasting glucose turnover but not peripheral insulin resistance in metabolic syndrome patients. *Clinical Nutrition,* Vol. 29, No. 6 (December 2010), pp. 801-807. ISSN 1202-3884

Reaven, G.M. (2005). The insulin resistance syndrome: definition and dietary approaches to treatment. *Annual Reviews of Nutrition,* Vol. 25, pp. 392-406. ISSN 0199-9885

Robertson M.D., Bickerton A.S., Dennis A.L., Vidal H., & Frayn K.N. (2005). Insulin - sensitizing effects of dietary resistant starch and effects on skeletal muscle and adipose tissue metabolism. *The American Journal of Clinical Nutrition,* Vol. 82, No. 3 (September 2005), pp. 559-567. ISSN 0002-9165

Robertson M.D., Currie J.M., Morgan L.M., Jewell D.P., & Frayn K.N. (2003). Prior short-term consumption of resistant starch enhances postprandial insulin sensitivity in healthy subjects. *Diabetologia,* Vol. 46, No. 5 (May 2003), pp. 659-665. ISSN 0012-186X

Salmerón J., Ascherio A., Rimm E.B., Colditz G.A., Spiegelman D., Jenkins D.J., Stampfer M.J., Wing A.L., & Willett W.C. (1997a). Dietary fiber, glycemic load, and risk of NIDDM in men. *Diabetes Care,* Vol. 20, No. 4 (April 1997), pp. 545-550. ISSN 0149-5992.

Salmerón J., Manson J.E., Stampfer M.J., Colditz G.A., Wing A.L., & Willett W.C. (1997b). Dietary fiber, glycemic load, and risk of non-insulin-dependent diabetes mellitus in women. *Journal of the American Medical Association,* Vol. 277, No. 6 (February 1997), pp. 472-477. ISSN 0098-7484

Schulze M.B., Schula M., Heidemann C., Schienkiewitz A., Hoffman K., & Boeing H. (2007). Fiber and magnesium intake and incidence of type 2 diabetes: a prospective study and meta-analysis. *Archives of Internal Medicine,* Vol. 167, No. 9 (May 2007), pp. 956-965. ISSN 0003-9926

Singh, B. & Saxena, A. (2010). Surrogate markers of insulin resistance: A review. *World Journal of Diabetes. Vol.* 1, No. 2, pp. 36-47. ISSN 1948-9358

Stolar M. (2010). Glycemic control and complications in type 2 diabetes mellitus. *American Journal of Medicine,* Vol. 123, No. 3 Suppl (March 2010), pp. S3-S11. ISSN 0002-9343

Tarini J. & Wolever T.M.S. (2010). The fermentable fibre inulin increases postprandial serum short-chain fatty acids and reduces free-fatty acids and ghrelin in healthy subjects. *Applied Physiology Nutrition and Metabolism,* Vol. 35, No. 1 (February 2010), pp. 9-16. ISSN 1715-5320

Taskinen M.R., Sane T., Helve E., Karonen S.L., Nikkila E.A., & Yki-Jarvinen H. (1989). Bedtime insulin for suppression of overnight free-fatty acid, blood glucose, and glucose production in NIDDM. *Diabetes,* Vol. 38, No. 5 (May 1989), pp. 580-588. ISSN 0012-1797

Tuomilehto J., Lindström J., Eriksson J.G., Valle T.T., Hämäläinen H., Ilanne-Parikka P., Keinänen-Kiukaanniemi S., Laakso M., Louheranta A., Rastas M., Salminen V., & Uusitupa M. (2001). Prevention of type 2 diabetes mellitus by changes in lifestyle among subjects with impaired glucose tolerance. *New England Journal of Medicine,* Vol. 344, No 18 (May 2001), pp. 1343-1350. ISSN 0028-4793

Utzschneider K.M., Tong J., Montgomery B., Udayasankar J., Gerchman F., Marcovina S.M., Watson C.E., Ligueros-Saylan M.A., Foley J.E., Holst J.J., Deacon C.F., & Kahn S.E. (2008). The dipeptidyl peptidase-4 inhibitor vildagliptin improves beta-cell function and insulin sensitivity in subjects with impaired fasting glucose. *Diabetes Care,* Vol. 31, No. 1 (January 2008), pp. 108-113. ISSN 0022-3166

van Dam R.M., Willett W.C., Rimm E.B., Stampfer M.J., & Hu F.B. (2002). Dietary fat and meat intake in relation to risk of type 2 diabetes in men. *Diabetes Care,* Vol. 25, No. 3 (March 2002), pp. 417-24. ISSN 0149-5992

Van de Werve W.G., Lange A., Newgard C., Mechin M.C., Li Y., & Berteloot A. (2000). New lessons in the regulation of glucose metabolism taught by the glucose 6-phosphatase system. *European Journal of Biochemistry,* Vol. 267, pp. 1533–1549. ISSN 0014-2956

Weickert M.O., Möhlig M., Schöfl C., Arafat A.M., Otto B., Viehoff H., Koebnick C., Kohl A., Spranger J., & Pfeiffer A.F.H. (2006). Cereal fiber improves whole-body insulin sensitivity in overweight and obese women. *Diabetes Care,* Vol. 29, No. 4 (April 2006), pp. 775-780. ISSN 0149-5992

Weickert M.O. & Pfeiffer A.F.H. (2008), Metabolic effects of dietary fiber consumption and prevention of diabetes. *The Journal of Nutrition,* Vol. 138, No. 3 (March 2008), pp. 439-442. ISSN 0022-3166

Williams D.E., Prevost A.T., Whichelow M.J., Cox B.D., Day N.E., Wareham N.J. (2000). A cross-sectional study of dietary patterns with glucose intolerance and other features of the metabolic syndrome. *British Journal of Nutrition.* Vol. 83, No. 3, (March 2000), pp. 257-266. ISSN 0007-1145

Wolever T.M. (1991). Small intestinal effects of starchy foods. *Canadian Journal of Physiology and Pharmacology*, Vol. 69, No. 1 (January 1991), pp. 93-99. ISSN 0008-4212

Part 4

Complications

10

Characteristics of Vitamin B12 Deficiency in Adult Chinese Patients with Type 2 Diabetes and the Implication of Metformin

Chan Chee Wun Joyce, Chan Hoi Yan Florence,
Wong Ho Nam Howard and Yeung Chun Yip
*Department of Medicine, Pamela Youde Nethersole Eastern Hospital, Hong Kong
China SAR*

1. Introduction

Vitamin B12 deficiency remains a worldwide health problem in the 21st century. The advent of metabolite assays in the last few decades further expands the population with subclinical or tissue deficiency and thus the magnitude of the problem. The increasing recognition of its association with the use of metformin raises another controversy for clinicians regarding detection and treatment of vitamin B12 deficiency. Since the clinical use of metformin in 1957, malabsorption of vitamin B12 in diabetic patients treated with metformin was first noted in 1969 (Berchtold et al., 1969). Subsequent studies revealed both short-term and long-term use of metformin induces malabsorption of vitamin B12 and causes decreased serum vitamin B12 concentrations in 10% to 30% of diabetic patients (Tomkin et al., 1971; Bauman et al., 2000; Wulffele el al., 2003; Hermann et al., 2004). A randomized placebo controlled Dutch trial recently reconfirmed this finding and demonstrated treatment with metformin for a mean of 4.3 years resulted not only in a 19% persistent and progressive reduction of mean serum vitamin B12 concentrations, but also raised serum homocysteine concentrations (de Jager et al., 2010). Other case-control and cross-sectional studies identified duration and dosage of metformin use as risk factors for vitamin B12 deficiency (Ting et al., 2006). It is believed that if individuals with type 2 diabetes receiving metformin develop low serum vitamin B12 concentrations, a stage of asymptomatic tissue deficiency, would eventually progress to symptomatic clinical deficiency, as evidenced by reports of megaloblastic anaemia caused by metformin-related vitamin B12 malabsorption, unless they are duly treated (Gilligan, 2002; Filioussi et al., 2003; Liu et al., 2006).
Metformin is now extensively used as the first line pharmacological agent for glycaemic control especially following the favourable results of the United Kingdom Prospective Diabetes Study (UKPDS 34) in 1998. This coupled with the rising incidence of type 2 diabetes in many parts of the world constitutes a driving force for relevant parties to make appropriate recommendations or guidelines concerning the detection and treatment of vitamin B12 deficiency among diabetic patients on metformin. Although the haematological and neurological manifestations of overt or clinical vitamin B12 deficiency are easy to diagnose, they are often overlooked and attributed to diabetic complications or aging among diabetic patients.

The present study attempts to address the issue from the end spectrum of the disorder - florid vitamin B12 deficiency in type 2 diabetic patients. Through description and analysis of the clinical manifestations of overt vitamin B12 deficiency in a cohort of adult Chinese patients with type 2 diabetes, and delineation of the underlying aetiology of vitamin B12 deficiency, the study aims to highlight the characteristics of vitamin B12 deficiency in type 2 diabetic patients, and to evaluate the implications of metformin use in relation to the development of vitamin B12 deficiency of undetermined origin in diabetic patients.

2. Materials and methods

2.1 Patient source and stratification

The patient source was from a longitudinal study of adult Chinese patients (≥ 18 years) presenting with megaloblastic anaemia and/or neurological deficits in association with low serum vitamin B12 levels serially encountered in a regional hospital in Hong Kong between May 1994 and October 2010 (Chan et al., 2008). According to whether they had type 2 diabetes as shown by the diagnostic codes in the medical records at the time of diagnosis of vitamin B12 deficiency, patients were stratified into diabetic and non-diabetic groups. Documentation of diagnosis of diabetes was at the discretion of in-charge physicians and the diagnostic criteria of World Health Organization (WHO, 1999) with fasting plasma glucose ≥7.0 mmol/L or 2-hour post prandial plasma glucose ≥11.1 mmol/L were adopted. Diabetes both with and without complications were included. Diabetic patients were further stratified according to whether they were on metformin at the time of diagnosis of vitamin B12 deficiency. Diabetic patients who had been on metformin for one or more years immediately before the diagnosis of vitamin B12 deficiency were counted as metformin users and assigned to the "on metformin" group. Other diabetic patients on dietary control, insulin, sulphonylureas, metformin for less than one year or longer period but having stopped in the one year before the diagnosis of vitamin B12 deficiency, were assigned to the "not on metformin" group.

2.2 Data collection and analysis

Baseline data were retrieved from patients' medical records and investigators' file of adult Chinese patients with vitamin B12 deficiency. Data entry included presenting clinical and laboratory features at the time of diagnosis of vitamin B12 deficiency; causes of vitamin B12 deficiency; medications including metformin, sulphonylureas, insulin, proton pump inhibitors (PPI), histamine 2 blockers (H2B), lipid lowering agents, antiplatelet agents, antihypertensive and cardiac agents; duration of metformin use; and duration of diabetic history.

The sequence of data analysis was shown in Box 1. (i) The presenting features and the causes of vitamin B12 deficiency were compared between patients with and without type 2 diabetes. The odds ratio (OR) of developing vitamin B12 deficiency of undetermined origin among diabetic patients to non-diabetic patients was determined. (ii) The presenting features and the causes of vitamin B12 deficiency were compared between type 2 diabetic patients "on metformin" and diabetic patients "not on metformin". The OR of developing vitamin B12 deficiency of undetermined origin among diabetic patients "on metformin" to patients "not on metformin" was determined. (iii) For diabetic patients with undetermined aetiology of vitamin B12 deficiency, the presenting features and the medications prescribed at the time of diagnosis of vitamin B12 deficiency were compared between those "on metformin" and those "not on metformin". (iv) The duration of metformin use in relation to the onset of vitamin B12 deficiency was studied among all diabetic patients on metformin, irrespective of the underlying aetiology of vitamin B12 deficiency.

Box 1: Flowchart of data analysis of patients with vitamin B12 deficiency

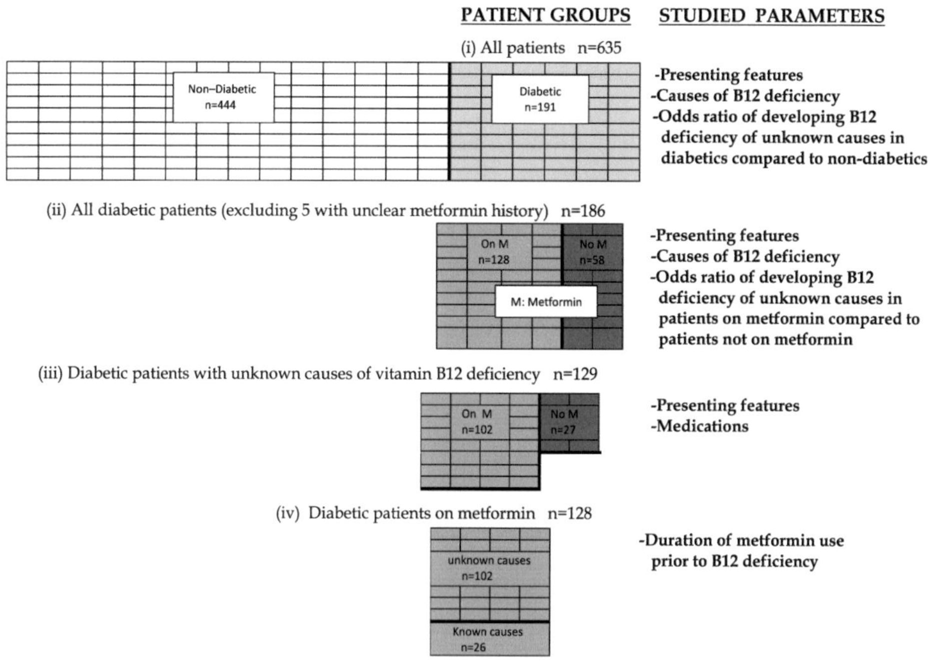

2.3 Definitions

Known causes of vitamin B12 deficiency include (i) pernicious anaemia (PA) defined by the presence of serum intrinsic factor (IF) antibody and/or by abnormal Schilling test compatible with immune loss of IF; (ii) probable PA (PPA) defined by the absence of demonstrable IF antibody, no performance of Schilling test, and the presence of at least 2 out of 3 immune features - gastric parietal cell (GPC) antibody, antithyroid antibodies, and histological evidence of autoimmune gastropathy (J.C.W. Chan & F.H.Y. Chan, 2011); (iii) gastrointestinal disorders such as total gastrectomy and terminal ileal resection or diseases e.g. Crohn's disease, ulcerative colitis; (iv) nutritional deficiency in strict vegetarians. Only after excluding PA and PPA, the first two overriding causes, gastrointestinal and nutritional causes are considered.

The cause of vitamin B12 deficiency is considered to be undetermined if none of the above conditions are present. Common predisposing factors for the development of vitamin B12 deficiency of undetermined causes include food cobalamin malabsorption, idiopathic gastric atrophy, Helicobacter pylori (HP) associated gastritis, use of PPI and H2B, metformin related malabsorption of vitamin B12, and a multitude of other conditions all of which currently lack easily available confirmatory tools and are diagnosed largely by exclusion. Known causes of vitamin B12 deficiency and the diagnostic approach to arrive at the conclusion of undetermined aetiology of vitamin B12 deficiency are summarized in Box 2.

2.4 Measurements

Serum cobalamin was measured with a fluorometric method using Abbott IMX analyzer (Abbott Laboratory, Chicago, IL) from 1994 to 2002; and with a chemiluminescent immunoassay using paramagnetic particles of Access Immunoassay System (Beckman Coulter, Fullerton, CA) from 2003 to 2010. Reference range for serum vitamin B12 level was 132–835 pmol/L from 1994 to 2002, and 180–914 ng/L from 2003 to 2010. To facilitate analysis, serum vitamin B12 levels in pmol/L were converted to ng/L by using the equation, 1 pmol/L=1.355 ng/L, (molecular mass of vitamin B12=1355 mol/g). Vitamin B12 deficiency was defined by serum vitamin B12 levels below 132 pmol/L or below 180 ng/L.

Box 2: Aetiology of vitamin B12 deficiency	
Known causes	Undetermined causes (diagnostic steps)
(i) pernicious anaemia	(i) exclusion of known causes
(ii) probable pernicious anaemia	(ii) examples of predisposing factors:
(iii) gastrointestinal disorders	food cobalamin malabsorption, gastric atrophy,
(iv) malnutrition	Helicobacter pylori infection, long-term ingestion of
	metformin, proton pump inhibitor, histamine 2 blocker

2.5 Statistical analysis

Statistical analyses were performed using the Statistical Package for the Social Sciences (SPSS Inc, Chicago, Illinosis, USA), version 15. Data were reported as means and standard deviation (SD), or as medians and interquartile range (IQR). The chi-square test was used for comparison between categorical variables, Student's t test for continuous variables of normal distribution, and Mann-Whitney U test for continuous data of skewed distribution. P values of less than 0.05 were considered to indicate statistical significance. Among patients with B12 deficiency, a chi-square analysis (two-tailed; two-by-two table) was used to estimate the crude OR of having B12 deficiency of undetermined origin among patients with type 2 diabetes to those without diabetes, and another chi-square analysis (two-tailed; two-by-two table) was used to calculate the crude OR of having B12 deficiency of undetermined origin among patients taking metformin to the diabetic patients not taking metformin. Multivariate analysis using stepwise forward logistic regression were used to identify risk factors independently associated with vitamin B12 deficiency of undetermined origin in all patients and in diabetic patients; and in diabetic patients on metformin and not on metformin. Extended Mantel-Haenzel chi-square analysis was performed for linear trend.

3. Results

Between May 1994 and October 2010, 635 adult Chinese patients (excluding 1 patient with type 1 diabetes and PA diagnosed at the age of 14 years old) were diagnosed to have overt vitamin B12 deficiency in a regional hospital in Hong Kong. At the time of diagnosis of vitamin B12 deficiency, 191 (30%) patients had type 2 diabetes, and 444 (70%) were non-diabetics.

3.1 Vitamin B12 deficiency: Type 2 diabetic and non-diabetic patients

Concerning the demographic features (Table 1), 37% of 191 diabetic patients and 44% of 444 non-diabetic patients were male (p=0.079), and the mean ages of diabetic and non-diabetic patients were 75.6 years (SD 9.1) and 72.3 years (SD 14.5) respectively (p=0.001). The clinical manifestations of vitamin B12 deficiency were less symptommatic in diabetic than non-diabetic patients, as evidenced by 34% of diabetic and 47% of non-diabetic patients having anaemia (p=0.002), and 3% of diabetic and 7% of non-diabetic patients having peripheral

	Number of patients (%)				
	With diabetes (n=191)	No diabetes (n=444)	p	adjusted OR	95% CI
Demographics					
Sex, male	70/191 (37)	196/444 (44)	0.079		
Mean age [SD], years	75.6 [9.1]	72.3 [14.5]	**0.001**		
Presenting features					
Anaemia	65/191 (34)	210/444 (47)	**0.002**		
PN/SCD[1]	5/191 (3)	30/444 (7)	**0.036**		
Dementia	15/191 (8)	41/444 (9)	0.574		
Laboratory findings					
Mean Haemoglobin [SD], g/L	9.8 [2.5]	9.0 [2.9]	**0.001**		
Mean MCV[2] [SD], fl	110.0 [12.1]	113.4 [15.4]	**0.003**		
Mean serum B12 level [SD], ng/L	85.8 [38.1]	80.0 [41.9]	**0.106**		
Intrinsic Factor Antibody +ve	49/191 (26)	248/444 (56)	**<0.001**		
GPC[3] Antibody +ve	73/191 (38)	245/444 (56)	**<0.001**		
Anti-thyroid antibody +ve	26/159 (16)	126/337 (37)	**<0.001**		
Thyrogastric features					
History of AITD[4]	4/191 (2)	29/444 (7)	**0.021**		
Biopsy proven gastric atrophy	25/80 (31)	86/196 (44)	**0.052**		
ECH[5]	0/80 (0)	6/196 (3)	0.114		
HP[6] +ve histology	10/80 (13)	16/196 (8)	0.263		
Aetiology of B12 deficiency					
Undetermined	129/191 (68)	132/444 (30)	**<0.001**	5.54	3.66 - 8.38
Known	62/191 (32)	312/444 (70)			
Pernicious anaemia	54/191 (28)	265/444 (60)	**<0.001**		
Probable pernicious anaemia	4/191 (2)	15/444 (3)	0.384		
Gastrointestinal surgery/disorder	2/191 (1)	24/444 (5)	**0.011**		

[1]peripheral neuropathy/subacute combined degeneration [2]mean corpuscular volume
[3]Gastric Parietal Cell, [4]autoimmune thyroid disease, [5]Enterochromaffin Cell Hyperplasia, [6]Helicobacter pylori

Table 1. Comparison of presenting features and causes of vitamin B12 deficiency: type 2 diabetic and non-diabetic patients

neuropathy and/or subacute combined degeneration of cord (p=0.036). Dementia was the presenting feature in 8% of diabetic and 9% of non-diabetic patients (p=0.574). The mean haemoglobin (Hb) concentrations of diabetic and non-diabetic patients were 9.8 g/L (SD 2.5) and 9.0 g/L (SD 2.9) respectively (p=0.001), and the mean mean corpuscular volume (MCV) of the two groups were 110.0 fl (SD 12.1) and 113.4 fl (SD 15.4) respectively (p=0.003). The mean serum vitamin B12 levels of diabetic and non-diabetic patients were 85.8 ng/L (SD 38.1) and 80.0 ng/L (SD 41.9) respectively (p=0.106). Serum IF antibody was detected in 26% of diabetic and 56% of non-diabetic patients (p<0.001); GPC antibody in 38% of diabetic and 56% of non-diabetic patients (p<0.001); and anti-thyroid antibodies in 16% of diabetic and 37% of non-diabetic patients (p<0.001). History of autoimmune thyroid disease (AITD) was obtained in 2% of diabetic and 7% of non-diabetic patients (p=0.021). Endoscopically proven gastric atrophy was detected in 31% of diabetic and 44% of non-diabetic patients (p=0.052), enterochromaffin cell hyperplasia (ECH) in 0% of diabetic and 3% of non-diabetic patients (p=0.114), and HP organisms in 13% of diabetic and 8% of non-diabetic patients (p=0.263). The underlying aetiology of vitamin B12 deficiency was undetermined in 68% of diabetic and 30% of non-diabetic patients (p<0.001); due to PA in 28% of diabetic and 60% of non-diabetic patients (p<0.001); PPA in 2% of diabetic and 3% of non-diabetic patients (p=0.384); related to gastrointestinal surgery or disorders in 1% of diabetic and 5% of non-diabetic patients (p=0.011); and malnutrition in 1% of diabetic and 2% of non-diabetic patients (p=0.484). The percentages of patients with vitamin B12 deficiency of undetermined origin, due to PA, and other known causes (PPA, gastrointestinal disorders, malnutrition) among diabetic and non-diabetic patients were shown in Figure 1. The crude OR of developing vitamin B12 deficiency of undetermined origin in type 2 diabetic patients compared with non-diabetic patients was 4.90 (95% CI, 3.41- 7.08). The adjusted OR (adjusted for sex, age, use of PPI/H2B) of developing vitamin B12 deficiency of undetermined origin in type 2 diabetic patients compared with non-diabetic patients was 5.54 (95% CI, 3.66 - 8.38).

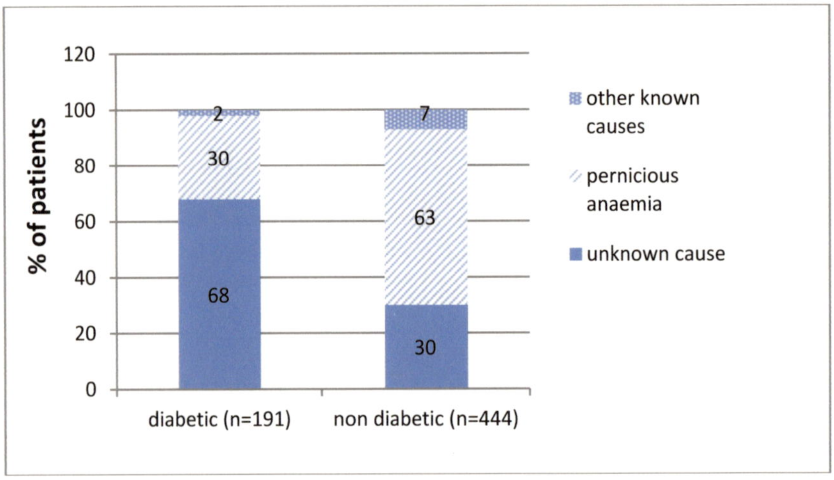

Fig. 1. Comparison of causes of vitamin B12 deficiency: type 2 diabetic and non-diabetic patients

3.2 Vitamin B12 deficiency: type 2 diabetic patients "on metformin" and "not on metformin"

Among the 191 patients with type 2 diabetes, 5 patients with unclear metformin history were excluded from analysis, and 186 patients - 128 (69%) "on metformin" and 58 (31%) "not on metformin" were analysed (Table 2). Of the 128 patients "on metformin", 30% were male, and of the 58 patients "not on metformin", 50% were male (p=0.008). The mean ages of patients "on metformin" and "not on metformin" were 75.3 years [SD 9.2] and 76.3 years [SD 9.2] respectively (p=0.463). Thirty one percent of patients "on metformin" and 36% of patients "not on metformin" presented with anaemia (p=0.505); 0.8% of patients "on metformin" and 7% of patients "not on metformin" had peripheral neuropathy and/or subacute combined degeneration of cord (p=0.017), and 9% of patients "on metformin" and 3% of "not on metformin" had dementia (p=0.156). The mean Hb concentrations of patients "on metformin" and "not on metformin" were 9.9 g/L [SD 2.4] and 9.7 g/L [SD 2.6] respectively (p=0.498), and the mean MCV 108.5 fl [SD 12.0] and 112.1 fl [SD 11.9] respectively (p=0.058). The mean serum

	Number of diabetic patients (%)				
	On metformin (n=128)	Not on metformin (n=58)	p	adjusted OR	95% CI
Demographics					
Sex, male	38/128 (30)	29/58 (50)	**0.008**		
Mean age [SD], years	75.3 [9.2]	76.3 [9.2]	0.463		
Presenting features					
Anaemia	40/128 (31)	21/56 (36)	0.505		
PN/SCD[1]	1/128 (0.8)	4/58 (7)	**0.017**		
Dementia	12/128 (9)	2/58 (3)	0.156		
Laboratory findings					
Mean Haemoglobin [SD], g/L	9.9 [2.4]	9.7 [2.6]	0.498		
Mean MCV[2] [SD], in fl	108.5 [12.0]	112.1 [11.9]	0.058		
Mean serum B12 level [SD], ng/L	90.3 [37.6]	76.7 [38.6]	**0.026**		
Intrinsic Factor Antibody +ve	20/128 (16)	24/58 (41)	**<0.001**		
Gastric Parietal Cell Antibody +ve	41/127 (32)	30/58 (52)	**0.012**		
Anti-thyroid Antibody +ve	15/115 (13)	11/42 (26)	**0.050**		
Thyrogastric features					
History of AITD[3]	3/128 (2.3)	1/58 (1.7)	0.787		
Biopsy proven gastric atrophy	8/48 (17)	13/28 (46)	**0.005**		
Enterochromaffin Cell Hyperplasia	0/48 (0)	0/28 (0)	-		
Helicobacter pylori +ve histology	8/48 (17)	2/28 (7)	0.236		
Aetiology of B12 deficiency					
Undetermined	102/128 (80)	27/58 (47)	**<0.001**	5.20	2.33-11.60
Known	26/128 (20)	31/58 (53)			
Pernicious anaemia	22/128 (17)	27/58 (47)	**<0.001**		
Probable pernicious anaemia	1/128 (0.8)	3/58 (5)	0.384		
Gastrointestinal surgery/disorder	1/128 (0.8)	1/58 (1.7)	0.011		
Nutritional	2/128 (1.6)	0/58 (0)	0.484		
Median diabetic duration [IQR], years	10 [6.5-11.5] (n=121)	4 [1.5-8.5] (n=41)	**<0.001**		

[1]peripheral neuropathy/subacute combined degeneration
[2]mean corpuscular volume [3]autoimmune thyroid disease

Table 2. Comparison of presenting features and causes of vitamin B12 deficiency: type 2 diabetic patients "on metformin" and "not on metformin"

B12 levels of patients "on metformin" and "not on metformin" were 90.3 ng/L [SD 37.6] and 76.7 ng/L [SD 38.6] respectively (p=0.026). Frequencies of IF antibody in the "on metformin" and "not on metformin" groups were 16% and 41% respectively (p<0.001), that of GPC antibody 32% and 52% respectively (p=0.012), and that of anti-thyroid antibodies 13% and 26% respectively (p=0.050). History of AITD was obtained in 2.3% of patients "on metformin" and 1.7% of patients "not on metformin" (p=0.787). Histological evidence of gastric atrophy was detected in 17% of patients "on metformin" and 46% of patients "not on metformin" (p=0.005), ECH in none of the patients in the two groups, and HP organisms in

17% of patients "on metformin" and 7% of patients "not on metformin" ($p=0.236$). The median duration of diabetic history for those "on metformin" (n=121) and "not on metformin" (n=41) were 10 years [IQR 6.5-11.5] and 4 years [IQR 1.5-8.5] respectively ($p<0.001$).

Of the 128 diabetic patients "on metformin" and 58 diabetic patients "not on metformin", the causes of vitamin B12 deficiency were undetermined in 80% of patients "on metformin" and in 47% of those "not on metformin" ($p<0.001$); due to PA in 17% of patients "on metformin" and 47% of "not on metformin" ($p<0.001$); PPA in 0.8% of patients "on metformin" and 5% of "not on metformin" ($p=0.384$); due to gastrointestinal disorders in 0.8% and 1.6% of patients "on metformin" and "not on metformin" respectively ($p=0.011$), and due to malnutrition in 1.5% and 0% of patients "on metformin" and "not on metformin" respectively ($p=0.484$). The percentages of patients with vitamin B12 deficiency of undetermined origin, due to PA, and other known causes (PPA, gastrointestinal disorders, malnutrition) among non-diabetic patients, diabetic patients "on metformin", and diabetic patients "not on metformin" were shown in Figure 2. The crude OR of developing vitamin B12 deficiency of undetermined origin in type 2 diabetic patients "on metformin" compared with diabetic patients "not on metformin" was 4.50 (95% CI, 2.30 - 8.82). The adjusted OR (adjusted for sex, age, use of PPI/H2B) of developing vitamin B12 deficiency of undetermined origin in type 2 diabetic patients "on metformin" compared with diabetic patients "not on metformin" was 5.20 (95% CI, 2.33 - 11.60).

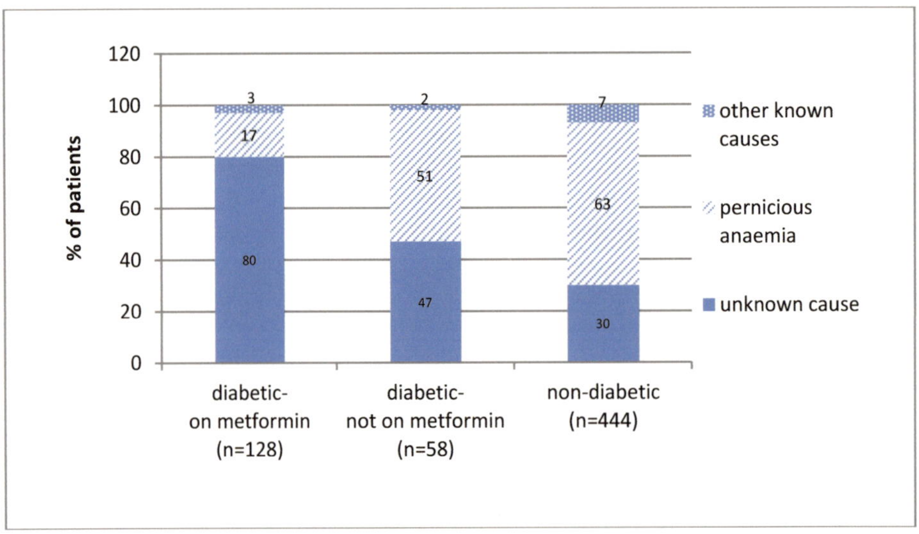

Fig. 2. Comparison of causes of vitamin B12 deficiency: diabetic patients on metformin and not on metformin, non-diabetic patients

3.3 Vitamin B12 deficiency of undetermined origin: "on metformin" and "not on metformin"

Of the 191 diabetic patients with vitamin B12 deficiency, 62 patients (including 5 with unclear metformin history) had known causes of vitamin B12 deficiency. Excluding these 62 patients, 129 diabetic patients had vitamin B12 deficiency of undetermined aetiology - 102 (79%) "on metformin" and 27 (21%) "not on metformin" at the time of diagnosis of vitamin B12 deficiency (Table 3). Thirty two percent of patients "on metformin" were male, and 44% of patients "not on metformin" were male (p=0.241). The mean ages of patients "on metformin" and "not on metformin" were 76.4 years [SD 8.2] and 77.1 years [SD 10.3] respectively (p=0.721). Anaemia was the presenting feature in 25% of patients "on metformin"

	Number of patients (%)		
	On metformin (n=102)	Not on metformin (n=27)	P
Demographics			
Sex, male	33/102 (32)	12/27 (44)	0.241
Mean age [SD], in years	76.4 [8.2]	77.1 [10.3]	0.721
Presenting features			
Anaemia	25/102 (25)	8/27 (30)	0.588
PN/SCD[1]	1/102 (1)	3/27 (11)	**0.007**
Dementia	9/102 (9)	1/27 (4)	0.376
Laboratory findings			
Mean Haemoglobin [SD], g/L	10.2 [2.2]	10.2 [2.4]	0.988
Mean MCV[2] [SD], fl	107.3 [11.1]	108.2 [11.3]	0.706
Mean serum B12 level [SD], ng/L	93.7 [38.1]	86.0 [43.5]	0.369
Gastric Parietal Cell Antibody +ve	24/101(24)	12/27 (44)	**0.034**
Anti-thyroid Antibody +ve	11/91 (12)	0/18 (26)	0.120
Thyrogastric features			
History of AITD[3]	1/102 (1)	0/27 (0)	0.606
Biopsy proven gastric atrophy	2/39 (5)	3/13 (23)	0.057
Enterochromaffic Cell Hyperplasia	0/39 (0)	0/13 (0)	-
Helicobacter pyloria +ve histology	8/39 (21)	1/13 (8)	0.290
Median diabetic duration [IQR] in years	10 [6-10] (n=99)	3.5 [1.3-6.8] (n=20)	**<0.001**
Diabetic medications			
Sulph[4]+metformin* Sulph[4] alone**	54/102 (53)*	11/27 (41)**	0.260
Insulin+metformin* Insulin alone**	9/102 (9)*	1/27 (4)**	0.376
Metformin alone	39/102 (38)	-	
Nil anti-diabetic medication	-	15/27 (55)	
Other concomitant medications			
PPI/H2B[5]	26/101 (26)	9/26 (35)	0.815
Anti-platelet agents	42/101 (42)	6/26 (23)	0.083
Lipid lowering agents	28/101 (28)	3/26 (12)	0.087
Hypertensive/cardiac agents	88/101 (87)	18/26 (69)	**0.028**

[1]peripheral neuropathy/subacute combined degeneration [2]mean corpuscular volume
[3]autoimmune thyroid disease
[4]sulphonylurea [5]proton pump inhibitor/ histamine 2 blocker

Table 3. Comparison of presenting features and medications of diabetic patients with vitamin B12 deficiency of undetermined aetiology: "on metformin" and "not on metformin"

and 30% of patients "not on metformin" (p=0.588), peripheral neuropathy/subacute combined degeneration of cord in 1% of patients "on metformin" and 11% of patients "not on metformin" (p=0.007), and dementia in 9% of patients "on metformin" and 4% of patients "not on metformin" (p=0.376). The mean Hb concentrations of those "on metformin" and "not on metformin" were 10.2 g/L [SD 2.2] and 10.2 g/L [SD 2.4] respectively (p=0.988), the mean MCV of the two groups were 107.3 fl [SD 11.1] and 108.2 fl [SD 11.3] respectively (p=0.706), and the mean serum vitamin B12 levels were 93.7 ng/L [SD 38.1] and 86.0 ng/L [SD 43.5] respectively (p=0.369). GPC antibody was detected in 24% of patients "on metformin" and 44% of patients "not on metformin" (p=0.034), and anti-thyroid antibodies in 12% and 26% of the two groups respectively (p=0.120). AITD occurred in 1% of patients "on metformin" and none of the patients "not on metformin" (p=0.606). Histology of gastric atrophy was detected in 5% of patients "on metformin" and 23% of patients "not on metformin" (p=0.057), ECH in none of the patients in the two groups, and histological evidence of HP organisms in 21% and 8% of the two groups respectively (p=0.290).

The median duration of diabetes for the "on metformin" (n=99) and "not on metformin" (n=20) patients were 10 years [IQR 6-10] and 3.5 years [IQR 1.3-6.8] respectively (p<0.001). Fifty three percent of the "on metformin" patients were also on sulphonylureas, and 41% of the "not on metformin" patients were on sulphonylurea alone (p=0.260). Nine percent of the "on metformin" patients were also on insulin, and 4% of the "not on metformin" patients were on insulin alone (p=0.376). Thirty eight percent of the "on metformin" patients were on metformin alone, and 55% of the "not on metformin" patients were not on any diabetic agents - 4 chronic renal insufficiency, 2 early deaths, 9 early stage of diabetes on dietary control alone (Table 3). Other concomitant medications of 101 (99%) "on metformin" and 26 (96%) "not on metformin" diabetic patients at the time of diagnosis of vitamin B12 deficiency were available for analysis. Twenty six percent of "on metformin" and 35% of "not on metformin" diabetic patients were on either PPI or H2B (p=0.815), 42% of "on metformin" and 23% of "not on metformin" diabetic patients were on antiplatelet agents, (p=0.083), 28% of "on metformin" and 12% of "not on metformin" diabetic patients were on lipid lowering agents (p=0.087), and 87% of "on metformin" and 69% of "not on metformin" diabetic patients were on antihypertensive agents and/or medications for ischaemic heart disease (p=0.028).

3.4 Duration of metformin use in relation to development of vitamin B12 deficiency

Of the 128 diabetic patients on metformin, 47 (37%) patients developed vitamin B12 deficiency of all causes within 1 to 5 years of metformin use, 71 (55%) within 6 to 10 years, and 10 (8%) after 10 years, as shown in Figure 3 (i). Among these 128 patients, 102 (80%) patients had vitamin B12 deficiency of undetermined aetiology, and 26 (20%) had known causes. Of the 102 patients with undetermined aetiology, 31 (30%) developed overt vitamin B12 deficiency within 1 to 5 years of metformin use, 63 (62%) within 6 to 10 years, and 8 (8%) beyond 10 years, up to 30 years. Of the 26 patients with known causes, 16 (62%) developed vitamin B12 deficiency within 1 to 5 years of metformin use, 8 (31%) within 6 to 10 years, and 2 (8%) after 10 years. The relationship between the duration of metformin use and the development of vitamin B12 deficiency of undetermined and known causes was shown in Figure 3 (ii). The Extended Mantel-Haenzel chi-square analysis for linear trend was 4.74 (p = 0.029 with one degree of freedom).

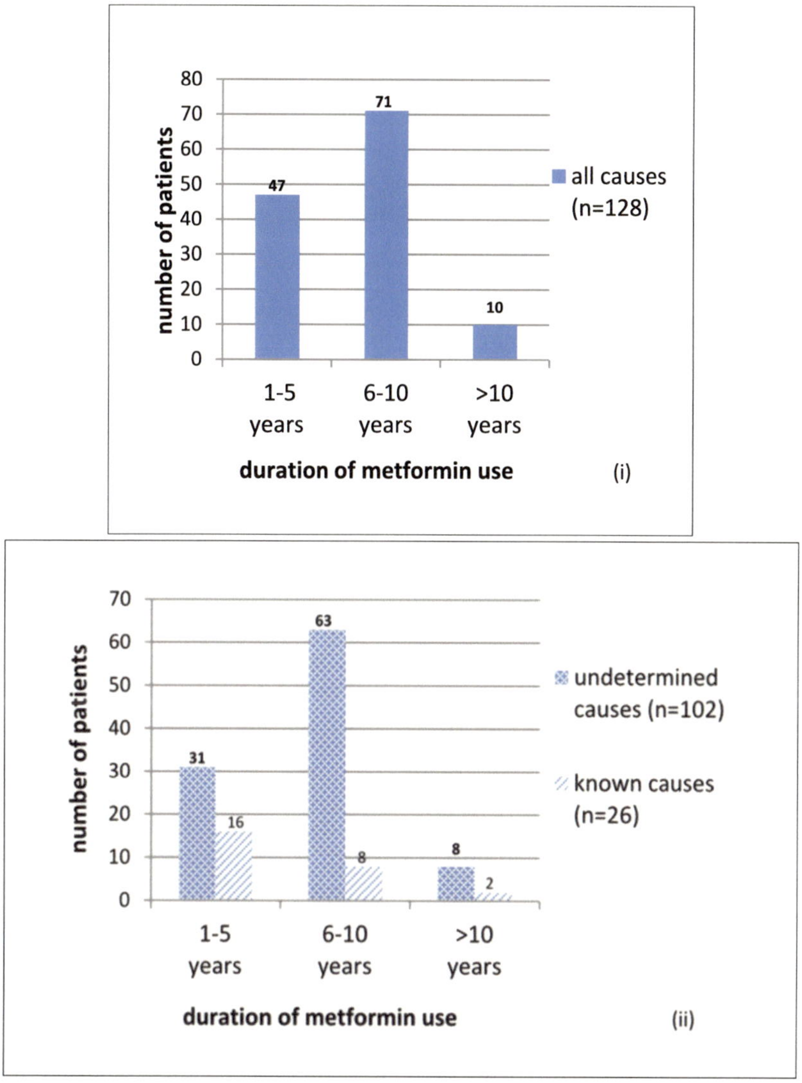

Fig. 3. Relationship between duration of metformin use and development of vitamin B12 deficiency (i) of all causes (ii) of undetermined and known causes

4. Conclusions

4.1 Characteristics of vitamin B12 deficiency in type 2 diabetic patients

The present study illustrates certain characteristics of vitamin B12 deficiency in adult Chinese patients with type 2 diabetes. Majority of the common causes of vitamin B12 deficiency encountered in the general population such as PA, gastrointestinal diseases and nutritional deficiency also occur in type 2 diabetic patients. The frequencies of occurrence of these causes however differ between diabetic and non-diabetic patients. Vitamin B12 deficiency of undetermined origin is more frequently encountered in diabetic than non-diabetic patients (68% versus 30%), whereas PA, the most common definitive cause of vitamin B12 deficiency, is more frequently detected in non-diabetic than diabetic patients (63% versus 30%). This preponderance of vitamin B12 deficiency of undetermined origin is even more conspicuous in diabetic patients on metformin than diabetic patients not on metformin (80% versus 47%). In this cohort of adult Chinese patients, the risk of developing vitamin B12 deficiency of undetermined origin is 5.5-fold higher in diabetic than non-diabetic patients, and diabetic patients taking metformin have a 5.2-fold higher risk of developing vitamin B12 deficiency of undetermined origin than patients not taking metformin.

This remarkable difference in the aetiological pattern of vitamin B12 deficiency between diabetic and non-diabetic patients accounts for the differences in the clinical manifestations of vitamin B12 deficiency between the two groups of patients. PA as an autoimmune disease causes profound gastric atrophy, IF depletion and vitamin B12 malabsorption, and is often accompanied by immune features; whereas conditions causing vitamin B12 deficiency of undetermined origin are often non-immune processes. They tend to cause a less severe degree of vitamin B12 malabsorption and have a paucity of immune features. Diabetic patients with vitamin B12 deficiency of undetermined origin thus generally have a less severe degree of vitamin B12 deficiency, a less severe degree of anaemia, and less autoimmune features such as GPC and antithyroid antibodies, AITD, and autoimmune gastropathy compared with non-diabetic patients, as shown in the study.

4.2 Implications of metformin use in type 2 diabetic patients

4.2.1 Evidence of association of metformin use with vitamin B12 deficiency

The finding of a greater proportion of type 2 diabetic patients especially those on metformin having vitamin B12 deficiency of undetermined origin in comparison with non-diabetic subjects implies the association of metformin use with vitamin B12 deficiency of undetermined origin. However, not all cases of vitamin B12 deficiency of undetermined origin are related to metformin. Vitamin B12 deficiency of undetermined origin actually has causative factors. Lack of easily available diagnostic tools bars the clarification or confirmation of these factors. In general, diagnostic approach to define the causes of vitamin B12 deficiency is first to look for nutritional deficiency and malabsorption syndromes notably PA and structural lesions of the stomach and intestine. These are the classical known causes of vitamin B12 deficiency. The previously less common or less well defined aetiologies of vitamin B12 deficiency, such as atrophic gastritis, gastric disease associated with Helicobacter pylori infection, gastric bypass for obesity, pancreatic insufficiency due to alcohol abuse, long-term use of metformin and acid-suppressive drugs like cimetidine, ranitidine, omeprazole, intestinal bacterial overgrowth, or even ageing and idiopathic, are principally diagnosed on clinical grounds and are grouped as vitamin B12 deficiency of undetermined origin, or now increasingly known as food cobalamin malabsorption, to be distinguished from the classical known causes (Clarke & Brown, 2003; Andres, 2008). Metformin-induced vitamin B12 deficiency is among one of the miscellaneous causes which are classified as "unknown" or "undetermined" simply because of lack of objective means to prove it as the sole agent or condition in the causation of vitamin deficiency.

The present cohort study, comprising 186 type 2 diabetic patients with 128 on metformin, serves only to provide indirect evidence that metformin use constitutes a risk factor for the development of vitamin B12 deficiency, among other "unknown" factors which may also be present in these diabetic patients. The methodology adopted by the study is traditional - exclusion of the classical known causes. In this context, the study has the advantage that as part of a previously reported longitudinal study of PA (Chan et al., 2008), all patients had documented vitamin B12 deficiency, had IF and GPC antibody assay performed, and had Schilling test done during the period when it was available. This diagnostic approach to arrive at the conclusion of metformin-induced vitamin B12 deficiency is similar to that cited in the other reports (Table 4, Table 5).

In addition, the study attempted to include medications other than metformin in the analysis of risk factors. Two principal categories of drugs that have been commonly reported to have interaction with vitamin B12 are biguanides and acid suppressive therapy. PPI and H2B have been shown to suppress acid secretion by parietal cells and impair the absorption of protein bound dietary vitamin B12 and thus contribute to the development of vitamin B12 deficiency (Howden, 2000; Ruscin et al., 2002; Force et al., 2003; den Elzen et al., 2008; Ali et al., 2009). The current evidence of vitamin B12 deficiency associated with long-term PPI use however is based on small nonrandomized retrospective studies (Steinberg et al., 1980; Marcuard et al., 1994; Termanini et al.,1998; Hirschowitz et al., 2008). Overall the current collective body of information supports the notion that prolonged use of PPI notably in the elderly and in persons on high doses of PPI is associated with increased risk of vitamin B12 deficiency (Thomas et al., 2010). In the present study, evaluation of medications prescribed at the time of diagnosis of vitamin B12 deficiency showed no significant differences in the utilization rates of PPI/H2B, between diabetic and non-diabetic patients, and diabetic patients "on metformin" and "not on metformin". There were also no significant differences in the utilization rates of other medications such as lipid lowering agents, anti-platelet agents, sulphonylureas and insulin between diabetic patients "on metformin" and "not on metformin". As all patients in one group were exposed to metformin compared to none in the other group, metformin in the study emerged as the most likely culprit for medication-related vitamin B12 malabsorption. The antihypertensive and cardiovascular agents were significantly more frequently used by diabetic patients "on metformin" than those "not on metformin" in the study. This could be related to the longer diabetic history and the associated more cardiovascular complications in the group of patients on metformin. Although there are studies reporting longer diabetic history might predispose to the development of vitamin B12 deficiency (Pfipsen et al., 2009), there is insufficient data for a definite conclusion to be drawn.

Literature search found further evidence of metformin related vitamin B12 malabsorption. Impaired vitamin B12 absorption in patients who had been treated with metformin for up to 3 months were first reported in 1969 (Berchtold et al., 1969). In the ensuing 4 decades, both observational and interventional studies unequivocally demonstrated the association between metformin use and vitamin B12 deficiency (Table 4). An observational study described malabsorption of vitamin B12 in 30% of diabetic patients during biguanide therapy (Adams et al., 1983). A cross-sectional study demonstrated a 22% prevalence of metabolically confirmed vitamin B12 deficiency in type 2 diabetic patients, with those on metformin exhibiting a statistically higher risk for B12 deficiency (Pflipsen et al., 2009). Another cross-sectional study demonstrated 6.9% of diabetic patients on metformin had low serum vitamin B12 level (Nervo et al., 2011). A case-control study demonstrated impaired gastrointestinal absorption in 30% and decreased serum B12 levels in 6% of patients in the metformin arm compared to none in the control arm (Tomkin et al., 1971). Another case-control study similarly demonstrated significant falls in the mean serum B12 levels in the metformin arm compared to the control arm (Bauman et al., 2000). A nested case-control study comparing diabetic patients on metformin with and without vitamin B12 deficiency

Authors Report year	Metformin duration	Metformin dosage	Outcome parameters	No. of patients on metformin	Study type
Tomkin 1971	4-6 y[1]	1.5-6g/d	*absorption B12↓ **serum B12↓	*21/71 (30%) **4/71 (6%)	[2]
		control	*no change*	*19 on S[5]*	
Adams 1983	1-6 y	1-3g/d	absorption B12 ↓	14/46 (30%)	[1]
Bauman 2000	3 months	0.85-2.55g/d	mean serum B12↓ serum holoTCII[2]↓	14	[2]
		control	*no change*	*7 on S[5]*	
Wulffele 2003	16 weeks	0.85-2.55g/d	mean serum B12↓: 16% HCy[3]↑: 8%	171	[3]
		placebo	*B12↓: 2%* *HCy↑: 4%*	*182 on I[6]*	
Hermann 2004	mean 5.2 y (range 1-18)	mean 2.2 g/d (range 0.85-3.4)	*serum B12↓ **serum HCy↑	*12/53 (23%) **7/53 (13%)	[2]
		control	*no change*	*31 on S[5] I[6] D[7]*	
Pongchaidecha 2004	>6months	-	mean serum B12 } P=0.011	88	[2]
		control	*serum B12*	*64§*	
Ting 2006	median 4 y (IQR 2-5)	2.0±0.7g/d	mean serum B12↓	155	[2]
	median 2 y (IQR 1-4)	*1.4±0.7g/d*	*serum B12 normal*	*310*	
Sahin 2007	6 weeks	-	mean serum B12↓	165	[2]
		control	*no change*		
Pflipsen 2009	-	-	serum B12↓ ±MMA[4], HCy↑	44/195†(22%)	[1]
Stehouwer 2010	4.3 y	2.05g/d	mean serumB12↓:19% serum HCy↑:26%	134	[3]
		placebo	*mean serum B12↓:0%* *serum HCy↑:20%*	*146 on I[6]*	
Nervo 2011	median 4 y (IQR 2-8.1)	1.7-2.55g/d	serum B12↓	10/144(6.9%)	[1]

[1]years [2]holotranscobalamin II [3]homocysteine [4]methylmalonic acid [5]sulphonylurea [6]insulin [7]diet
[1] observational / cross-sectional study [2] case control cohort study [3] randomized placebo controlled study
† ± metformin § no metformin

Table 4. Studies investigating associations between metformin use and vitamin B12 deficiency

indicated both the dose and the duration of metformin use are risk factors for vitamin B12 deficiency (Ting et al., 2006). Other cross-sectional cohort studies in Sweden, Thailand and Turkey also pointed to patients on metformin had lower serum B12 levels compared with thenon-exposed control group (Hermann et al., 2004; Pongchaidecha et al., 2004; Sahin et al., 2007). Effects of short-term (16 weeks) and long-term (52 months) treatment with metformin on the serum concentrations of vitamin B12 in type 2 diabetic patients were investigated by a Dutch randomized placebo controlled trial and showed both short- and long-term use of metformin increased the risk of vitamin B12 deficiency (Wulffele et al., 2003; Stehouwer et al., 2010). All these studies defined vitamin B12 deficiency based on biochemical markers and did not evaluate the clinical importance.

Concerning reports on the clinical manifestations of metformin-related vitamin B12 deficiency in diabetic patients (Table 5), there are case reports of megaloblastic anaemia related to long-term metformin treatment causing vitamin B12 deficiency (Callaghan et al., 1980; Gilligan, 2002; Liu et al., 2006; Lin et al., 2007). A case series showed metformin-related megaloblastic anaemia accounted for 6% (10/162) of all vitamin B12 deficiency patients (Andres et al., 2002), and another case series revealed a 9% prevalence (54/600) of megaloblastic anemia in diabetic patients taking long-term biguanides (Filioussi et al., 2003). Neurological deficits due to vitamin B12 deficiency manifest chiefly as peripheral neuropathy, subacute combined cord degeneration, and cognitive impairment. There are case reports of subacute combined degeneration and peripheral neuropathy related to metformin therapy (Liu et al., 2006; Bell, 2010), and a prospective case-control study demonstrating diabetic patients with concurrent symptomatic peripheral neuropathy had lower serum B12 levels and more severe neuropathy in the metformin treatment group in comparison with non-metformin treated patients (Wile & Toth, 2010).

Authors Report year	**Metformin duration**	**Metformin dosage**	**Presenting features**	**No. of patients on metformin**	**Tests**	**Metformin off/ continued**	**B12**	**Study type**
Callaghan 1980	8 y[1]	1g/d	MA[2]	1	Schill[5]	continued	inj[10]	[4]
Gilligan 2002	5 y	-	MA	1	Schill IF[6]	off	oral	[4]
Andres 2002	8.9±3.4 y range 3-10	2.015± 0.45g/d range 1.4-2.5	MA	10	Schill IF	continued:8 off:2	inj:4 oral:6	[5]
Filioussi 2003	11.8±3.6 y	-	MA	54/600 (9%)	GPC[7]	continued	Route NM	[5]
Liu 2006	*>10 y	- -	*SCD[3], dementia	1	IF	off	inj	[4]
	**8 y		**MA	1	IF GPC	off	inj	
Lin 2007	6 y	1g/d	MA DVT[4]	1	GPC	off	inj	[4]
Wile 2010	>6 months	total 3389.5g	mean B12 ↓, more severe neuropathy	59				[6]
		control	*normal B12, less severe neuropathy*	*63 †*				
Bell 2010	3 y	-	peripheral neuropathy	1	IF CD[8]	NM[9]	inj	[4]

[1]years [2]megaloblastic anaemia [3]subacute combined degeneration [4]deep vein thrombosis [5]Schilling test [6]intrinsic factor antibody [7]gastric parietal cell antibody [8]celiac disease ruled out [9]not mentioned [10]injection †on sulphonylurea/insulin [4] case report [5] case series [6] prospective case control study

Table 5. Reports of metformin-related symptomatic vitamin B12 deficiency

B12 malabsorption associated with long-term metformin treatment (Callaghan et al., 1980; Gilligan, 2002; Liu et al., 2006; Lin et al., 2007). A case series showed metformin-related megaloblastic anaemia accounted for 6% (10/162) of all established vitamin B12 deficiency patients (Andres et al., 2002), and another case series revealed a 9% prevalence (54/600) of megaloblastic anemia in diabetic patients taking long-term biguanides (Filioussi et al., 2003).

Neurological deficits due to vitamin B12 deficiency manifest chiefly as peripheral neuropathy, subacute combined cord degeneration, and cognitive impairment. There are case reports of subacute combined degeneration and peripheral neuropathy related to metformin therapy (Liu et al., 2006; Bell, 2010), and a prospective case-control study demonstrating diabetic patients with concurrent symptomatic peripheral neuropathy had lower serum B12 levels and more severe neuropathy in the metformin treatment group compared with non-metformin treated patients (Wile & Toth, 2010).

4.2.2 Duration and dosage of metformin use in relation to onset of vitamin B12 deficiency

From the present study, for diabetic patients on metformin, about 30% developed vitamin B12 deficiency of undetermined origin within 5 years of metformin use, and 60% within 6 to 10 years; and for those with known causes especially those with PA, 60% within the first 5 years, and 30% within 6 to 10 years. The main determining factor in the latter group of patients was probably the known cause, e.g. PA, and whether metformin use contributed to or hastened the development of vitamin B12 deficiency in these patients is difficult to determine at this stage. Due to the retrospective nature of data collection concerning diabetic control and medications, precise analysis of metformin duration and dose in relation to the development of vitamin B12 deficiency is beyond the capacity of the present study. One practical message is that clinicians should be aware of the development of vitamin B12 deficiency with both short-term and long-term use of metformin ranging from 1 year to beyond 10 years. An equally important message corollary to this is that known causes of vitamin B12 deficiency such as PA occur in diabetic patients as in non-diabetic subjects, and the same diagnostic approach to delineate the underlying cause of vitamin B12 deficiency should be adopted for diabetic patients as for other patients in general.

From the reports in the literature (Table 4), diminished absorption of vitamin B12, manifested as decreased serum B12 levels, occurred as early as 3 to 4 months after the use of metformin (Bauman et al., 2000; Wulffele et al., 2003). Symptomatic deficiency of the vitamin, according to most reports (Table 5), occurred 5 to 10 years after the use of metformin. This is in line with the established knowledge that the body store of vitamin B12 is huge (2500 μg) in comparison to daily loss/requirement (1-2 μg) (Carmel, 2008), and depletion of the pre-existing body store vitamin thus takes 12 to 15 years. The process of exhaustion of body store will be hastened in the presence of other predisposing factors for vitamin B12 deficiency such as partial gastrectomy.

Two recent reports concerning metformin-related vitamin B12 deficiency suggested need for improved management of such patients. The increased risk of vitamin B12 deficiency with metformin use was re-emphasized by a nested case-control study of Chinese patients (Ting et al., 2006). It showed correlation between the dose and duration of metformin use with vitamin B12 deficiency. Compared with those receiving metformin for less than 3 years, the adjusted OR was 2.39 (95% CI, 1.46-3.91) for those using metformin for 3 years or more. After excluding subjects with borderline vitamin B12 concentrations, the metformin dose remained the strongest independent predictor of vitamin B12 deficiency. Each 1-g/day increment in metformin dose conferred an OR of 2.88 (95% CI, 2.15-3.87) of developing vitamin B12 deficiency. In a prospective randomized placebo controlled trial, the Dutch scientists found the fall in serum B12 levels with metformin persists and becomes more apparent with time (Stehouwer et al., 2010). It is reasonable to assume that harm will eventually occur in some patients with metformin-induced low vitamin B12 levels.

4.2.3 Treatment of metformin-induced vitamin B12 deficiency

There is no consensus on optimal treatment of metformin-induced vitamin B12 deficiency. In the present study, metformin was continued unless there were other reasons for discontinuation or switching to other anti-diabetic therapy such as renal insufficiency or poor glycaemic control. Vitamin B12 replacement was given intramuscularly, daily, monthly, and then 3-monthly as maintenance. Most authors of the case reports/series (Table 5) treated their patients' metformin-induced megaloblastic anaemia with vitamin B12 either orally or parenterally at 1000 μg daily or on alternate days initially, and continued metformin therapy (Callaghan et al., 1980; Andres el al., 2002; Filioussi et al., 2003). In all these cases the anaemia responded but the neuropathy of one patient persisted (Bell, 2010).

In general, two aspects of treatment have to be considered. Vitamin B12 replacement is mandatory and can be given either intramuscularly or orally. Parenteral route may be preferred for subjects with neurological deficits due to the potential risk of irreversibility. The rationale for oral vitamin B12 replacement is that there is evidence for an alternative pathway of vitamin B12 absorption that does not require IF or the presence of an intact ileum (Berlin et al., 1968; Kuzminski et al., 1998; Andres et al., 2008). For both routes of administration, large doses of crystalline cobalamin in the range of 1000 μg should be given. The duration of vitamin B12 supplementation depends on the removal of the triggering factor. If metformin is continued, appropriate vitamin B12 replacement should be administered. Although malabsorption of vitamin B12 is reversible 2 to 8 weeks after stopping metformin therapy (NeLM, 2005), withdrawal of metformin is not mandatory in view of its efficacy and safety, and most of the complications of vitamin B12 deficiency are remediable apart from irreversible damage to the central and peripheral nervous system which may occur if treatment is delayed.

Up to now, the mechanism of metformin-related vitamin B12 malabsorption is still not fully understood. Metformin causes fall in blood glucose primarily through suppression of hepatic gluconeogenesis, enhancement of insulin sensitivity, and reduction of gastrointestinal absorption of glucose. This action is achieved through reduction of efficiency of ion exchange across cell membranes which is brought about through activation of AMP-activated protein kinase and perhaps other enzymes. This mode of action also underlies the untoward side effects of increased intestinal motility and lactic acidosis. Whether the process of malabsorption of vitamin B12 is also similarly mediated is unclear. Currently the most likely mechanism is impaired uptake of vitamin B12-intrinsic factor complex at the ileal cell membrane receptors. This uptake has been shown to be a calcium dependent process (Bauman et al., 2000). The hydrophobic tail of metformin extends into the hydrocarbon core of cell membrane and the protonated metformin group gives a positive charge to the membrane surface and displaces divalent cations. Thus by altering the membrane potentials and affecting the divalent cation membrane functions, especially those calcium-dependent ones, metformin may act as a calcium channel blocker. This postulation is supported by studies showing reversal of malabsorption by increasing calcium intake (Bauman et al., 2000). Other studies showed the malabsorption might be related to decreased IF secretion (Adams et al., 1983), or delay in intestinal transit and bacterial overgrowth in diabetic patients. Some studies however failed to show bacterial overgrowth in such patients (Bauman et al., 2000). Further research is required to clarify the mode of metformin-induced malabsorption of vitamin B12.

4.3 Future direction

The prevalence of vitamin B12 deficiency is expected to increase with time in view of the ageing population and the more widespread use of sensitive metabolite assays to detect subtle cobalamin deficiency. Among the population over the age of 60, the prevalence of metabolically confirmed vitamin B12 deficiency ranges from 12% to 23% (Pennypacker et al., 1992; Lindenbaum et al., 1994; Johnson et al., 2003). Type 2 diabetes, at the same time, is becoming more common almost everywhere in the world. The global prevalence of type 2 diabetes is 2.8% (171 million people) in 2000 (Wild et al., 2004), 6.6% (285 million) in 2010, and will be reaching 7.8% (438 million) in 2030 (The Diabetes Atlas, 2009). The global prevalence of age-standardized adult diabetes, according to a recent large international study, was 9.8% (8.6-11.2) for men, and 9.2% (8.0-10.5) for women in 2008 (Danaei et al., 2011). In Hong Kong, the prevalence of type 2 diabetes in elderly subjects above the age of 60 is estimated to range between 9.8% (Woo et al., 1987) and 10.7% (Kung et al., 1996), and the age-standardized prevalence of type 2 diabetes for the 35-64 age group was 9.5% for men and 10.2% for women (Lam et al., 2000).

(new paragraph) Concerning anti-diabetic therapy, metformin remains one of the two oral anti-diabetic drugs in the WHO model list of essential medicine in 2010, in spite of a large array of new therapeutic agents available in the pharmaceutical market. It is the only anti-diabetic drug that has been conclusively shown to prevent the cardiovascular complications of diabetes. The drug remains active after months or years of therapy and its efficacy is little dependent on the residual effective β-cell mass. It causes less weight gain and fewer hypoglycaemic attacks compared with sulphonylureas and insulin. It is now recommended as the initial therapy for type 2 diabetes by the National Institute for Health and Clinical Excellence of the United Kingdom, the American Diabetes Association, and the European Association for the Study of Diabetes. As metformin has been available in the United Kingdom since 1958, in Canada since 1972, in the United States since 1995, and for over 40 years in Hong Kong, the pool of diabetic patients with metformin-induced vitamin B12 deficiency, diagnosed or undiagnosed, could be considerable in the present era. Concomitant occurrence of two comorbid conditions, diabetes and vitamin B12 deficiency, in one subject is apparently undesirable. Florid deficiency of vitamin B12 is accompanied and actually preceded by reciprocal rise of homocysteine levels imposing an increased risk of cardiovascular complications (Hoogeveen et al., 2000; The Homocysteine Studies Collaboration, 2002). Neurological deficits, one of the major manifestations of vitamin B12 deficiency can often be diagnostically confused with diabetic neuropathy, one of the long-term microangiopathic complicaitons of diabetes. Clinicians should therefore have a high index of suspicion for metformin-induced vitamin B12 deficiency in diabetic patients.

To prevent vitamin B12 deficiency, it is reasonable to consider formulating appropriate screening strategy for diabetic patients on metformin. According to the WHO's criteria, a condition is worthwhile screening if it is an important health problem, if there are simple tests available to detect the condition at an early and treatable stage, and if effective and safe treatment is available (Wilson & Junger, 1968). The condition of vitamin B12 deficiency fulfills these criteria. Before such screening guidelines are available, appropriate preventive measures may be instituted. These may include monitoring of vitamin B12 levels at regular intervals such as annually or biannually; or giving vitamin B12 prophylactically as dietary supplement or more conveniently as annual injection at 1000 μg, a dose sufficient to cover vitamin B12 needs for at least a year.

5. References

Adams, J.F.; Clark, J.S.; Ireland, J.T.; Kesson, C.M. & Watson, W.S. *Malabsorption of Vitamin B12 and Intrinsic Factor Secretion During Biguanide Therapy*. Diabetologia. (1983); 24:16-18

Ali, T.; Roberts, DN. & Tierney, WM. *Long term safety concerns with proton pump inhibitors*. Am J Med (2009);122(10):896-903.

Andres, E.; Noel, E. & Goichot, B. *Metformin-associated vitamin B12 deficiency*. Arch Intern Med.(2002);162(19):2251-2252.

Andres, E. & Dali-Youcef, N. *An update on cobalamin deficiency in adults*. Q J Med. (2008);102(1):17-28.

Bauman, WA.; Shaw, S.; Jayatilleke, E.; Spungen, AM. & Herbert, V. *Increased intake of calcium reverses vitamin B12 malabsorption induced by metformin*. Diabetes Care (2000);23(9):1227-1231.

Bell David, SH. *Metformin-induced vitamin B12 deficiency presenting as a peripheral neuropathy*. Southern Medical Journal. (2010);103(3):265-267.

Berchtold, P.; Bolli, P.; Arbenz, U. & Keiser, G. *Disturbance of intestinal absorption following metformin therapy (observations on the mode of action of biguanides)*. Diabetologia (1969);5:405-412.

Berlin, H.; Berlin, R. & Brante, G. *Oral treatment of pernicious anemia with high doses of vitamin B12 without intrinsic factor*. Acta Med Scand. (1968);184(4):247-258

Callaghan, TS.; Hadden, DR. & Tomkin, GH. *Megaloblastic anaemia due to vitamin B12 malabsorption associated with long-term metformin treatment*. BMJ (1980); 280(6225): 1214-1215.

Carmel, R. *How I treat cobalamin (vitamin B12) deficiency*. Blood. (2008);112(6):2214-2221.

Chan, JCW.; Liu, HSY.; Kho, BCS.; Lau, TKH.; Li, VL.; Chan, FHY.; Leong, IS.; Pang, HK.; Lee, CK. & Liang, YS. *Longitudinal study of Chinese patients with pernicious anaemia*. Postgrad Med J (2008);84(998):644-650.

Chan, J. & Chan, HYF. *Usefulness of thyrogastric immune features as predictors of pernicious anaemia that lacks intrinsic factor antibody*. Int. Jnl. Lab. Hem (2011);33:400-408

Clarke, R. & Brown DL. *Vitamin B12 deficiency*. Am Fam Physician. (2003);67(5):979-986.

Danaei, G.; Finucane, MM.; Lu, Y.; Singh, GM.; Cowan, MJ.; Paciorek, CJ.; Lin, JK.; Farzadfar, F.; Khang, YH.; Stevens, GA.; Rao, M.; Ali, MK.; Riley, LM.; Robinson, CA.; Ezzati, M.; Global Burden of Metabolic Risk Factors of Chronic Diseases Collaborating Group (Blood Glucose). *National, regional, and global trends in fasting plasma glucose and diabetes prevalence since 1980: systematic analysis of health examination surveys and epidemiological studies with 370 country-years and 2.7 million participants*. Lancet (2011); 378(9785): 31-40.

de Jager, J.; Kooy, A.; Lehert, P.; Wulffele, MG.; van der Kolk, J.; Bets, D.; Verburg, J.; Donker, AJM. & Stehouwer, CDA. *Long term treatment with metformin in patients with type 2 diabetes and risk of vitamin B12 deficiency: randomized placebo controlled trial*. BMJ (2010); 340:c2181.

den Elzen, WP.; Groeneveld, Y.; de Ruijter, W.; Souverijn, JH.; le Cessie, S.; Assendelft, WJ. & Gussekloo, J. *Long-term use of proton pump inhibitors and vitamin B12 status in elderly individuals*. Aliment Pharmacol Ther. (2008);27(6):491-497.

Evans, JM.; Donnelly, LA.; Emslie-Smith, AM.; Alessi, DR. & Morris, AD. *Metformin and reduced risk of cancer in diabetic patients.* BMJ. (2005);330(7503):1304-1305.

Filioussi, K.; Bonovas, S. & Katsaros, T. *Should we screen diabetic patients using biguanides for megaloblastic anaemia?* Australian Family Physician (2003);32(5):383-384.

Force, RW.; Meeker, AD.; Cady, PS.; Culbertson, VL.; Force WS. & Kelley, CM. *Ambulatory care increased vitamin B12 requirement associated with chronic acid suppression therapy.* Ann Pharmacother (2003);37(4):490-493.

Gilligan, MA. *Metformin and vitamin B12 deficiency.* Arch Intern Med (2002);162:484-485.

Hermann, LS.; Nilsson, BO. & Wettre, S. *Vitamin B12 status of patients treated with metformin: a cross-sectional cohort study.* Br J Diabetes Vasc Dis (2004);4:401-406.

Hirschowitz, BI.; Worthington, J. & Mohnen, J. *Vitamin B12 deficiency in hypersecretors during long-term acid suppression with proton pump inhibitors.* Aliment Pharmacol Ther. (2008);27(11):1110-1121.

Hoogeveen EK.; Kostense, PJ.; Jakobs, C.; Dekker, JM.; Nijpels, G.; Heine, RJ.; Bouter, LM. & Stehouwer, CD. *Hyperhomocysteinemia increases risk of death, especially in type 2 diabetes: 5-year follow-up of the Hoorn Study.* Circulation. (2000);101(13):1506-1511.

Howden, CW. *Vitamin B12 levels during prolonged treatment with proton pump inhibitors.* Journal of Clinical Gastroenterology. (2000);30(1):29-33.

Johnson, MA.; Hawthorne, NA.; Brackett, WR.; Fischer, JG.; Gunter, EW.; Allen, RH. & Stabler, SP. *Hyperhomocysteinemia and vitamin B12 deficiency in elderly using Title IIIc nutrition services.* Am J Clin Nutr (2003);77:211-220.

Kung, AWC.; Janus, ED. & Lau, C. *The prevalence of diabetes mellitus and its effect in elderly subjects in Hong Kong.* Hong Kong Med J (1996);2:26-33.

Kuzminski, AM.; Del Giacco, EJ.; Allen, RH.; Stabler, SP. & Lindenbaum, J. *Effective treatment of cobalamin deficiency with oral cobalamin. Blood.* (1998);92(4):1191-1198.

Lam, TH.; Liu, LJ.; Janus, ED.; Lam, KS.; Hedley, AJ. *Fibrinogen, other cardiovascular risk factors and diabetes mellitus in Hong Kong: a community with high prevalence of type 2 diabetes mellitus and impaired glucose tolerance,* Diabet. Med. (2000);17 (11): 798–806.

Lin, HY.; Chung, CY.; Chang, CS.; Wang, ML.; Lin, JS. & Shen, MC. *Hyperhomocysteinemia, deep vein thrombosis and vitamin B12 deficiency in a metformin-treated diabetic patient.* J Formos Med Assoc. (2007);106(9):774-778.

Lindenbaum, J.; Rosenberg, IH.; Wilson, P.; Stabler, SP. & Allen, RH. *Prevalence of cobalamin deficiency in the Framingham elderly population.* Am J Clin Nutr (1994);60:2-11.

Liu, KW.; Dai, LK. & Woo, J. *Metformin-related vitamin B12 deficiency.* Age and Ageing (2006);35(2):200-201.

Marcuard, SP.; Albernaz, L. & Khazanie, PG. *Omeprazole therapy causes malabsorption of cyanocobalamin (vitamin B12).* Ann Intern Med. (1994);120(3):211-215.

NeLM. (2005) *What effect does metformin have on vitamin B12 levels?* http://www.druginfozone.nhs.uk/Record%20Viewing/viewRecord.aspx?id=560841

Nervo, M.; Lubini, A.; Raimundo, FV.; Faulhaber, GA.; Leite, C.; Fischer, LM. & Furlanetto, TW. *Vitamin B12 in metformin-treated diabetic patients: a cross-sectional study in Brazil.* Rev Assoc Med Bras. (2011);57(1):46-49.

Pflipsen, MC.; Robert, C.; Saguil, A.; Seebusen, DA.; Seaquist, D. & Topolski, R. *The Prevalence of Vitamin B12 Deficiency in Patients with Type 2 Diabetes: A Cross-Sectional Study.* J Am Board Fam Med (2009);22:528-534

Pennypacker, LC.; Allen, RH.; Kelly, JP.; Matthews, J. & Stabler, SP. *High prevalence of cobalamin deficiency in elderly populations.* J Am Geriatr Soc (1992);40:1197-1204.

Pongchaidecha, M.; Srikusalanukul, V.; Chattananon, A. & Tanjariyaporn, S. *Effect of metformin on plasma homocysteine, vitamin B12 and folic acid: a cross-sectional study in patients with type 2 diabetes mellitus.* J Med Assoc Thai. (2004);87(7):780-787.

Ruscin, JM. Page RL 2nd, Valuck, RJ. *Vitamin B12 deficiency associated with histamine (2)-receptor antagonists and a proton-pump inhibitor.* Ann Pharmacother. (2002); 36(5):812-816.

Sahin, M.; Tutuncu, NB.; Ertugrul, D.; Tanaci, N. & Guvener, ND. *Effects of metformin or rosiglitazone on serum concentrations of homocysteine, folate, and vitamin B12 in patients with type 2 diabetes mellitus.* J Diabetes Complications. (2007);21(2):118-123.

Steinberg, WM.; King, CE. & Toskes, PP. *Malabsorption of protein-bound cobalamin but not unbound cobalamin during cimetidine administration.* Dig Dis Sci. (1980);25(3):188-191.

Termanini, B.; Gibril, F.; Sutliff, VE.; Yu, F.; Venzon, DJ. & Jensen, RT. *Effect of long-term gastric acid suppressive therapy on serum vitamin B12 levels in patients with Zollinger-Ellison syndrome.* Am J Med. (1998);104(5):422-430.

The Diabetes Atlas. International Diabetes Federation. Third Edition. Brussels: International Diabetes Federation; 2009.

The Homocysteine Studies Collaboration. *Homocysteine and risk of ischemic heart disease and stroke.* JAMA. (2002);288(16):2015-2022.

Thomas, AB.; Sauve, MD.; Kassam, N. & Kamitakahara, H. *Safety of the long-term use of proton pump inhibitors.* World J Gastroenterol.(2010);16(19):2323-2330.

Ting, RZW.; Szeto, CC.; Chan, MHM.; Ma, KK. & Chow, KM. *Risk factors of vitamin B12 deficiency in patients receiving metformin.* Arch Intern Med (2006);166(18):1975-1979.

Tomkin, GH.; Hadden, DR.; Weaver, JA. & Montgomery, DAD. *Vitamin-B12 status of patients on long-term metformin therapy.* BMJ (1971); 2(5763): 685-687.

UK Prospective Diabetes Study Group: *Effect of intensive blood-glucose control with metformin on complications in overweight patients with type 2 diabetes (UKPDS 34).* Lancet (1998); 352(9131):854-865.

Wild, S.; Roglic, G.; Green, A.; Sicree, R. & King, H. *Global prevalence of diabetes: estimates for 2000 and projections for 2030.* Diabetes Care. (2004);27(5):1047–1053.

Wile, Daryl. & Toth, Cory. *Association of metformin, elevated homocysteine, and methylmalonic acid levels and clinically worsened diabetic peripheral neuropathy.* Diabetes Care (2010); 33(1):156-161.

Wilson, JMG. & Junger, G. *Principles and practice of screening for disease.* Geneva, Switzerland: World Health Organization; (1968);65(4):281-393.

Woo, J.; Swaminathan, R.; Cockram, C.; Pang, CP.; Mak, YT.; Au, SY. & Vallance-Owen, J. *The prevalence of diabetes mellitus and an assessment of methods of detection among a community of elderly Chinese in Hong Kong.* Diabetologia (1987);30(11):863-868.

World Health Organization, *Definition, Diagnosis and Classification of Diabetes Mellitus and its Complications, Report of a WHO Consultation. Part 1.* Diagnosis and Classification of

Diabetes Mellitus, Geneva, Department of Noncommunicable Disease Surveillance, (1999).

Wulffele, MG.; Kooy, A.; Lehert, P.; Bets, D.; Ogterop, JC.; Borger Van Der Burg, B.; Donker, AJM. & Stehouwer, CDA. *Effects of short-term treatment with metformin on serum concentrations of homocysteine, folate and vitamin B12 in type 2 diabetes mellitus: a randomized, placebo-controlled trial.* Journal of Internal Medicine (2003);254(5):455-463.

11

Assessment of Microcirculation and the Prediction of Healing in Diabetic Foot Ulcers

Jarrod Shapiro and Aksone Nouvong
Western University of Health Sciences, College of Podiatric Medicine
United States of America

1. Introduction

Globally, diabetes mellitus has grown to pandemic proportions, affecting 194 million people worldwide and is expected to increase in prevalence to 344 million by the year 2030 (Wild, et al., 2004). Of these patients, between 2 and 6% will develop a diabetic foot ulcer (DFU) yearly (Ramsey, et al., 1999). The onset of a DFU often precipitates a complex chain of events that may lead to limb loss. Infected DFUs account for 20% of hospital visits for this patient population (Bouter, et al. 1993) and precede roughly 85% of lower extremity amputations in patients with diabetes (Pecoraro, et al. 1990). The long-term outcome for a diabetic patient after a major limb amputation is grave with 50% of these patients deceased at 5 years (Moulik, et al. 2003). Additionally, the cost to treat this disease places a significant strain on the health-care system. The cost to manage these foot disorders is estimated at several billion dollars annually (Wild, et al. 2004), while the individual cost of a major limb amputation is estimated at almost $45,000 (Apelqvist, et al. 1994). With the combination of excessive cost to treat diabetes complications coupled with the major detrimental health effects on individual patients, it is necessary to develop and employ new technological methods to predict healing of diabetic foot ulcers.

Once a diabetic patient develops a pedal ulceration it becomes incumbent on the physician to evaluate the ulcer's healing potential. Much research has focused on the prediction of diabetic foot ulcer healing. Clinically, it has been shown that a 50% decrease in area over a 4-week period with standard wound care adequately predicts ulcer healing at 12 weeks (Sheehan, et al., 2003). The disadvantage of this method, however, is the delay in treatment that occurs as a result of the natural time deferment in this process. As such, newer technologies have utilized the determination of microcirculation to predict ulcer healing. This chapter focuses on the application of these new technologies to determine microvascular circulation and predict diabetic foot ulcer healing.

Large artery (macrocirculatory) disease has been well documented elsewhere with disease at the infrapopliteal region (Bembi, et al. 2006) causing loss of tissue perfusion and critical limb ischemia and gangrene. Various noninvasive vascular testing modalities exist to determine large vessel luminal disease. These include dual mode ultrasound, segmental leg pressures, ankle brachial indices, pulse volume recordings, toe pressures, and toe brachial indices. The above tests have been found to yield useful clinical data regarding large vessel disease and often function as safe precursors to more advanced imaging techniques such as magnetic resonance arteriography. These methods also assist with surgical revascularization planning. However, the options for assessment of microvascular disease are comparatively sparse. This chapter will focus on the following noninvasive modalities to evaluate microvascular disease and predict ulcer healing: Transcutaneous Oxygen Pressure, Skin Perfusion Pressure, Laser Speckle Perfusion Imaging, and Hyperspectral Imaging.

2. Peripheral arterial disease and the pathophysiology of microvascular disease in diabetes

The pathogenesis of macrocirculatory disease has been discussed in depth elsewhere. Microcirculation includes the capillaries, arterioles, and venules. These microvessels are arranged in two horizontal network patterns with a superficial subpapillary plexus and a deeper cutaneous plexus with capillary blood flow providing nutrition and arteriovenous shunts that serve a thermoregulatory function (Chao & Cheing, 2009). The nutritional capillaries are organized into functional units within the papillary layer of the dermis. A precapillary sphincter is situated just upstream of the capillary which controls vasodilation and constriction (LaFontaine, et al., 2006). Arteriovenous anastomoses exist between the arterioles and venules to allow normal shunting of blood under physiologic conditions. The internal vessel lumen is lined with a single-layer-thick endothelium. This endothelium lies on a basement membrane which is normally thicker in the foot than other body locations due to the increased hydrostatic pressure associated with stance (LaFontaine, et al., 2006). Blood flow to the skin runs through this arteriovenous system supplying nutrition, oxygen, and regulating temperature through an increase or decrease of blood flow to the dermal papilla.

Blood flow to the skin is controlled by the peripheral sympathetic nervous system via vasodilatory cholinergic and vasoconstrictor adrenergic nerve fibers (Chao & Cheing, 2009) as well as vasoactive substances such as nitric oxide. Additionally, the endothelial basement membrane regulates blood flow and the local inflammatory response via vasoactive substances (Guerci, et al. 2001).

The pathogenesis of microvascular disease in diabetics is complex and multifactorial. Hyperglycemia is considered the most important risk factor (LaFontaine, et al., 2006) and is noted to occur in two stages, a reversible functional stage and a structural adaptation and remodeling stage leading to a thickened basement membrane and capillary failure (LaFontaine, et al., 2006). The hemodynamic hypothesis of microangiopathic disease was first described by Parving, et al (Parving, et al. 1983). Blood flow dysregulation, caused by neuropathic changes to the sympathetic nerve fibers, is mediated by hyperglycemia. The resulting stimulation of the polyol pathway decreases nitric oxide production, increasing blood flow and capillary pressure. This increased pressure leads to thickening of the basement membrane which resists vasodilation and increases capillary permeability with ensuing chronic edema.

A second mechanism that has gained experimental support is the "capillary steal syndrome" (Uccioli, et al. 1992). This is thought to result from sympathetic denervation with chronic vasodilation, resulting in an increased blood flow through the arteriovenous shunt away from the arterioles in the papillary dermis. As blood moves more rapidly toward the postcapillary venule, nutrition, metabolite, and oxygen exchange are significantly reduced (Boulton, et al, 1982).

It is unknown which pathway is dominant or if another mechanism is responsible, though there is most likely a combination of both pathogenic pathways that end with functional ischemia, reduced nutritional capacity, and increased metabolic end products that function together to limit healing capacity in the face of skin ulceration.

3. Current methods to assess healing potential in diabetic foot ulcers

Large vessel disease is evaluated through several noninvasive methods including dual mode ultrasound, segmental leg pressures, ankle brachial indices, pulse volume recordings, toe pressures, toe brachial indices, magnetic resonance angiography, and computed tomographic angiography. However, these modalities only characterize blockages of large arteries and do not assist with prediction of direct wound healing on the lower extremity. Contemporary microvascular technologies utilize the above pathogenic principles to evaluate microangiopathic changes and predict ulcer healing. The following discussion will review the currently available methods to clinically assess microvascular blood flow and predict the healing potential of diabetic foot ulcers.

4. Transcutaneous oxygen pressure

Physiology of test. Transcutaneous oxygen pressure (TcPO2) measures excess oxygen diffusion from red blood cells as they pass through the capillary circulation. This pressure reflects the metabolic state of the adjacent interstitial spaces. TcPO2 is measured via electrochemical reduction at a cathode placed against the skin.
Method. Transcutaneous oxygen pressures are measured by placing a heated probe against the skin. The standard 44 degrees Celsius causes vasodilation and a local reactive hyperthermia (Figures 1 and 2). Oxygen defusing across the skin and toward the cathode in the probe is reduced. This reduction is proportional to the number of oxygen molecules (Mathieu and Mani 2007) and is measured as oxygen pressure. Common locations of measurement include the dorsum of the foot, anteromedial calf approximately 10 cm below the patella, and the thigh 10 cm above the patella. The subclavicular region is often used as a reference point due to its close anatomic location to coronary perfusion and low likelihood of arterial insufficiency. Pressure measurements may be enhanced by having the patient exercise, increasing the metabolic demand and need for oxygen. Placing the leg in a dependent position additionally augments oxygenation, providing further information about the arterial reserves available. TcPO2 measurement may also be performed in patients in which arterial claudication is suspected. In this situation normal oxygen metabolic demands are sufficiently supplied. However, when stress is applied to the extremity, oxygen demands increase and exceed the oxygen supplied by the now insufficient arterial flow (Franzeck, et al. 1982). To test this, transcutaneous oxygen tension measurements may be performed while the patient exercises. It is also important to consider that resting TcPO2 measurement is more likely to diagnose disease in more severe occlusions due to the lack of metabolic demand when the patient is at rest during the examination. Byrne, et al. compared transcutaneous oxygen measurement with angiography. They found TcPO2 to have a sensitivity of 100% following exercise but falling to 77% at rest (Byrne, et al. 1984). This striking drop in sensitivity argues for standard exercise TcPO2 testing.
Interpretation of Findings. Normal limb TcPO2 values are 50- 60mmHg, though values greater than 55mmHg at any site regardless of age are considered normal (Cina, et al, 1984). Wound healing is considered unimpaired at pressures less than 40mmHg (White, et al. 1982). Pressures of 20mmHg are seen in legs with rest pain, ischemic ulcers, and/or gangrene, while pressures below 20mmHg usually require amputation (Oh, et al. 1987) (Table 1).

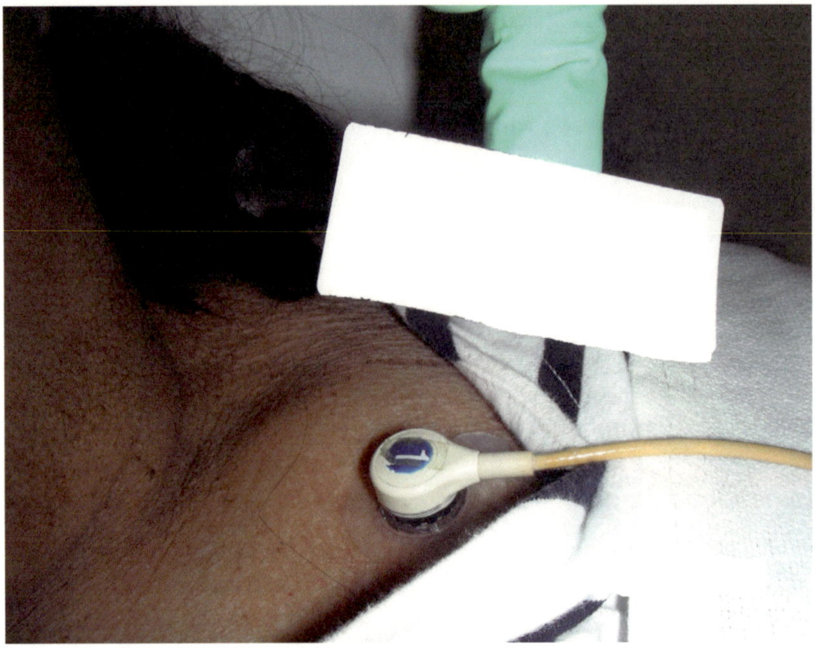

(a)

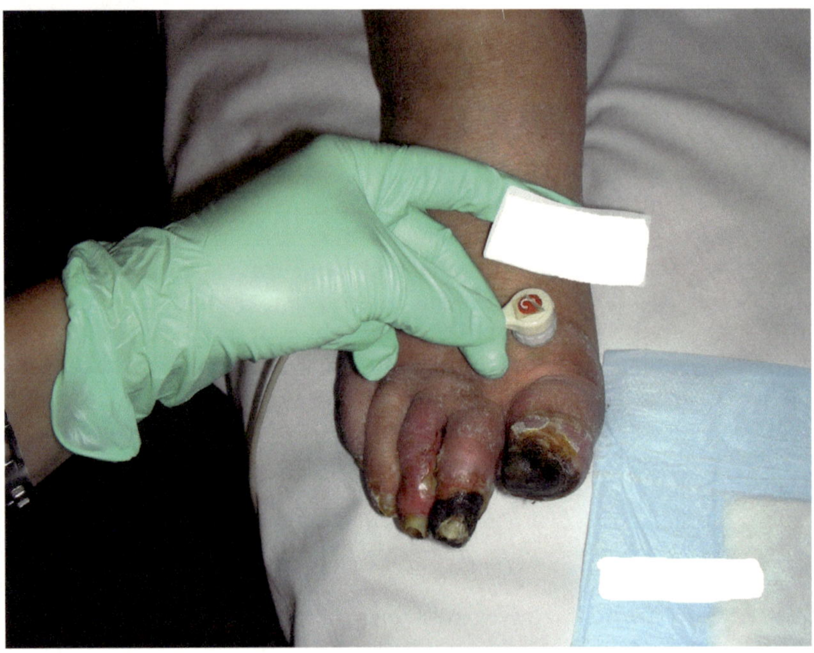

(b)

Fig. 1. Transcutaneous oximetry measurement technique. (a) chest and (b) foot.
Courtesy of Casa Colina Centers for Rehabilitation Wound Care and Hyperbaric Medicine Program.

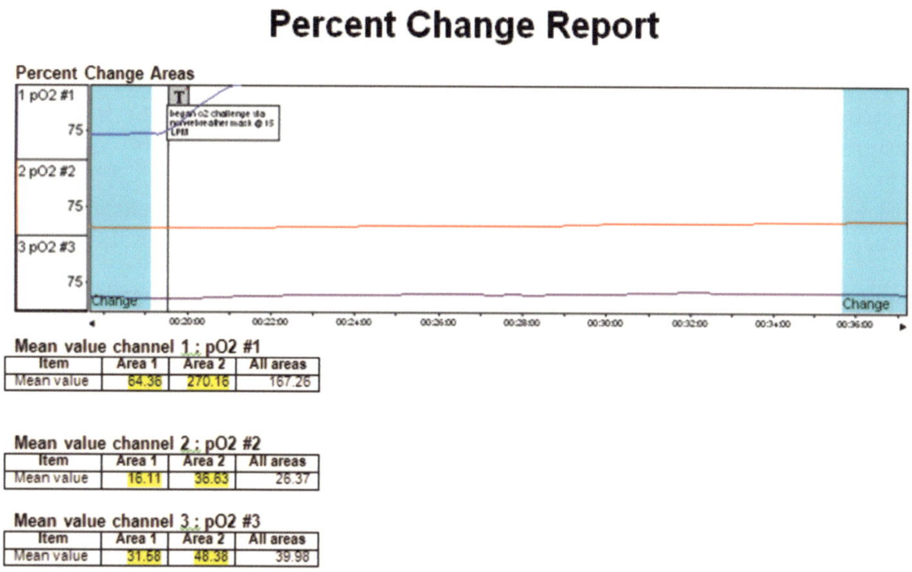

Fig. 2. Standard TCPO2 report. Courtesy of Casa Colina Centers for Rehabilitation Wound Care and Hyperbaric Medicine Program.

TcPO2 Value	Interpretation
>50 mmHg	Normal
40mmHg	Unimpaired wound healing
<30 mmHg	Impaired wound healing
20mmHg	Predicted rest pain, ischemic ulceration, gangrene.
<20mmHg	Amputation likely

Table 1. Transcutaneous oxygen values and associated clinical interpretation.

As noted above, TcPO2 measurement is most clinically relevant for assessing oxygenation in patients with more advanced arterial occlusion or performing the test with exercise. Additionally, since the results are not affected by sclerosis of the tunica media of arteries this is a viable test in patients with diabetes and renal disease (Hauser, et al. 1984). TcPO2 may also be used in conjunction with hyperbaric oxygen therapy.

Several limitations exist with the use of TcPO2. TcPO2 cannot be measured under certain physical conditions (edema, dry flaky skin, maceration, callused or plantar skin, cellulitis, or skin over bones and tendons) (Dooley, et al. 1996). These conditions tend to decrease the sensitivity of the probe to detect skin perfusion. Since the electrode probe is placed on intact adjacent skin rather than directly on the wound itself this method does not measure oxygen tension within the wound. The need to warm the extremity causes temperature differences between sites and subjects leading to false readings. TcPO2 is reliable in the normal but not in the low range, resulting in a high false positive rate for critical limb ischemia (Byrne, et al. 1984). Mechanical pressures on the electrode alter the TcPO2 value. Additionally, a significant amount of time is necessary to obtain pressure measurements with calibration, sensor maintenance and skin preparation delaying a reliable reading upwards of 45 minutes. TcPO2 is therefore site restrictive and operator sensitive.

Ulcer healing predictive value. TcPO2 has a wound healing predictive accuracy of 83% and is unaffected by diabetic status or chronic renal failure (Padberg, et al., 1996). In reference to the appropriate time to perform lower extremity salvage surgery using TcPO2 measurements after surgical intervention for arterial occlusion, Arroyo et al. found an optimal waiting period of at least three days and preferably one week before intervention (Arroyo, et al. 2002). In regards to predicting amputation healing Katsamouris and colleagues found that a level of 40mmHg at the anterior skin surface was predictive of successful healing after partial foot and lower leg amputations (Katsamouris, et al. 1984). Similarly, Ballard and colleagues successfully used TcPO2 measurements to determine the severity of foot ischemia and guide treatment. They found that a transmetatarsal TcPO2 level of 30mmHg or greater successfully predicted healing with conservative care in 31/36 (86%) of diabetic patients (Ballard, et al. 1995).

5. Skin perfusion pressure

Physiology of test. Skin perfusion pressure (SPP) utilizes a laser doppler and pressure cuff to evaluate reactive hyperemia. SPP measures the pressure at which blood flow first returns to the capillary during the controlled release of occlusive pressure.

Method. A laser sensor is placed on the desired location while a pressure cuff is placed at the ankle. The cuff is inflated until occlusion of the arterial flow to the extremity occurs and is then released. As arteriolar flow is restored and the subsequent reactive hyperemia occurs, the laser sensor reads the resulting arteriolar pressures.

Interpretation of Findings. Skin perfusion pressures greater than 40mmHg are considered non-ischemic while marginal ischemia is noted between 30 and 40mmHg. The wound is unlikely to heal below a pressure of 30mmHg (Castronuovo, et al., 1997).

The advantages of SPP are the following: it can be used in the presence of edema and in the plantar foot, no calibration is needed, no maintenance is required, no skin warming is necessary, and it is faster than TcPO2 measurement (2-3 minutes per site).

The limitations of SPP are that it provides data regarding the limited area of skin under the sensor. Multiple separate readings are necessary to obtain a global understanding of pedal microvasculature.

Ulcer healing predictive value. SPP predicts a 90% healing ability above 30mmHg (Castronuovo, et al., 1997) and has a 100% negative predictive value (Adera, et al. 1995). In patients with critical limb ischemia SPP was 80% accurate in diagnosing this condition (Castronuovo, et al., 1997). Similarly, Faris and colleagues found SPP was useful in predicting healing of ulcers or gangrene of the feet in 35 of 40 diabetic patients with levels above 40mmHg. Conversely healing was unlikely if the SPP was less than 40mmHg (Faris, et al. 1985). Yamada, et al. studied a larger cohort of 211 patients with ischemic limbs. However, this cohort was not restricted to diabetic patients alone. As with the above mentioned studies, this group also found a threshold of 40mmHg as predictive of healing ulceration or gangrene but with a slightly lower sensitivity and specificity (72% and 88%, respectively) (Yamada, et al. 2008). In 85 limbs of 71 patients referred to a vascular laboratory, skin perfusion pressure measurement was found to correlate closely with toe pressure measurements (Tsai, et al. 2000), allowing substitution of SPP for toe pressures. This is a significant benefit in certain circumstances since it may be impractical to determine toe pressures due to the commonality of wounds on the toes.

6. Hyperspectral Imaging (HSI)

Physiology of test. Skin with wounds requires a greater amount of oxygen, without which healing will not occur. Hence, both oxygen delivery (measured by oxyhemoglobin) and oxygen extraction (measured by deoxyhemoglobin) into the wounded tissue can function as indicators of a wound's capacity to heal. This is done with the use of hyperspectral imaging (CombiVu-R System, HyperMed, Waltham, MA) which uses a spectral separator to vary the wavelength of light admitted to a detector. Red blood cells in the skin are struck with this variable light which is reflected back toward the detector. Since the wavelengths of light absorbed and emitted by oxygenated red blood cells (RBCs with oxyhemoglobin) differs by that emitted by deoxygenated red blood cells (RBCs with deoxyhemoglobin) the machine is able to detect the respective levels of these molecules with a high level of accuracy (Gillies, et al 2003, Greenman, et al. 2005). The data is then compared using a computer with standardized data for these molecules, and an image is provided with a color bar legend for comparison, and colored scans are used to demonstrate levels of oxygenation (Gilles, et al. 2003).

Method. Patients are placed supine, and scans are obtained from various areas of the lower extremity, including the wound site. The imaging technology does not require contact with the skin. An approximately 30 second scan is obtained at a 12 inch distance from the site in question. Images are displayed on a computer screen with a color bar for comparison. Oxyhemoglobin levels are associated with varying colors while deoxyhemoglobin is demonstrated by varying levels of brightness. Numerical values are also placed on the color bar, measured in AUs (astronomical units) (Figures 3 and 4).

Interpretation of Findings. A healing index has been suggested for the use of ulcer healing prediction based on the ratio of oxyhemoglobin to deoxyhemoglobin. Higher levels of both molecules correlate with a greater potential for healing (Khaodhiar, et al., 2007). In general a healing index greater than zero predicts an ulcer will heal while a negative healing index demonstrates an ulcer that is unlikely to heal.

Hyperspectral imaging provides multiple advantages including the lack of contact with skin, global examination of lower extremity microvascular supply, immediate accurate ulcer healing prediction, use on glabrous and nonglabrous skin, and ease of use and interpretation with a healing index.

Disadvantages of HSI are that few studies currently exist to fully validate the use of this modality. A thicker border surrounding the wound decreases the ability of HSI to discriminate well from poorly vascularized tissues. It is currently recommended to use a border thickness of 0.5 to 1 cm (Nouvong, et al., 2009).

Ulcer healing predictive value. Khaodhiar and colleagues found the following ulcer healing predictive values in a pilot study of HSI: sensitivity 93%, specificity 86%, positive predictive value 93%, and negative predictive value 86% (Khaodhiar, et al., 2007). A larger prospective clinical study by Nouvong, et al. found similar prediction values of 86% sensitivity, 88% specificity, and 96% positive predictive value (Nouvong, et al., 2009). This modality compares strongly with clinical observations to predict wound healing. Sheehan and colleagues in their study of clinical healing indicators found a 91% sensitivity, 58% specificity, 58% positive predictive value, and 91% negative predictive value using the percent change in area over a four week time period to predict ulcer healing (Sheehan, et al., 2003). Comparing HSI with clinical indicators demonstrates hyperspectral imaging is superior to following the clinical course in predicting the potential healing and nonhealing of diabetic foot ulcers.

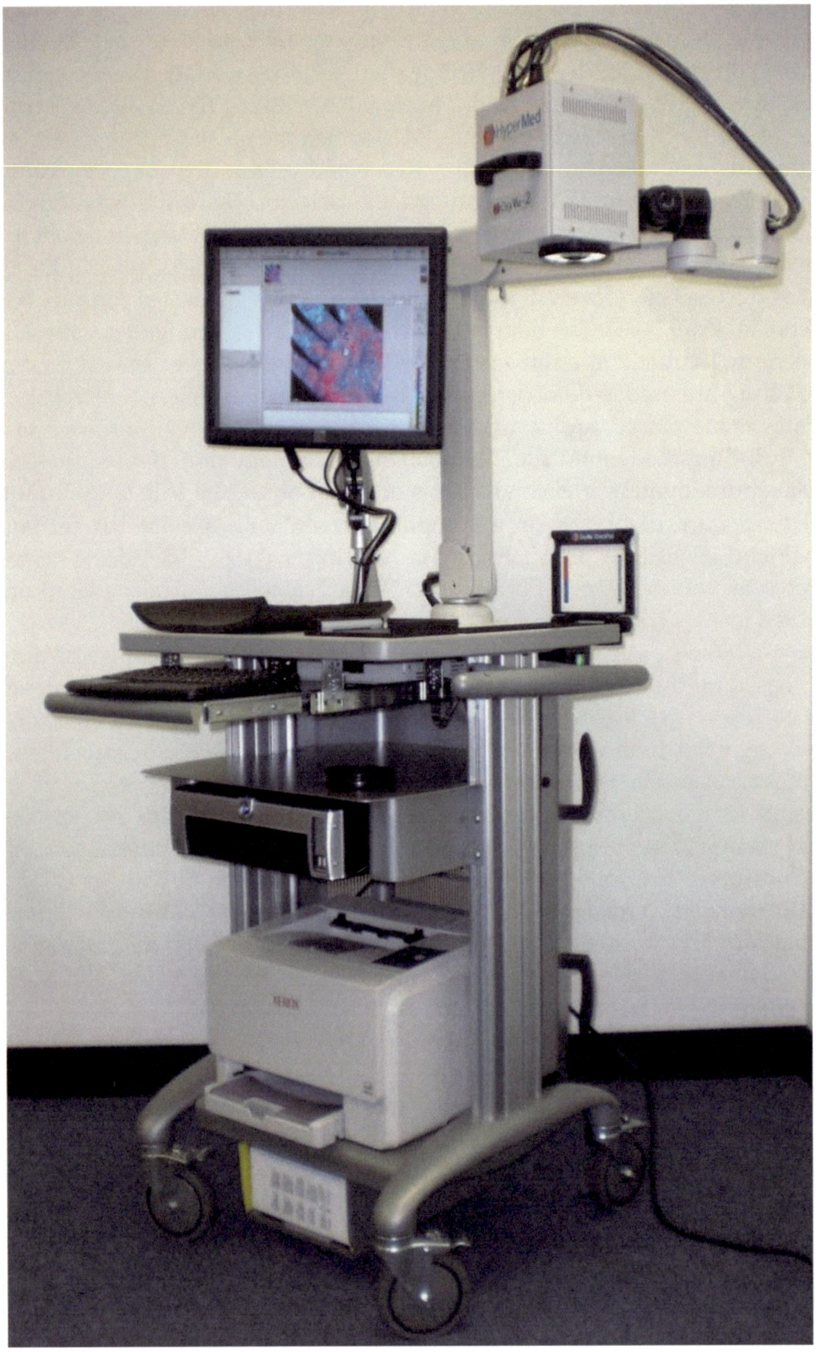

Fig. 3. Hyperspectral imaging system.

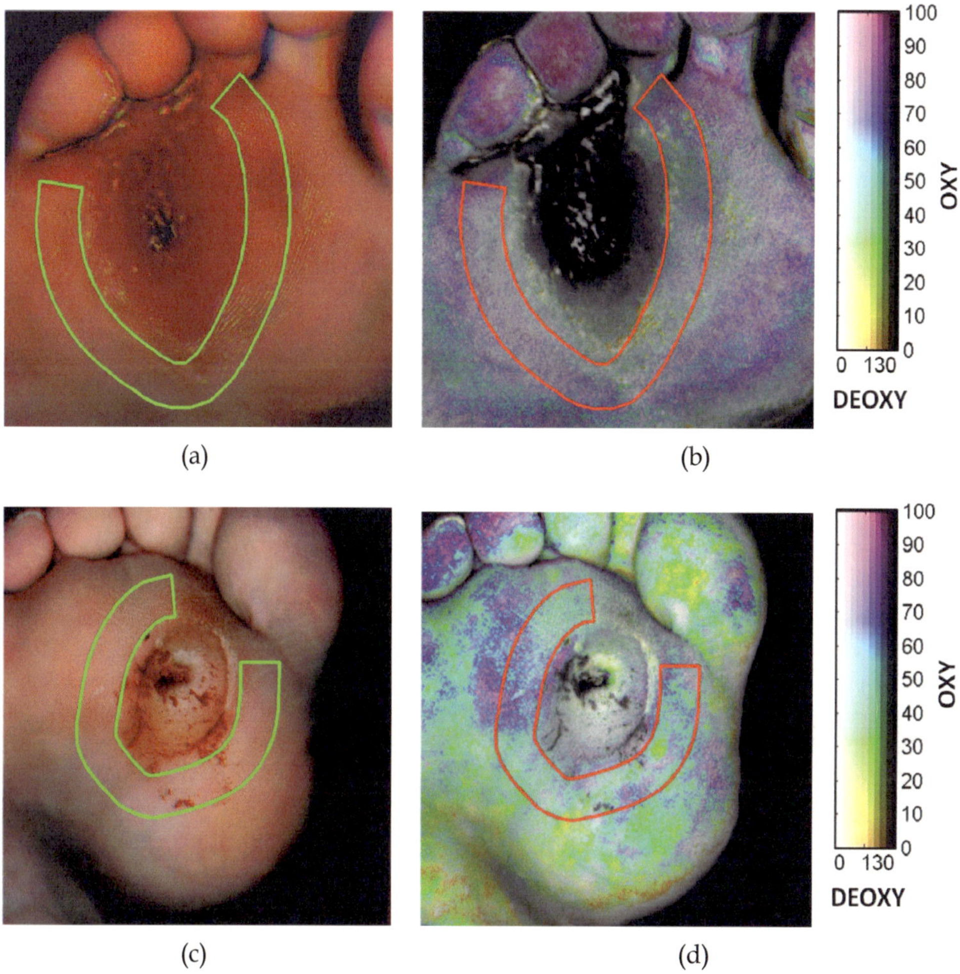

Fig. 4. (a) visible and (b) hyperspectral images of a healing diabetic foot ulcer and (c) visible and (d) hyperspectral images of non-healing diabetic foot ulcer.

7. Future directions for microcirculation testing

The assessment of microangiopathic disease is a new science with early clinical applications. As new technologies are developed physicians will increasingly be able to extract information about the vascular status of potentially ischemic areas while providing a greater understanding of the pathophysiology of the diabetic lower extremity.

Laser Speckle Perfusion Imaging. This new technology employs the principle of laser scatter contrast imaging. In this technique a laser illuminates an area of tissue which produces a backscattered light. This light forms a pattern of light and dark areas called a speckle pattern (Draijer, et al. 2009). In 2007 a new device, the Full-Field Laser Perfusion Imager (FLPI) (Moor Instruments, Essex, UK), was released for commercial use (McGuire & Howdieshell, 2010). This device images skin to a depth no greater than 1 mm and results in images of blood flow within the skin (McGuire and Howdieshell 2010). The presence or absence of blood in the microvasculature indicates the ability to heal. This new technology is advantageous in providing real-time video images of microvascular blood flow (Thompson and Andrews 2010) and represents the potential future ability to view the dynamic microvascular environment within the skin. Future research is necessary to determine the predictive value of laser speckle perfusion imaging in wound healing and amputation level prediction.

8. References

Adera H, et al. Prediction of amputation wound healing with skin perfusion pressure. Journal of Vascular Surgery, May 1995; 21(5): 823-828.

Apelqvist J, et al. Diabetic foot ulcers in a multidisciplinary setting: An economic analysis of primary healing and healing with amputation. Journal of Internal Medicine, May 1994; 235(5): 463-471.

Arroyo C, et al. Optimal waiting period for foot salvage surgery following limb revascularization. Journal of Foot and Ankle Surgery, July 2002; 41(4): 228-232.

Ballard J, et al. A prospective evaluation of transcutaneous oxygen measurements in the management of diabetic foot problems. Journal of Vascular Surgery, Oct 1995; 22(4): 485-492.

Bembi V, et al. Prevalence of peripheral arterial disease in a cohort of diabetic patients. Southern Medical Journal, June 2006; 99(6): 564-569.

Bouter K, et al. The diabetic foot in Dutch hospitals: epidemiological features and clinical outcome. European Journal of Medicine, Apr 1993; 2(4): 215-218.

Byrne P, et al. The use of transcutaneous oxygen tension measurements in the diagnosis of peripheral vascular insufficiency. Annals of Surgery, Aug 1984; 200(2): 159-165.

Cina C, et al. Utility of transcutaneous oxygen tension measurements in peripheral arterial occlusive disease. Journal of Vascular Surgery, Mar 1984; 1(2): 362-371.

Chao C and Cheing G. Microvascular dysfunction in diabetic foot disease and ulceration. Diabetes Metabolism Research and Reviews, 2009; 25: 604-614.

Dooley J, et al. Use of transcutaneous pressure of oxygen in the evaluation of edematous wounds. Undersea Hyperbaric Medicine, Sep 1996; 23(3): 167-174.

Draijer M, et al. Review of laser speckle contrast techniques for visualizing tissue perfusion. Lasers in Medical Science, 2009; 24: 639-651.

Faris I, et al. Skin perfusion pressure in the prediction of healing in diabetic patients with ulcers or gangrene of the foot. Journal of Vascular Surgery, July 1985; 2(4): 536-540.
Franzeck U, et al. Transcutaneous PO2 measurements in health and peripheral arterial occlusive disease. Surgery, Feb 1982; 91(2): 156-163.
Gillies R, et al. Systemic effects of shock and resuscitation monitored by visible hyperspectral imaging. Diabetes Technology and Therapeutics, July 2004; 5(5): 847-855.
Greenman R, et al. Early changes in the skin microcirculation and muscle metabolism of the diabetic foot. Lancet, Nov 2005; 366: 1711-1717.
Guerci B, et al. Endothelial dysfunction and type 2 diabetes. Diabetes Metabolism, 2001; 27(4): 4360447.
Hauser C, et al. Superiority of transcutaneous oximetry in noninvasive vascular diagnosis in patients with diabetes. Archives of Surgery, Jun 1984; 119(6): 690-694.
Katsamouris A, et al. Transcutaneous oxygen tension in selection of amputation level. The American Journal of Surgery, Apr 1984; 147: 510-517.
La Fontaine J, et al. Current concepts in diabetic microvascular dysfunction. Journal of the American Podiatric Medical Association, May 2006; 96(3): 245-252.
Mathieu D and Mani R. A review of the clinical significance of tissue hypoxia measurements in lower extremity wound management. Lower Extremity Wounds, 2007; 6(4): 273-283.Nov 2010; 164(1): e201-e212.
McGuire P and Howdieshell T. The importance of engraftment in flap revascularization: confirmation by laser speckle perfusion imaging. Journal of Surgical Research,
Moulik P, et al. Amputation and mortality in new-onset diabetic foot ulcers stratified by etiology. Diabetes Care, Feb 2003; 26(2): 491-494.
Oh P, et al. The predictability of the success of arterial reconstruction by means of transcutaneous oxygen tension measurements. Journal of Vascular Surgery, Feb 1987; 5(2): 356-362.
Padberg F, et al. Transcutaneous oxygen (TcPO2) estimates probability of healing in the ischemic extremity. Journal of Surgical Research, Feb 1996; 60(2): 365-369.
Parving H, et al. Hemodynamic factors in the genesis of diabetic microangiopathy. Metabolism, Sept 1983; 32(9): 943-949.
Pecoraro R, et al. Pathways to diabetic limb amputation. Basis for prevention. Diabetes Care, May 1990; 13(5): 513-521.
Ramsey, S, et al. Incidence, outcomes, and cost of foot ulcers in patients with diabetes. Diabetes Care, March 1999; 22 (3): 382-387.
Sheehan P, et al. Percent change in wound area of diabetic foot ulcers over a 4-week period is a robust predictor of complete healing in a 12-week prospective trial. Plastic and Reconstructive Surgery, June 2006; 117(7 suppl): 239S-244S.
Thompson O and Andrews M. Tissue perfusion measurements: multiple-exposure laser speckle analysis generates laser Doppler-like spectra. Journal of Biomedical Optics, Mar 2010; 15(2): 027015-1 - 027015-7.
Tsai F, et al. Skin perfusion pressure of the foot is a good substitute for toe pressure in the assessment of limb ischemia. Journal of Vascular Surgery, July 2000; 32(1): 32-36.
Uccioli L, et al. Lower limb arterio-venous shunts, autonomic neuropathy and diabetic foot. Diabetes Research and Clinical Practice, May 1992; 16(2): 123-130.

Wild, S, et al. Global prevalence of diabetes: estimates for the year 2000 and projections for 2030. *Diabetes Care,* May 2004; 27 (5): 1047-1053.

White, et al. Noninvasive evaluation of peripheral vascular disease using transcutaneous oxygen tension. American Journal of Surgery, July 1982; 144(1): 68-75.

Yamada T, et al. Clinical reliability and utility of skin perfusion pressure measurement in ischemic limbs - comparison with other noninvasive diagnostic methods. Journal of Vascular Surgery, Feb 2008; 47(2): 318-323.

12

Association Between the Hypertriglyceridemic-Waist Phenotype in Mothers and in Their Offspring

Valeria Hirschler
Hospital Durand
Argentina

1. Introduction

The hypertriglyceridemic-waist phenotype(Htg-WP), the combination of an increased waist circumference and hypertriglyceridemia, could be a useful and inexpensive screening tool to identify people who are at an increased risk of coronary artery disease and type 2 diabetes. (1-3). The concept of the Htg-WP was introduced by Lemieux and colleagues who suggested that this simple phenotype could be a useful marker for cardiovascular risk and a better predictor of cardiovascular disease. (4)

Imaging studies using techniques such as computed tomography or magnetic resonance imaging have shown that, among equally obese individuals, those with an excess of intra-abdominal or visceral adipose tissue have metabolic abnormalities and are at an increased risk for coronary artery disease and type 2 diabetes (5,6). The systematic measurement of waist circumference has been proposed as a crude anthropometric correlate of intra-abdominal adiposity (7). Because waist circumference cannot fully discriminate intra-abdominal from subcutaneous abdominal adiposity, it has been previously suggested that the presence of elevated triglyceride levels could be used as a marker of metabolic abnormalities in people with an increased waistline(4,8).

An association between parental metabolic syndrome and metabolic syndrome in their offspring has been observed among Korean adolescents (9). Family risk factors include their genetic history as well as their shared environment (9). Parents are in a key position to shape the environments of children, and there is an increasing interest in the contribution of parental behaviors to cardiovascular risk. Maternal feeding practices have received particular attention as a risk factor for childhood OB. A previous study of our group showed that mother's waist circumference predicted their child's metabolic syndrome (10); however, as maternal Htg-WP includes two metabolic disorders, it could increase risk of her child's cardiovascular risk. As far as we know, there are no large studies in elementary school children showing the role that maternal Htg-WP plays in relation to the development of children's Htg-WP. The objective of this study was to determine the association between mothers' Htg-WP and the presence of Htg-WP in their offspring.

2. Methods

Data were collected cross-sectionally from 1009 children between the ages of 5 and 15 years in 6 elementary schools between April 2007 and March 2008. The schools were randomly selected from 42 schools from the west side of Buenos Aires suburbs. Measurement of BMI, waist circumference, blood pressure, and serum glucose, lipids, and insulin were obtained in mothers and their offspring. Given the fact that the prevalence of OW/OB was approximately 33% among children in a similar population (11), the sample size was estimated to achieve that percentage with an error lower than 0.05. The sample size consistent with this error was 340 children. Five hundred and ninety-five children (296 boys) and their mothers were examined, which means that the sample error was less than 0.04.

Exclusion criteria included: missing BMI and blood pressure information, missing lipid profile and glucose information, not being the biological offspring of their mothers, the informed consent not being signed, self-reported pregnancy at the time of the examination, not being in the fasting state for at least 10 hours, known diabetes or other chronic disease, and the use of medication that alters blood pressure or glucose or lipid metabolism. Only one child per family was included; because most families had more than one child, we randomized the sample to determine which child would be included. Originally 1009 children and their mothers were recruited from six elementary schools. All the offspring who attended on the day of the evaluation were examined (n=1009). To include only one child per mother, we assigned a random number to each child with uniform distribution. We chose the highest random number from the generated variable. This was the selection based on the random number assignment. As a result, 369 siblings were excluded from the study. Furthermore, one child taking a thyroid medication, eight who declined to participate, 16 missing BMI information, and 29 mothers with missing serum lipid and glucose measurements were also excluded. All subjects were examined by the same physician. The study was approved by the Human Rights Committee of Durand Hospital in Buenos Aires. Each parent gave written informed consent, and children gave assent after an explanation of the study and before its initiation.

Sociodemographic characteristics included age and level of parental education and the presence or absence of a refrigerator or a dirt floor. Questionnaires for socio-economic status have been described in detail elsewhere (11).

Measurements of height, weight, and waist circumference in mothers and in their offspring were determined as previously described (10). Because children BMI varies according to age and gender we standardized the values for age and sex by converting them to a *z*-score according to the Centers for Disease Control and Prevention (CDC) growth charts (12). The children were classified as normal weight (BMI<85 percentile) OW, (85<BMI<95percentile) or OB (BMI>95 percentile) per CDC norms (12). The physical examination also included determination of the stage of puberty according to the Tanner criteria (13). Three separate blood pressure measurements were recorded by a trained technician using a random-zero sphygmomanometer after the participant was seated at rest for five minutes. The averages of the three measurements of systolic and diastolic blood pressures were used (14).We used the National Heart, Lung and Blood Institute's recommended cutoff point for hypertension (14).

Risk factors for cardiovascular disease were defined using the same cut off as Cook et al (15) used: central OB (waist circumference >90th percentile); fasting triglycerides >110 mg/dL; HDL-C <40 mg/dL; blood pressure>90th percentile for age, sex, and height; and fasting glucose >100 mg/dL.

Maternal Htg-WP was defined as a waist circumference of 85 cm or more and a triglyceride level of 132 mg/dL(1.5 mmol/L)or higher (16). The Htg-WP in children was defined using the same cut off for waist circumference and triglycerides as Cook et al used (15).

Homeostasis model assessment of insulin resistance (HOMA-IR) was performed. The equation for HOMA-IR was:

fasting insulin (in μU/L) × fasting glucose (in mmol/L)/22.5(17).

Baseline blood samples were obtained from subjects while they were fasting to measure glucose, insulin, and lipid levels. Plasma glucose was assayed by the glucose oxidase technique, and serum lipids were measured with a Modular P analyzer (Hitachi High Technologies Corp., Tokyo, Japan). Serum insulin levels were determined by radioimmunoassay (Diagnostic Products, Los Angeles, CA), and insulin did not cross-react with proinsulin or C-peptide (percentage coefficient of variance, 5.2–6.8%).

3. Results

Characteristics of children

Physical and metabolic profiles are shown in table 1. Five hundred and ninety five children (296 males) aged 9.0 ± 1.9 years were examined. One hundred and five (17.6%) children

	Mothers (595)	Offsping(595)
Age (years)	35.8± 7.0	9.0 ± 1.9
BMI (kg/m2)	27.3± 5.9	18.7 ± 3.5
z-BMI (per CDC)		0.6 ± 1.0
WC (cm)	89 ± 13	65± 11
Systolic BP (mmHg)	111± 16	96± 13
Fasting glucose (mg/dL)	79± 18	78 ± 8
TC(mg/dL)	174± 37	152± 26
TG (mg/dL)	81(58-117)	51(67-90)
HDL-C (mg/dL)	52± 12	50± 12
Fasting insulin (μIU/mL)	5.7 (3.7-8.4)	4.9 (2.8-7.4)
HOMA -IR	1.0 (0.7-1.6)	0.9(0.5-1.4)
OW	182(30.6%)	110 (18.5%)
OB	158 (26.6%)	105 (17.6%)
Centrally OB	364 (61.2%)	91 (15.3%)
High blood pressure	57(9.8%)	38 (6.4%)
High fasting glucose	19(3.2%)	5 (0.8%)
High triglyceride	103(17.3%)	75(12.6%)
Low HDL-C	276 (46.4%)	129 (21.7%)
Htg-WP	93(15.6%)	32(5.4%)

Waist circumference (WC),blood pressure (BP), total Cholesterol (TC), triglyceride (TG) Data are mean ±SD or median (interquartile range) for continuous variables and percentage for categorical variables . Significance: *p<0.05; **p<0.001. Children's cardiovascular risk is defined by the following features: WC≥90th percentile, fasting glucose level ≥100 mg/dL, BP ≥90th percentile, TG ≥110 mg/dL, and HDL-C ≤40 mg/dL.

Table 1. Clinical and Metabolic Characteristics of 595 family members

were obese, and 110 (18.5%) overweight. There was not a significant difference in the prevalence of overweight or obesity between genders. Sixty seven percent, 21.2%, 10.3%, and 1.2% were at Tanner stage 1, 2, 3, and 4 respectively. The prevalence of Htg-WP was 5.4% (n=32) in children.

Approximately 40% of the children had at least 1 risk factor for cardiovascular disease and 13% had 2 or more risk factors. The risk factors of low HDL (129/595; 21.7%), central obesity (95/595; 15.3%) and high triglycerides (75/595; 12.6%), were common while hypertension (39/595; 6.4%) and impaired fasting glucose (5/595; 0.8%) were infrequent. One child had diabetes and none had all 5 risk factors. There was no significant difference in the prevalence of individual risk factors and in the prevalence of Htg-WP between boys and girls. There was not a significant difference in the distribution of Tanner stages between the group with and that without Htg-WP. The mean z BMI was higher ($p<0.001$) in the Htg-WP group (z BMI=1.9 $\pm$ 0.3) than in the group without Htg-WP (z BMI=0.6 $\pm$ 0.9).

Characteristics of the Mothers

Physical and metabolic profiles are presented in table 1. The average maternal BMI was 27.3 which indicates that, as a group, they were overweight. Approximately 27% of the mothers were obese (BMI >30), and 30.6% overweight (25<BMI<30). The educational backgrounds of the mothers were as follows: 1.2% had no formal education, 30% had completed elementary school, 52% had completed high school and 17% had university and/or advanced degrees. Participants came from a low and a middle socio-economic class. Overweight and obesity were more common ($p=0.003$) in mothers with a lower level of education (divided into high school or less and more).

Approximately 70% of mothers had at least 1 risk factor for cardiovascular disease, 34% had 2 or more risk factors. The risk factors of low HDL –C (276/595; 46.4%), central obesity (306/595;51.4%) and high triglycerides (103/595; 17.3%) were common while hypertension (47/595; 8%) and impaired fasting glucose (19/595; 3.2%) were less frequent. Four mothers had diabetes and only one mother had all 5 risk factors. Htg-WP was present in 15.6% (93) overall, 2% (5) of the normal, 17.6% (32) of the overweight, and 35.4% (56) of the obese group ($P < 0.01$). There was not a significant difference in the educational backgrounds in the group with and without Htg-WP. The mean BMI (32.0 vs 26.4; $p<0.01$) and mean age (39.8 vs 35.0; $p<0.01$) were higher in the group with Htg-WP than without Htg-WP.

Children's characteristics according to the presence of Htg-WP in their mothers

The prevalence of obesity was significantly higher in children with obese mothers than in the group of children whose mothers were not obese (27.2%vs 14.2%, $p<0.001$), respectively. The prevalence of obesity was significantly higher in children with mothers with Htg-WP than in the other group (29%vs 15.5%, $p=0.002$) , respectively. The prevalence of Htg-WP was significantly higher in children with mothers with Htg-WP than in the group of children with mothers without Htg-WP(16.1%vs 3.4%, $p<0.001$) , respectively.

Children of mothers with Htg-WP had values of z-BMI, waist circumference, systolic blood pressure, diastolic blood pressure, total cholesterol, triglycerides, insulin, and HOMA-IR which were higher ($p<0.01$) than those for the children of mothers without Htg-WP (Figure 1 and Table 2). Compared with children whose mothers did not have Htg-WP, the OR in children with maternal Htg-WP was [OR, 4.5 (95% CI 1.7-11.4)] for offspring's Htg-WP adjusted for age, Tanner stage, gender, maternal HOMA-IR, offspring's HOMA-IR, and offspring's hypertension. When socioeconomic class was included in the model, results did not change. The stepwise regression analysis showed that the most strongly predictive value of increased offspring's hypertriglyceridemic waist was maternal increased hypertriglyceridemic waist. Therefore, compared with children whose mothers did not have Htg-WP, children of mothers with Htg-WP were four and a half times more likely to have Htg-WP.

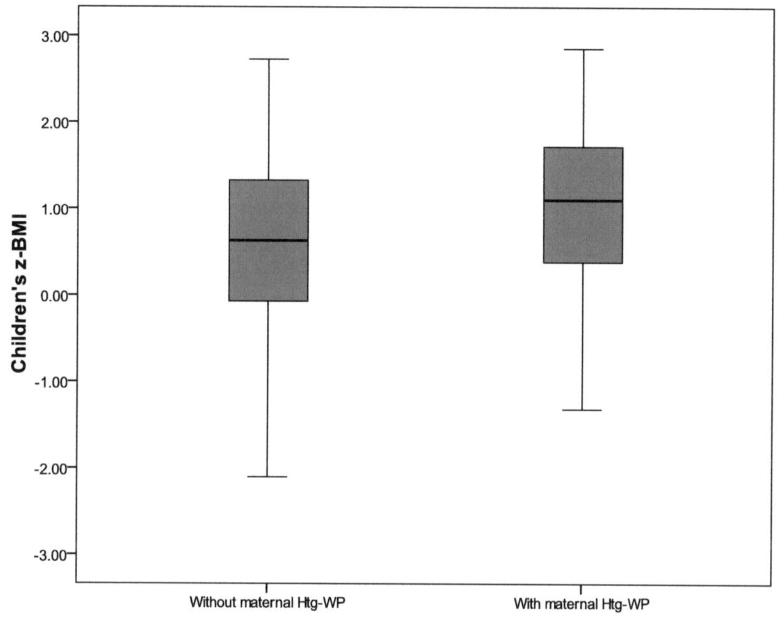

Panel A

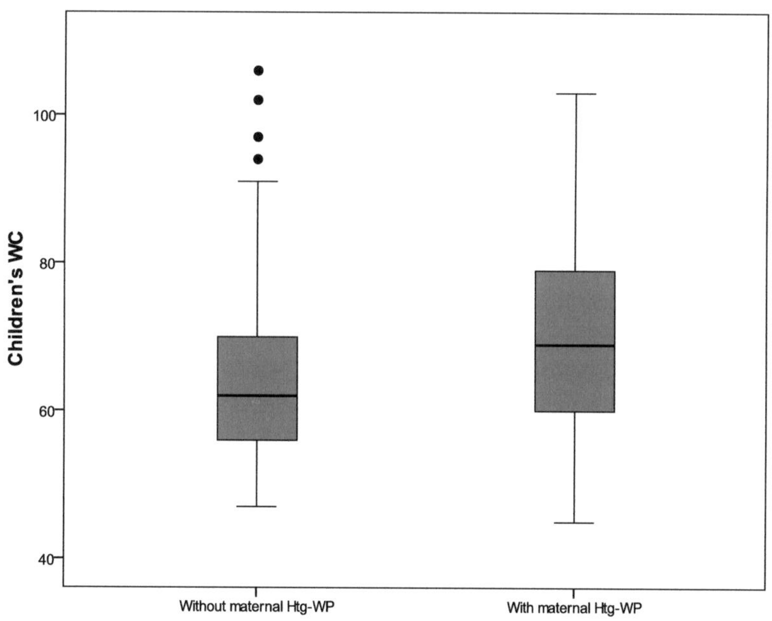

Panel B

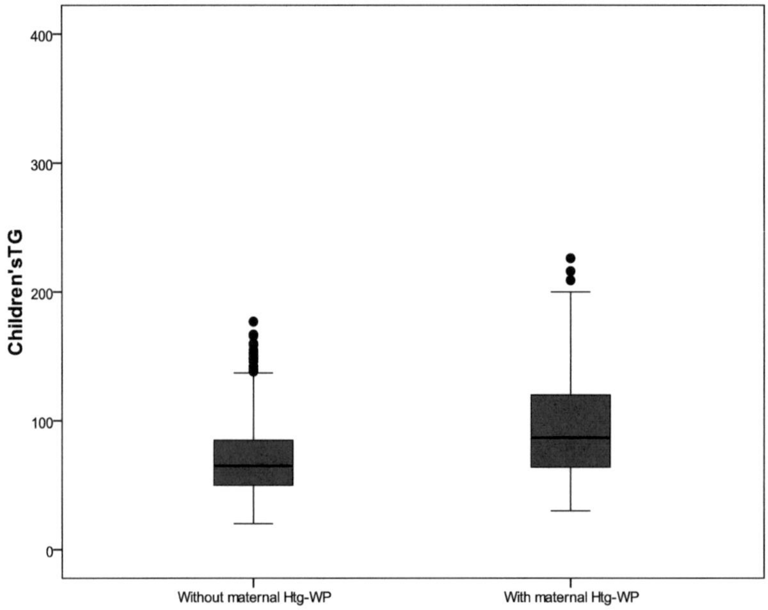

Panel C

Fig. 1. Boxplot: the boxes define the 25th and 75th percentiles, and enclose the median; the extensions define the range of values. Median values and interquartile range for children's z-BMI, children's WC and children's TG are presented separately for children without and with mothers with Htg-WP in Panel A, panel B and panel C, respectively. Waist circumference (WC) and triglyceride (TG)

4. Discussion

In this cross sectional analysis of school children and their mothers, our main finding was that Htg-WP in children was highly correlated with the maternal status of Htg-WP. We have previously demonstrated the association between maternal waist circumference and metabolic syndrome (a cluster of metabolic abnormalities that include glucose intolerance, central obesity, dyslipidemia, and hypertension) in their offspring (10). The maternal status of Htg-WP defined as an elevated waist circumference $\geq$85 cm in women) along with an elevated plasma triglyceride concentration (defined as a level $\geq$177 mg/dl) has been proposed and shown to be a stronger marker of cardiovascular risk and a better predictor of cardiovascular disease (4) than the waist circumference alone (18). As far as we know, there have not been large studies in elementary school children showing the association between maternal Htg-WP and their children's Htg-WP. We found that compared to children whose mothers did not have high Htg-WP, children whose mothers had high Htg-WP were approximately four and a half times more likely to have high Htg-WP adjusted for confounding variables consistent with known familial associations of high Htg-WP and cardiovascular disease.

The prevalence and severity of obesity has been increasing in children and adolescents, as well as in adults (19,20). Excess body fat in children is associated with insulin resistance and predicts development of the metabolic syndrome in adulthood (21). This research showed a high prevalence of overweight and obesity in children (35%) and in their mothers (57%). The

	Mothers without Htg-WP	Mothers with Htg-WP	P values
n (%)	502(84.4)	93 (15.6)	
Age (years)	8.9±1.9	9.4±1.8	0.237
Z-BMI	0.6±1.0	0.9±1.0	0.004*
BMI (Kg/m²)	18.5±3.4	19.9±3.9	0.001*
Waist (cm)	64±10	70±12	<0.001*
DBP (mmHg)	57±10	61±8	0.001*
SBP (mmHg)	95±13	100±13	0.001*
TC (mg/dL)	151±26	157±27	0.041*
HDL-C (mg/dL)	50±12	47±11	0.073
TG (mg/dL)	65(50-85)	87(63-121)	<0.001*
Glucose (mg/dL)	78±8	79±7	0.07
Insulin (uUI/ml)	4.8 (2.6-7.1)	5.4 (3.3-9.0)	0.03*
HOMA-IR	0.9 (0.5-1.4)	1.0 (0.6-1.8)	0.02*

Waist circumference (WC) ,blood pressure (BP), total Cholesterol (TC), triglyceride (TG) Data are means or median (interquartile range)±SD or percent. Group 1 (normal waist circumference and normal triglycerides; waist circumference≤85 cm in women and triglycerides ≤132mg/dL, n =317); group 2 (high waist circumference and high triglycerides; waist circumference ≥85 cm in women and triglycerides ≤132mg/dL, n =278). Significance: *p<0.05

Table 2. Characteristics of offspring according to the presence of Htg-WP in their mothers

increasing prevalence of obesity in children could be due to interactions between genetic and environmental factors (22). Recent changes in nutritional and physical activity patterns are considered to have produced changes in the fatness of children (22).Garn et al (23) suggest that childhood eating and exercise patterns are modeled after parental behaviors, and that parental behavior serves as the basis for developing and changing the health habits of children. A recent study showed that parental leanness confers significant protection against development of overweight in children, whereas parental obesity is associated with a prevalence of overweight in their children more than double that for children of lean parents (24). Excessive BMI gains of parents during childhood and adulthood were associated with a higher BMI and risk of obesity in the offspring (25). Substantial evidence now exists which demonstrates the importance of obesity in childhood in creating the metabolic conditions for cardiovascular disease and type 2 diabetes in young adulthood (26). Consistent with this study, we found that the prevalence of obesity was significantly higher in children whose mothers were obese than in the other group. An important epidemiologic aspect of cardiovascular risk in children is the tracking of these risk factors over time. Such tracking has been demonstrated in a number of studies, most notably the Muscatine Study and Bogalusa Heart Study (27, 28) which had demonstrated the presence of early lesions of coronary heart disease in the heart vessels of children and adolescents.

Despite the strong association of obesity, especially central obesity, to metabolic and cardiovascular disease, not all obese individuals carry the same metabolic and cardiovascular risk (18). Waist circumference is a simple and inexpensive marker of abdominal adiposity, but not all people with an increased waistline are at increased risk of coronary artery disease. The Htg-WP is a simple and inexpensive marker to help identify patients with intraabdominal obesity who have a deteriorated cardiometabolic risk profile and are thus at increased risk of coronary artery disease. An additional advantage is that the phenotype can be determined easily, without additional and expensive testing. Plasma triglyceride levels are available from any standard lipid profile obtained in clinical practice, and waist circumference can be measured at no cost. Therefore, elevated plasma triglyceride levels have been proposed as a marker of the metabolic alterations associated with excess intra-abdominal adiposity, such as ectopic fat deposition (liver, skeletal and epicardial fat) and insulin resistance (4). The association between mothers' obesity and morbidity and their children's obesity justifies looking for various markers of adiposity in all mothers. Parental obesity is a strong predictor of obesity in children (29,30). According to these studies, we showed that children of mothers with Htg-WP had significantly higher levels of z-BMI, waist circumference, blood pressure, insulin, and triglycerides than children whose mothers did not have Htg-WP. A previous study of our group showed that mother's waist circumference predicted her child's metabolic syndrome (11) consistent with known familial associations of OB and type 2 diabetes. However, maternal Htg-WP (the cluster) and its association with Htg-WP in their offspring have not been previously investigated. This study shows that children of mothers with Htg-WP had mean values of cardiovascular risk factors which were significantly higher than those for the children of mothers without Htg-WP. Furthermore, compared with children whose mothers did not have Htg-WP, children of mothers with Htg-WP were four and a half times more likely to have Htg-WP. As familial transmission is a risk factor for future cardiovascular disease, it is important to evaluate familial factors in order to identify strategies for the prevention and management of future diseases.

This study has several potential limitations. First, it is a cross-sectional study. Our data only show the association with present risk factor conditions but do not directly predict the future risk of cardiovascular events. Second, the fact that only mothers were included in the sample might decrease the power of the study. Third, we used criteria (Htg-WP) that has not been previously established for children. The final limitation was that as the sample was drawn from Buenos Aires neighborhoods of a middle and low socioeconomic level, it cannot be viewed as representative of Buenos Aires as a whole. However, it can be seen as representative of a large portion of Buenos Aires.

The strengths of our study include the large school age population-based sample, which was more likely to represent the general population, the high response rate of the children, the use of Tanner staging for measurement of puberty, the collection of fasting blood samples, and the use of multiple regression models, which allowed investigators to account for the complex interrelationships between these physiologic traits and potential confounders such as gender, pubertal development, children's HOMA-IR and maternal BMI.

5. Conclusions

Markers for an increased risk of cardiovascular disease are already present in children consistent with known familial associations of cardiovascular risk. This study demonstrates the importance of maternal Htg-WP in predicting children's Htg-WP even after adjustment for confounding variables. This criterion (Htg-WP) could be an easy and inexpensive tool to predict future cardiovascular disease. Health awareness efforts must include children whose mothers had Htg-WP and advocate lifestyle changes which may be easier to achieve in this group before they develop cardiovascular disease ant type 2 diabetes. Longitudinal studies should be conducted to confirm these findings.

6. References

[1] Bos G, Dekker JM, Heine RJ. Non-HDL cholesterol contributes to the "hypertriglyceridemic waist" as a cardiovascular risk factor: the Hoorn study. *Diabetes Care* 2004;27:283-4. 13.

[2] LaMonte MJ, Ainsworth BE, DuBose KD, et al. The hypertriglyceridemic waist phenotype among women. *Atherosclerosis* 2003;171:123-30. 14.

[3] Solati M, Ghanbarian A, Rahmani M, et al. Cardiovascular risk factors in males with hypertriglycemic waist (Tehran Lipid and Glucose Study). *Int J Obes Relat Metab Disord* 2004;28:706-9.

[4] Lemieux I, Pascot A, Couillard C, et al. Hypertriglyceridemic waist: A marker of the atherogenic metabolic triad (hyperinsulinemia; hyperapolipoprotein B; small, dense LDL) in men? *Circulation* 2000;102:179-84.

[5] Sironi AM, Gastaldelli A, Mari A, et al. Visceral fat in hypertension: influence on insulin resistance and beta-cell function. *Hypertension* 2004;44:127-33.

[6] Arsenault BJ, Lachance D, Lemieux I, et al. Visceral adipose tissue accumulation, cardiorespiratory fitness, and features of the metabolic syndrome. *Arch Intern Med*2007; 167:1518-25.

[7] Pouliot MC, Després JP, Lemieux S, et al. Waist circumference and abdominal sagittal diameter: best simple anthropometric indexes of abdominal visceral adipose tissue accumulation and related cardiovascular risk in men and women. *Am J Cardiol* 1994;73:460-8.

[8] Lemieux I, Poirier P, Bergeron J, et al. Hypertriglyceridemic waist: a useful screening phenotype in preventive cardiology? *Can J Cardiol* 2007;23(Suppl B): 23B-31B.

[9] Park HS, Park JY, Cho SI. Familial aggregation of the metabolic syndrome in Korean families with adolescents. Atherosclerosis. 2006;186:215-21.

[10] Hirschler V, Roque M, Calcagno ML, Gonzalez C, Aranda C. Maternal waist circumference and the prediction of children's metabolic syndrome Arch Pediatr Adolesc Med. 2007 ;161:1205-10.

[11] Hirschler V, Oestreicher K, Maccallini G, Aranda C Relationship between obesity and metabolic syndrome among Argentinean elementary school children. Clin Biochem. 2010;43:435-41.

[12] Kuczmarski R, Ogden C, Guo SS, Grummer-Strawn LM, Flegal KM, Mei Z, Wei R, Curtin LR, Roche AF, Johnson CL .: 2000 CDC growth charts for the United States: methods and development. Vital Health Stat 2002; 11:1–190.

[13] Tanner JM: Growth at Adolescence: With a General Consideration of the Effects of Hereditary and Environmental Factors upon Growth and Maturation from Birth to maturity, 1962, 2nd ed. Oxford, UK: Blackwell Scientific.

[14] National High Blood Pressure Education Working Group on High Blood Pressure in Children and Adolescents. The Fourth Report on the Diagnosis, evaluation and treatment on High Blood Pressure in Children and Adolescents. Pediatrics 2004; 114: 555-76.

[15] Cook S, Weitzman M, Auinger P, Nguyen M, Dietz WH. Prevalence of a metabolic syndrome phenotype in adolescents. Arch Pediatr Adolesc Med. 2003;157:821–827.

[16] Blackburn P, Lemieux I, Lamarche B, et al. Type 2 diabetes without the atherogenic metabolic triad does not predict angiographically assessed coronary artery disease in women. *Diabetes Care* 2008;31:170-2.

[17] Matthews DR, Hosker JP, Rudenski AS, Naylor BA, Treacher DF, Turner RC. Homeostasis model assessment: insulin resistance and ß-cell function from fasting plasma glucose and insulin concentrations in man. Diabetologia 1985;28:412-4198.

[18] Thamer C, Rittig K, Balletshofer B, Machicao F, Fritsche A, Haring HU. Identification and characterization of metabolically benign obesity in humans. Arch Intern Med 2008;168:1609–1616.

[19] Ogden CL, Carroll MD, Curtin LR, McDowell MA, Tabak CJ, Flegal KM. Prevalence of overweight and obesity in the United States, 1999- 2004. JAMA 2006; 295:1549–55.Wang Y, Beydoun MA.

[20] The obesity epidemic in the United States—gender, age, socioeconomic, racial/ethnic, and geographic characteristics:a systematic review and meta-regression analysis. Epidemiol Rev 2007; 29:6–28.

[21] Sun SS, Liang R, Huang TT, et al. Childhood obesity predicts adult metabolic syndrome: the Fels Longitudinal Study. J Pediatr 2008;152:191–200.

[22] Biro FM, Wien M. Childhood obesity and adult morbidities. Am J Clin Nutr. 2010; 91:1499S-1505S.

[23] Garn SM, Sullivan TV, Hawthorne VM. Fatness and obesity of the parents of obese individuals. Am J Clin Nutr. 1989;50:1308–1313.

[24] Semmler C, Ashcroft J, van Jaarsveld CH, Carnell S, Wardle J: Development of overweight in children in relation to parental weight and socioeconomic status. Obesity (Silver Spring) 2009;17:814–820.

[25] Li L, Law C, Lo Conte R, Power C: Intergenerational influences on childhood body mass index: the effect of parental body mass index trajectories. Am J Clin Nutr 2009;89:551–557.

[26] Ford AL, Hunt LP, Cooper A, Shield JP. What reduction in BMI SDS is required in obese adolescents to improve body composition and cardiometabolic health? Arch Dis Child. 2010; 95:256-61.

[27] Lauer RM, Lee J, Clarke WR. Factors affecting the relationship between childhood and adult cholesterol levels: the Muscatine Study. *Pediatrics*.1988; 82:309 –318.

[28] Webber LS, Srinivasan SR, Wattigney WA, Berenson GS. Tracking of serum lipids and lipoproteins from childhood to adulthood: the Bogalusa Heart Study. *Am J Epidemiol*. 1991; 133:884-899.

[29] Burke V, Beilin LJ, Dunbar D: Family lifestyle and parental body mass index as predictors of body mass index in Australian children: a longitudinal study. Int J Obes Relat Metab Disord 2001;25:147–157.

[30] Francis LA, Lee Y, Birch LL: Parental weight status and girls' television viewing, snacking, and body mass indexes. Obes Res 2003;11:143–151.

13

The Bidirectional Relationship Between Psychiatry and Type 2 Diabetes Mellitus

Menan Rabie
Ain Shams University,
Egypt

1. Introduction

The relationship between DM and Psychiatry is becoming obvious and may be traced through a huge research material over the last few decades. However the nature of the relationship is still an unanswered question: is there a causal relationship or is it a mere comorbidity? As the relationship is becoming more and more complicated with the discovery of antipsychotic induced DM all over the world, biologically based research is still needed to clarify the obscure areas of this relationship.

2. Psychological stress predisposing to DM

Diabetes mellitus has reached epidemic proportions and affects more than 220 million individuals worldwide (WHO, 2009). These figures are expected to rise to 366 million by 2030 (Wild et al., 2004). In more developed societies, among obese white adolescents 4% had diabetes and 25% had abnormal glucose tolerance (Sinha et al, 2002). Some 90% of diabetic individuals have type 2 (non-insulin-dependent) diabetes mellitus, and within this category no more than 10% can be accounted for by monogenic forms such as maturity-onset diabetes of the young (Fajans et al, 2001) and mitochondrial diabetes (Maassen et al, 2004) or late-onset autoimmune diabetes of the adult, which is actually a late-onset type 1 diabetes (Pozzilli and Di Mario, 2001).Thus, most diabetes in the world is accounted for by "common" type 2 diabetes, which has a multifactorial pathogenesis caused by alterations in several gene products.

To understand the cellular and molecular mechanisms responsible for type 2 diabetes it is necessary to conceptualize the framework within which glycaemia is controlled. Insulin is the key hormone for regulation of blood glucose and, generally, normoglycaemia is maintained by the balanced interplay between insulin action and insulin secretion. Importantly, the normal pancreatic β cell can adapt to changes in insulin action—ie, a decrease in insulin action is accompanied by upregulation of insulin secretion (and vice versa). (Bergman 1989) Deviation from this hyperbola, such as in the patients with impaired glucose tolerance and type 2 diabetes occurs when β-cell function is inadequately low for a specific degree of insulin sensitivity. Thus, β-cell dysfunction is a critical component in the pathogenesis of type 2 diabetes. This concept has been verified not only in cross-sectional studies but also longitudinally. (Weyer, et al, 1999)

Although lifestyle and overeating seem to be the triggering pathogenic factors, genetic elements are also involved in the pathogenesis of type 2 diabetes. Positive family history confers a 2-4 fold increased risk for type 2 diabetes. 15–25% of first-degree relatives of patients with type 2 diabetes develop impaired glucose tolerance or diabetes. The lifetime risk (at age 80 years) for type 2 diabetes has been calculated to be 38% if one parent had type 2 diabetes. (Pierce et al, 1995) If both parents are affected, the prevalence of type 2 diabetes in the offspring is estimated to approach 60% by the age of 60 years.(Tattersal and Fajans, 1975)

Since dizygotic twins share the environment (both intrauterine and extrauterine) but only 50% of their genes, concordance rates in monozygotic twins in excess of those in dizygotic twins have been used to distinguish genetic from non-genetic contributions. In individuals older than 60 years, concordance rates for diabetes were 35–58% in monozygotic twins, compared with 17–20% in dizygotic twins. (Kaprio *et al.*,1992; Newman et al, 1987). Inclusion of impaired glucose tolerance markedly increased the concordance in monozygotic twins to 88%. (Henkin et al, 2003). Nevertheless, concordance rates in monozygotic twins might produce an underestimate of genetic effects, because the monochorionic intrauterine nutrition of monozygotic twins has been shown to result in growth retardation compared with dizygotic twins. And low birthweight itself is associated with increased risk of type 2 diabetes later in life. (Beck-Nielsen et al 2003; Hales and Barker, 1992; Hattersley and Tooke, 1999)

The exact causes of type 2 diabetes are still not clear. Since the 17th century, it has been suggested that emotional stress plays a role in the etiology of type 2 diabetes mellitus. So far, review studies have mainly focused on depression as a risk factor for the development of type 2 diabetes mellitus. Yet, chronic emotional stress is an established risk factor for the development of depression. Results of longitudinal studies suggest that not only depression but also general emotional stress and anxiety, sleeping problems, anger, and hostility are associated with an increased risk for the development of type 2 diabetes. Conflicting results were found regarding childhood neglect, life events, and work stress. Moreover, a considerable number of depressed patients suffer from high levels of diabetes-specific emotional stress (Pouwer et al., 2005; Kokoszka et al., 2009). Important factors contributing to the increasing prevalence of type 2 diabetes are obesity, physical inactivity, and an increase in the number of individuals older than 65 years (Wild et al., 2004).

Interestingly, stress has long been suspected as having important effects on the development of diabetes. More than 400 years ago, the famous English physician Thomas Willis (1621-1675) noted that diabetes often appeared among persons who had experienced significant life stresses, sadness, or long sorrow (Willis, 1675). One of the first systematic studies testing Willis's hypothesis was described in 1935, by the American psychiatrist Dr. W. Menninger, who postulated the existence of psychogenic diabetes and described a "diabetic personality" (Menninger, 1935). More recently, numerous studies have been performed, elucidating the role of emotional stress as a risk factor for the development of type 2 diabetes. The majority of these studies focus on depression. However, there is growing evidence that other forms of emotional stress contribute to the development of type 2 diabetes as well.

Nowadays, the term "stress" is commonly used in the psychological, biological, and medical sciences. The concept of stress has been developed in the 1930s by the endocrinologist Hans Selye. In 1950, he has defined stress as "the nonspecific response of the body to any demand," with the body going through three universal stages of dealing with the stressor:

the alarm phase (Cannon's fight-or-flight), the resistance phase (in which resistance to the stress is built), and the exhaustion phase (when the duration of stress is sufficiently long), together encompassing the "general adaptation syndrome." A more recent stress theory by McEwen (1998) is based on Selye's general adaptation syndrome, but incorporates additionally the notion that the body anticipates a stress response by shifting the homeostatic set point (allostasis, or stability through change). This comes at a price though, because shifting a set point of one system (e.g., blood pressure) affects other physiological systems (e.g., kidney function), a concept which is known as allostatic load.

However, the meaning of the word "stress" has changed during the past decades. Currently, stress usually refers to the consequence of the failure of an organism to respond appropriately to emotional or physical threats, whether actual or imagined (Bao et al., 2008). Stress symptoms commonly include a state of alarm. Signs of stress can be defined at a cognitive, emotional, physical or behavioral level. Cognitive signs are for example poor judgment, low self-esteem, poor concentration, and negative cognitions. Emotional signs include moodiness or even depression, feeling of anxiety, excessive worrying, irritability, agitation, and feeling lonely or even isolated. Physical symptoms are for example aches and pains, diarrhea or constipation, nausea, dizziness, chest pain, and rapid heart rate. Behavioral symptoms of stress can for example include: eating too much or not enough, sleeping too much or not enough, social withdrawal, procrastination or neglect of responsibilities, increased alcohol, nicotine, or drug consumption, and nervous habits such as pacing about or nail-biting.

Although the stress response of the body functions to maintain stability or allostasis, a long-term activation of the stress system can have serious, negative consequences for the body (Bao et al., 2008). Based on nine prospective epidemiological studies, Knol et al. (2006) were the first to conclude that depression increases the risk for type 2 diabetes by 37%. Two years later, Mezuk et al. (2008) were able to include a total of 13 studies that investigated depression as a risk factor for diabetes, representing 6,916 incident cases. In that meta-analytic review, the risk for incident diabetes was 60% higher in depressed participants, compared to non-depressed controls.

Engum (2007) has tested anxiety as a risk factor for the development of diabetes, using data from a large Norwegian prospective population-based study (n=37,291). Both baseline anxiety and depression were associated with an increased risk for the development of type 2 diabetes at 10 years follow-up. Among participants with a high level of depression/anxiety at both baseline and follow-up, the risk of type 2 diabetes was even higher (Engum, 2007).

Persons who had experienced significant life events during the past five years had a 1.6-fold increased risk to have type 2 diabetes compared to those who had not experienced life events. Interestingly, data from the Hoorn Study showed that life events were positively associated with the Waist-Hip-Ratio, an important risk factor for diabetes and cardiovascular disease (Mooy et al., 2000). Visceral adiposity does not seem to be the main link between stress and development of type 2 diabetes. Goodwin and Stein (2004) used data from the National Comorbidity Survey (n=5,877). In particular, a history of childhood neglect was associated with a higher risk of diabetes and this risk was higher among women, after adjustment for age, gender, race, marital status, income, and education. The first prospective study in this area has been described by Räikkönen et al. (2007) who used data from the Healthy Women Study (n=523) to test whether psychosocial factors predict the risk for the development of the metabolic syndrome. These researchers found that among this group of middle-aged women, baseline depressive symptoms, feeling frequently intensely angry, tensed or stressed, and very stressful life events were all associated with an increased risk to develop the metabolic syndrome during the 15-year follow-up.

Several prospective studies have tested the hypothesis that "general emotional stress" is associated with an increased risk for the development of type 2 diabetes. Rod et al. (2009) analyzed data from the Copenhagen City Heart Study, involving 7,066 women and men, finding that particularly stressed men but not women were more than two times as likely to develop diabetes during follow-up. Interestingly, participants who had reported high levels of stress compared to those with low levels of stress were less likely to quit smoking, more likely to become physically inactive, and less likely to stop drinking during follow-up: all these factors are known to be associated with an increased risk for type 2 diabetes. In another Japanese study by Toshihiro et al. (2008) among 128 male Japanese with impaired glucose metabolism, a high score on a questionnaire assessing "stress in daily life" was associated with an increased risk for the development of type 2 diabetes after a 3-year follow-up. Golden et al (2005) have conducted a longitudinal cohort study of 11,615 non-diabetic adults aged 48-67 years at baseline. Anger, particularly anger temperament, appeared to be associated with onset of type 2 diabetes. Additional analyses showed that particularly a higher caloric intake and adiposity but not smoking behaviors and physical activity were potential mediators of this association. Finally, Zhang et al. (2006) analyzed data from 643 non-diabetic men with a mean age of 63 years, and found that the persons who reported a high level of stress and high hostility were more likely to have higher insulin resistance levels. This result is in line with earlier studies by Surwit et al. (2002) and Raikkonen et al. (2003). In the study by Zhang et al., the association between hostility and insulin resistance was mediated by the stress hormone norepinephrine (Zhang et al., 2006).

Excessive overtime, probably due to over commitment to work has been reported to be associated with 4-fold higher risk of type 2 diabetes in Japanese men, independent of other risk factors (Kawakami et al., 1999). However, in the same study, job strain (defined as high work overload and low job control) was not significantly associated with incident diabetes. In the Whitehall II Prospective Study (Kumari et al., 2004), an imbalance in effort-reward, suggestive of significant work stress, was associated with a higher risk to develop diabetes in men but not in women. In a large (n=33,336) population-based sample, tense working situation related working stress was associated with onset of diabetes after, on average, 5 years, in women but not in men (Norberg et al., 2007). Burn-out, resulting from chronic work stress, has also been studied as a risk factor for the development of type 2 diabetes. Another study that was based on data from the Whitehall II Study (1991-2004) tested whether stress at work was associated with an increased risk of type 2 diabetes, in a sample of 5,895 middle aged civil servants (Heraclides et al., 2009). In that study, "psychosocial stress at work" appeared to be an independent predictor of the onset of type 2 diabetes among women, during a follow-up period of 15 years, but not in men. The strong association in the female group remained stable and decreased with only 20% after adjustment for life events, health behaviors, obesity, potentially confounding, and mediating factors (Heraclides et al., 2009).

Poor sleep can be an important indicator of emotional stress. On the one hand, emotional stress can easily affect different aspects of sleep, such as initiation of sleep, sleep duration, and sleep quality. Conversely, sleeping problems may not only be a consequence of emotional stress, but are often experienced as a significant source of stress. In their recent systematic review and meta-analysis, Cappuccio et al. (2010) tested whether habitual sleep disturbances were associated with a higher incidence of type 2 diabetes. They included 10 studies, comprising a total of 107.756 male and females. Follow-up durations of the studies ranged from 4 to 32 years. It appeared that short duration of sleep (less than 5 to 6 hours per night) increased the risk for type 2 diabetes. Difficulties in initiating sleep also increased the risk for the onset of type 2 diabetes. Interestingly, persons with a long duration of sleep, more than 8-9 hours per night were at increased risk for incident type 2 diabetes. Difficulty in maintaining sleep was associated with an 84% higher risk to develop type 2 diabetes. A high body mass index (BMI) is an important potential confounder in studies that investigate sleeping problems and incidence of type 2 diabetes. Overweight is a major risk factor for type 2 diabetes that can also contribute to snoring problems and sleep apnea (and thus to sleeping problems). Therefore all 10 studies that were included in the meta-analysis of Cappuccio adjusted their analyses for BMI.

Emotional stress can increase the risk for the development of type 2 diabetes through different pathways. The first pathway is via behavioral mechanisms. Emotional stress was found to be associated with unhealthy lifestyle behaviors, i.e., inadequate eating behaviors in terms of quality and quantity of food, low exercise levels, smoking and alcohol abuse (Bonnet et al., 2005; Rod et al., 2009). All these factors are well-known risk factors for the development of type 2 diabetes. The second pathway is via physiological mechanisms. Chronic stress reactions and depression are often characterized by long term activation of the hypothalamic-pituitary-adrenal axis and the sympathetic nervous system which were found to be associated with the development of abdominal obesity, and this may explain why depression or chronic stress increases the risk of diabetes (Björntorp, 2001; Vogelzangs et al., 2008).

Chronic stress can also initiate changes in immune system activity. There is experimental and clinical evidence that a rise in the concentration of pro-inflammatory cytokines and glucocorticoids, particularly cortisol, in response to chronic stress, both contribute to the behavioral changes associated with depression (Leonard and Myint, 2009). In addition, activation of the immune system can provoke neuroendocrine and neurotransmitter changes that are similar to those provoked by physical or psychological stressors (Anisman, 2009). Sleep disturbance and depression were also associated to hypercytokinemia and activated innate immunity (Pickup, 2004). Interestingly, Pickup (2004) also described convincing evidence that an ongoing cytokine-induced acute-phase response is closely involved in the pathogenesis of type 2 diabetes. Thus, inflammatory processes may be a common antecedent of stress vulnerability, depression, and type 2 diabetes, which can develop in parallel or in succession. Although the above-mentioned potential pathways give a slight indication of what is happening, we still know very little about the mechanisms by which different forms of emotional stress increase the risk of diabetes incidence and progression.

In general, the above described research findings support the notion that different forms of emotional stress are associated with an increased risk for the development of type 2 diabetes, particularly depression, general emotional stress, anxiety, anger/hostility, and sleeping problems. Conflicting results were found regarding childhood neglect/abuse, life events, and work stress. In several papers, childhood traumata and life events have been linked with higher odds of type 2 diabetes, but these studies were all limited by a cross-sectional design. Moreover, results from longitudinal studies in that area had conflicting results. A longitudinal study based on data from the Healthy Women Study showed that persons who had experienced life events were at increased risk for the metabolic syndrome, including impaired fasting glucose (Räikkönen et al., 2007), while another longitudinal study (Kumari et al. ,2004) found no significant association between life events and incident diabetes.

3. DM predisposing to Psychiatric disorders

Chronic diseases e.g. Diabetes Mellitus commonly pose a heavy weight on the patients' resilience and psychological well being, and eventually affect their mental health negatively. Numerous studies have suggested that certain psychiatric disorders occur with increased frequency among adults with type 2 diabetes mellitus for several reasons (Anderson et al, 2001; Peyrot and Rubin 1997): diabetes is considered as one of the most psychologically and behaviorally demanding of the chronic medical illnesses. Because 95% of the management of diabetes is conducted by the patient himself, a diagnosis of diabetes can lead to increased levels of anxiety, depressive symptoms, and lowered self-esteem. This is often true in individuals who are predisposed to psychiatric disorders or those with limited social supports (Llorente et al, 2006). Further, the increased co-occurrence of diabetes and psychiatric disorders may be due to the medical consequences of diabetes, e.g. dementia.

At present, there is no cure, and people with diabetes have multiple self-care tasks such as administering insulin injections and oral medication, implementing specific diet, exercise, weight reduction, and injection sites regimens. Between one-third and one-half of patients with diabetes do not achieve targets for good metabolic control (which includes glycaemic levels as well as lipids, blood pressure, and weight control). Type 2 Diabetes (T2DM) is a progressive condition, so that even with optimized intensive medical regimens in controlled settings glycaemic control continues to worsen over time A significant proportion of patients have clinically relevant difficulties with managing their self-care regimen despite receiving intensive medical, educational, and nursing input such as multiple injection regimens, continuous subcutaneous insulin infusion pumps, and structured education programmes for carbohydrate counting and insulin adjustment. There is now substantial evidence that certain aspects of self-management and suboptimal glycaemic control are associated with a variety of psychiatric and psychological problems. For instance, for people with T2DM, insulin therapy is associated with weight gain, which leads to a negative effect on body image and contributes to resistance to uptake of insulin treatment. (Ismail, 2009)

Depression is the most common psychiatric disorder associated with diabetes, and may occur at several stages of the natural history of diabetes. It is twice as common in diabetes as in the general population, with a pooled prevalence of 9% using diagnostic interviews and 26% using depressive symptom scores on self-report scales. Prevalence rates increase as the condition progresses, similar to those observed for other chronic medical conditions such as cardiovascular disease (Anderson et al, 2001). In a systematic review of mainly secondary analyses of retrospective community cohorts, depression was associated with an increased risk of 37% for subsequent diabetes (predominantly type 2) in adults, (Knol et al, 2006) suggesting a temporal association between the two conditions. There is around a three-fold increased risk of depression in people with diabetes complications (de Groot et al, 2001, Shehatah et al, 2010). There is a two to five fold increased risk of death in prospective cohort studies (Egede et al, 2005, Katon, *et al.* 2005). Elderly patients with T2DM and those with complications seem to represent a high-risk group. (Makine et al, 2009, Lustman et al, 2000, Lustman and Clouse, 2005, Zhang et al, 2005). A study by Shehatah et al, (2010), confirms the association of depression with complications of diabetes. Type 2 diabetic participants reporting the presence of at least one diabetic complication scored significantly higher on the BDI-II than participants with no complications. (Shehatah et al, 2010)

Depression in diabetes is underdetected, underdiagnosed, and undertreated. For instance, a US study of more than 9000 primary care patients with diabetes found a recognition rate for major depression of 51%; less than half (43%) of these depressed patients were given one or more antidepressant prescriptions, and a small proportion (6.7%) were offered four or more psychotherapy sessions during a 12-month period. (Katon *et al.*, 2004). It has yet to be seen whether the introduction of screening for depression in diabetes and heart disease in primary care in the UK has led to improved depression outcomes.

About 10% of the patients with type 2 diabetes suffer from "subthreshold" or "subclinical" depression (Ali et al, 2006). This subtype is characterized by pervasive depressive symptoms, not meeting all criteria for the psychiatric diagnosis of a depressive disorder. Subthreshold depression is clinically relevant and has been identified as a risk factor for subsequent major depressive disorder (Cuijpers and Smit, 2004). In addition, it has also been recently pointed out in research outcomes that most diabetes patients that have high levels of depressive symptoms are not clinically depressed (Fisher et al, 2007) and that screening for depression seems reasonable for both depression and emotional problems (Hermanns et al, 2006).

Depression has a doubling effect on disability. Quality of life is reduced with respect to psychological, physical, and occupational functioning. (Moussavi et al., 2007; Schram et al., 2009; Pouwer et al., 2010). In people with diabetes, depression has been associated with hyperglycemia (Tilburg et al 2001, Roy et al 2007); lower levels of diabetes self-care (Tilburg et al 2001); complications, including coronary/cardiovascular disease (Olson et al 2000, Kinder et al 2002), neuropathy (deGroot et al 2001, Lustman et al 1997), and retinopathy (Roy et al 2007, deGroot et al 2001); and increased mortality (Zhang et al 2005). Diabetes-related burdens are perceived as more severe, and satisfaction with diabetes treatment is lower, when depression is present. Patients with depression and diabetes were less physically active, were more likely to smoke tobacco, had less healthful eating habits, and adhered less to diabetes treatment (Gonzalez et al, 2007) Depression is associated with a negative appraisal of insulin therapies in those who are insulin naive, (Makine et al, 2009) and this could delay diabetes treatment such as initiation of insulin therapy in type 2 diabetes. In a handful of selected clinic samples, the course of depression appears to be of longer duration, with more recurrences and of greater severity in people with diabetes. Diabetes is a costly condition, and co-morbid depression adds to the health care costs; in one study in the USA, there was a four-fold increase. (Ismail, 2009)

In an earlier study Pouwer et al (2005) have found that diabetes-specific emotional problems, such as feelings of guilt or anxiety when the patient gets off track with the diabetes management (26–56%), concerns about food (26–41%), fear of hypoglycaemia(21–62%) or worries about complications (29–74%) were particularly common in patients with high levels of depression symptoms. Diabetes-specific emotional problems might be a chronic source of stress that can contribute to the onset of (new episodes of) major depression. Yet the reversed causation might also be true; depressed patients may experience their diabetes more frequently as a burden, as a result of their comorbid depressive disorder. Most of the research done on depression in diabetes has focused on depression symptomatology and used only self-report measures of depression. As inclusion of diabetes-specific issues during psychotherapy could increase treatment success.

Several studies have examined the relative correlation of depressed mood to glycemic control compared to the contribution of other psychosocial factors such as adherence to prescribed regimen, coping strategies, and perception of control over diabetes to glycemic control. Lustman et al (1997) examined the relative contribution of nortriptyline and improvement in depression on glycemic control. While nortriptyline showed negative effects (hyperglycemic) on blood glucose levels, reduction in depressive symptoms had a positive effect (hypoglycemic) on blood glucose levels. Adherence with diabetes regimen was hypothesized by the authors to account for the relationship between depressive symptoms and HbA1c although small sample sizes prevented empirical validation of this hypothesis.

The direction of the relationship between depression, behavior, and glycemic control remains unclear. Depression may be the precipitant of poor glycemic control or the result of failed efforts to improve blood glucose control. A cycle of effects may occur where feelings of disappointment about poor glycemic control may affect adherence to one's prescribed regimen, in turn worsening glycemic control. Longitudinal studies that track the course of disease, psychiatric comorbidity, and glycemic control at multiple points in time are needed to distinguish the trajectory of impacts among these variables. Lustman et al (1997) reported five year follow-up data for patients undergoing a randomized clinical trial of antidepressant treatment, documented worsened glycemic control in patients with recurrent major depression compared to baseline. Measures of adherence to a prescribed regimen during the follow-up period were not reported, thus leaving open the question of the direction of impacts on glycemic control.

Depression can be effectively treated in diabetic patients through pharmacotherapy, cognitive-behavioral therapy, and collaborative care. Depression interventions may also improve glycemic control and survival. (Lustman et al, 1998, 2000, Katon et al, 2004, Bogner et al, 2007). However, effective treatment of depressive symptoms accompanying diabetes is limited by low rates of detection and treatment. Jones and Doebbeling concluded that depression screening for diabetes patients remains below those of patients without diabetes (Jones and Doebbeling, 2007).

Some studies indicate that the major problems for a large group of diabetes patients could be addressed with the usage of psychotherapeutic methods, for example a cognitive behavioral therapy. The lack of statistically significant differences in the rate of complications among the studied groups may indicate that other factors, instead of complications, might be the most important determinants of the emotional well-being of people with diabetes. Examples of these factors may be personality, social support, life events, etc… diabetes-specific emotional problem are common in patients with high levels of depressive symptoms. "Worrying about the future and the possibility of serious complications" appeared to be among the most common diabetes-specific emotional problems (Pouwer et al, 2005), worrying about hypoglycaemia was also frequently endorsed as a significant problem in the present sample.

As diabetes-specific emotional problems were particularly common in depressed patients with diabetes, we believe that psychiatrists should not only have good biomedical knowledge about diabetes, its complications and its management, but also about the diabetes-specific forms of distress that are common in depressed patients with T2DM.

The handful of randomized controlled trials that have tested an antidepressant against placebo has included nortriptyline, fluoxetine, sertraline, and paroxetine. All suggest that antidepressants are effective in improving major depression but not mild depression.

Sertraline has been shown to reduce the risk of relapse of depression in diabetes. (Lustman *et al.*, 2006)

A number of complex interventions have combined psychological and pharmacological treatments in comparison with standard care. The psychological components of these treatments included combining antidepressants with problem-solving training, (Williams *et al.*, 2004, Katon *et al.*, 2004,), counseling (Stiefel *et al.*, 2008)or interpersonal therapy, (Bogner, et al, 2007) given according to patients' preferences or following a predefined algorithm. The methodological quality of these studies was better than that of the single-treatment interventions. There appears to be evidence that combined interventions improve depression outcomes but not glycaemic control. (Bogner, et al, 2007) These findings raise more questions than answers, for instance whether, and how, complex interventions for depression should include therapeutic components to improve diabetes self-care.

One interesting speculation is that depression and type 2 diabetes may have common origins. Shared developmental factors, environmental and genetic, may influence the onset of both. (Farmer *et al.*, 2008). Another suggestion is that dopamine reward systems are linked to obesity and a second suggestion is that dopamine reward systems are linked to obesity and impulsive disorders. (Wang *et al.*, 2001). Also, the well-known hypothesis that depressive disorders and chronic stress are accompanied by increased activity of the hypothalamic-pituitary-adrenal system, which increases cortisol and catecholamine levels, is receiving attention as they are associated with central adiposity. There is accumulating evidence that inflammatory factors such as high-sensitivity C-reactive protein and interleukin-6 are on the causal pathway to insulin resistance and emerging evidence that they may be increased in depression and related disorders. (Danese et al, 2007). Hyperglycaemia may activate the sympathetic nervous system. Hyperglycaemia and hypoglycaemia may also lead to microvascular cerebrovascular disease, which may manifest as a depressive syndrome and/or increase the susceptibility for depression. (Ismail, 2009)

Importantly, there are two studies in the literature reporting hippocampal volume loss in T2DM (den Heijer et al., 2003 and Gold et al., 2007). Given the role of the hippocampus in HPA axis feedback regulation (Jacobson and Sapolsky, 1991) and the close link between cortisol and glucose metabolism (Khani and Tayek, 2001), it is not all that surprising there is also some indication for HPA axis disturbances in T2DM, although the order of events remains unclear. Both unstimulated plasma levels (Lee et al., 1999), as well as dexamethasone-suppressed cortisol levels (Bruehl et al., 2007) have been shown to be elevated in T2DM (Andrews et al., 2002). In addition, elevated evening free cortisol salivary levels have been observed in T2DM relative to controls (Liu et al., 2005).

Several mechanisms could account for hippocampal damage in T2DM, among which are, for example, the formation of toxic advanced glycation end-products (Rojas and Morales, 2004), increased production of superoxides via increased intracellular glucose metabolism (Brownlee, 2001), and endothelial dysfunction (Tooke and Hannemann, 2000).

This corroborates the findings of two previous reports in healthy young (Pruessner et al., 2007) and older adults (Pruessner et al., 2005)

The hippocampus may have a role in the regulation of the HPA axis, which extends beyond the feedback regulation of the axis (de Kloet, 2000 and Herman et al., 2005). Studies on HPA axis have focused on the hippocampus as a regulatory entity with a *negative* feedback function or as a target structure for cortisol, and have generally yielded negative associations between hippocampal volume and cortisol levels (smaller volumes associated with higher cortisol levels).

T2DM, in addition to its recognized associated complications such as stroke, retinopathy, microvascular abnormalities, and neuropathy (Stumvoll et al., 2005), is also linked to cognitive dysfunction (Strachan et al., 1997 and Ryan and Geckle, 2000), with recent or declarative memory being the cognitive domain most frequently affected (Grodstein et al., 2001 and Gold et al., 2007), declarative memory impairments (Bruehl et al., 2007) and associated hippocampal volume reduction in late middle-aged and elderly patients with T2DM (Gold et al., 2007). Volume reductions of medial temporal lobe (MTL) structures, including the hippocampus and amygdala, have been reported in T2DM independent of atherosclerosis (den Heijer et al., 2003), hypertension and dyslipidemia even in individuals with well controlled diabetes of relatively short duration (Gold et al., 2007). The MTL structures, and in particular the hippocampus, have been shown to be highly vulnerable to damage (Cervos-Navarro and Diemer, 1991; Convit et al., 2003), and although the number of reports remains relatively small, it appears that they are affected by the metabolic dysregulation present in T2DM (Convit et al., 2003).

The reports of MTL abnormalities in T2DM have primarily come from gray matter volumetric assessments; however, the status of the MTL white matter remains unclear. WM assessment in T2DM has predominantly focused on gross overt structural changes, which is often accomplished using semi-quantitative methods (van Harten et al., 2006 and Manschot et al., 2007).

Emotional stimuli, particularly those of negative valence, are known to promote memory processing by, among other mechanisms, heightened arousal and attention (Kensinger, 2007). It has been shown that among women, brain activation associated with emotional arousal tends to be left lateralized and that stronger associations are found between emotional memory and activation of the left amygdale (Canli et al., 2002). Whether the observed blunted memory enhancing effects are related to amygdala dysfunction among these patients remains to be explored.

Another possible mechanism may be due to impaired cerebral perfusion and vasomotor reactivity, which has been demonstrated in diabetes (Novak et al., 2006) and which may result in diminished metabolic substrate delivery, particularly during periods of brain activation, thus contributing to the damage in T2DM (Convit, 2005).

Several prospective studies have found that obesity in middle age, as well as diabetes in later life, can increase the risk for developing dementia in at least two different ways. (Gustafson et al., 2003; Arvanitakis et al., 2004; Whitmer et al, 2005). First, animal studies have suggested that depletion of the neuronal insulin receptor mimics some aspects of the neurodegeneration seen in Alzheimer's disease. (de la Monte and Wands, 2005). This provides support for the idea that Alzheimer's disease may be caused in part by neuronal insulin resistance. Second, the presence of multiple cardiovascular risk factors at midlife substantially increases the risk of late-life dementia in a dose-dependent manner, (Whitmer et al, 2005), and T2DM is associated with a twofold increased risk of vascular dementia. (Hassing et al, 2002)

Although currently no guidelines exist regarding routine screening for cognitive disorders in older adults, memory deficits are not a part of normal aging. A clinician must have a high index of suspicion, particularly in an older patient who starts "forgetting" appointments, stops checking fingersticks, or inconsistently takes/refills prescriptions. Older adults who report memory problems merit a cognitive assessment. A cognitive screening instrument allows the provider to objectively document the deficit, and monitor the course of impairments. A laboratory dementia work-up, with complete blood count, metabolic profile,

rapid plasma reagin, thyroid function tests, B12, and folate serum levels, should also be completed to rule out treatable causes of cognitive impairment. (Llorente et al, 2006)
Additionally, the majority of patients with dementia will develop behavioral disturbances, including insomnia, agitation, and aggression, and as many as one-third will experience psychotic symptoms. Medical causes of memory problems, and associated behavioral disturbances, are important to consider in the older person with diabetes. Delirium, the sudden onset of impaired attention with a waxing and waning course, and, at times, associated visual hallucinations and agitation, may have multiple causes. In the patient with diabetes, hypoglycemia and hyperglycemia, as well as electrolyte and volume disturbances, and urinary or respiratory tract infections must be ruled out. Many medications taken commonly by older adults can result in cognitive impairment. These medications include those that have significant anticholinergic side effects (ie, opioids, diphenhydramine, olanzapine and conventional antipsychotics, incontinence medications, antispasmodics, antiparkinsonian medications, benzodiazepines, and histamine receptor antagonists. (Llorente et al, 2006)
In addition to poor self-care and greater health service use, mortality is also high in this group. In a population-based study of the elderly, adjusted 6-year relative risks of mortality in those with cognitive impairment and in those with diabetes were similar: 1.68 (1.53-1.86) and 1.62 (1.44-1.83), respectively. While no interaction was found between cognitive impairment and diabetes on risk of mortality, the proportion surviving with both illnesses after 6 years was approximately 50%.1
There have been few reports that other psychiatric disorders may coexist with depression in diabetes. Anecdotally, such coexistence is a common problem, but more epidemiological surveys are needed to confirm this observation. (Das-Munshi et al, 2007) Although studied less extensively, prevalence rates of anxiety disorders (Grigsby et al, 2002) and eating problems.(Mannucci et al, 2002, 2005, Allison *et al.*, 2007) are also increased in diabetes compared with those in healthy controls. As these disorders tend to co-occur with depression in the general population, this is likely also to be the case in diabetes. The implications of multiple psychiatric morbidities in diabetes for the prognosis and management of depression, as well as of the diabetes, also remains unknown but is likely to be deleterious. (Ismail, 2009)

4. Psychiatric medications predisposing to DM

An iatrogenic problem relating psychiatric disorders to diabetes is the use of psychotropic medications which cause changes in the glucose tolerance test and were sometimes accused of causing T2DM and other metabolic hazards, called "the metabolic syndrome".
New generation "atypical" antipsychotic medications carry an increased risk of weight gain and new-onset T2DM (American Diabetes Association, 2004, Department of Veterans Affairs, 2002, Melkerson and Dahl, 2004, Cohen, 2004, Jin et al., 2002, Wirshing et al., 2002 and Caro et al., 2002). While the association between atypical antipsychotics and these metabolic side effects is clear, especially in patients with schizophrenia, information about comparative risks of weight gain and diabetes between specific atypical medications, the exact relationship between weight gain and diabetes, and comparative risks for patients with diagnoses other than schizophrenia remain important areas of concern (Kornegay et al., 2002, Koro et al., 2002, Kropp et al., 2004 and Beliard et al., 2003).

Olanzapine, risperidone, and quetiapine are the most frequently prescribed atypical antipsychotic medications. (Leslie and Rosenheck 2004). They found the risk for new-onset diabetes in schizophrenia patients was highest for clozapine (2.03%), with lower risks for quetiapine (0.80%), olanzapine (0.63%), and risperidone (0.05%) compared to a reference cohort of patients on haloperidol. Characteristics of the sample population such as older age, polypharmacy, and pre-existing obesity may increase the risk for development of diabetes. Costs of additional weight gain and DM on health, quality of life, survival, and health care expenditures are enormous (Wolf and Colditz, 1998 and Nasrallah, 2002).

In a study conducted by Lambert et al (2006), subjects in all groups developed newly diagnosed DM at a higher rate (10 to 130 per 1000) than the annual incidence reported by the U.S. Department of Health and Human Services (2002) among the general U.S. population (6.3 per 1000). Olanzapine subjects had a higher rate of new-onset DM than that reported in a previous study: 7.3% over a 12–24 month follow-up period (Leslie and Rosenheck, 2004). This difference may in part be due to the high prevalence of pre-existing obesity in study subjects increasing DM risk. On average the study population was near the cutoff for Class I Obesity and 42% met criteria for Class I Obesity at baseline. (McTigue, 2003). Clearly, patients prescribed olanzapine should receive careful laboratory monitoring for DM and relying on weight assessment alone is inadequate. Patients with additional risk factors, such as older age or pre-existing obesity should be very closely monitored for new-onset diabetes by baseline and repeat assessments of glucose status (fasting serum glucose, HbA1c).

Among the 13 large sample retrospective studies based on prescription or safety monitoring databases, eight compared the risk of developing DM directly or indirectly between AAP and conventional antipsychotics as groups. Seven of these reports (Sernyak et al., 2002; Koro et al., 2002; Gianfrancesco et al., 2002; Kornegay et al., 2002; Hedenmalm et al., 2002; Buse et al., 2003 and Fuller et al., 2003) suggested that certain atypical agents or atypicals as a group had a significantly increased risk of new-onset DM (or increased odds ratio for the case-control studies) compared to conventional antipsychotics. In evaluating the risk for new-onset DM among individual atypical agents, 8 of these 13 studies compared the risk among individual atypical agents or relative to conventional agents or non-users of antipsychotics. Seven of these studies (Caro et al., 2002; Sernyak et al., 2002; Koro et al., 2002; Gianfrancesco et al., 2002; Gianfrancesco et al., 2003a; Gianfrancesco et al., 2003b and Fuller et al., 2003) suggested that olanzapine was associated with a significantly greater risk of developing DM than either risperidone or non-users of antipsychotics. On the other hand, only one study (Buse et al., 2003) found that the risk of developing DM was significantly lower in patients taking olanzapine than in patients taking risperidone, and also found no difference between clozapine and haloperidol in the risk of new-onset DM. Two other studies which included clozapine found no increased DM risk (Lund et al., 2001 and Wang et al., 2001), while Sernyak et al. (2002) and Gianfrancesco et al. (2002) both suggested that patients on clozapine had a greater risk of developing DM than those on conventional antipsychotics or non-users of antipsychotics. The report by Biswasl et al. (2001) found only eight cases of diabetes among 8858 patients onolanzapine between 1996 and 1998 reported by responding clinicians to a pharmacovigilance questionnaire.

Among the clinical studies, five found that the use of olanzapine was associated with a significantly greater risk of increasing blood glucose or insulin levels compared to those on risperidone or a control group (Melkersson and Hulting, 2001; Newcomer et al., 2002; Wirshing et al., 2002; Meyer, 2002 and Lindenmayer et al., 2003). Similarly, five clinical

studies that evaluated clozapine suggested that glucose levels or other markers of glucose/insulinhomeostasis were significantly increased in the clozapine group compared to groups on conventional antipsychotics or controls (Melkersson et al., 1999;Melkersson and Hulting, 2001; Newcomer et al., 2002; Wirshing et al., 2002 and Lindenmayer et al., 2003), while, the difference did not reach significance in the Hagg study (Hagg et al., 1998).
While ziprasidone has been available in the U.S. for 3 years, and aripiprazole for about a year, there are limited published data aside from that used in support of the submission to the FDA and a small number of studies. Kato and Goodnick (2001) published a review of the effects of AAP on lipid and glucose levels, and noted that ziprasidone appeared to be neutral in its effects on serum glucose. Kingsbury et al. (2001) published data from the cohort of 37 patients who were switched from various atypical and typical antipsychotics to ziprasidone, and noted no significant changes in serum glucose levels or weight, although there was improvement in serum total cholesterol and triglycerides. Cohen et al. (2003) also noted a non-significant decrease of 3.6 mg/dl among 40 persons with mental retardation after 6 months of ziprasidone treatment. Aripiprazole also appears to be metabolically neutral in its effects on serum glucose and lipids, but these data have only been published as part of a review of its safety profile (Goodnick and Jerry, 2002). Case reports and retrospective database analyses suggest that conventional and atypical antipsychotics are associated with significant increases in fasting glucose concentrations. This hyperglycemia can result in new-onset T2DM, metabolic acidosis or ketosis, and even hyperglycemia-related deaths. Most cases of new-onset T2DM occur within the first 6 months of treatment and are often, although not always, associated with significant weight gain or obesity. A family history for diabetes is also associated with an increased risk.
Several mechanisms of glucose dysregulation have been proposed to explain this association. The medications most associated with diabetes are also those that induce the greatest amount of weight gain. There are patients who develop diabetes, however, in the absence of weight gain, so other causes must be sought. These drugs may disrupt hypothalamic regulation of glucose serum levels through hypothalamic dopamine antagonism. Additionally, elevated insulin levels have been found in 46% of clozapine-treated patients, compared with 21% of those receiving conventional medicines (Melkersson et al, 1999) and 71% of a small sample of olanzapine-treated patients, suggesting that insulin resistance is a possible mechanism.
Johnson et al. (2005) found that in vitro low concentrations of olanzapine and clozapine (both potent muscarinic antagonists) inhibited cholinergics-induced insulin secretion by blocking muscarinic M3 receptor activity. risperidone and ziprasidone had no such effects. These findings suggest an added role for potent anticholinergic activity as a contributing factor for development of diabetes. This is consistent with early findings of a higher association between low-potency conventional antipsychotics and increased weight gain. The low-potency drugs, in general, are much more anticholinergic than high-potency medications.
The results of analysis of diabetic vs. nondiabetic patients suggest that use of phenothiazines, olanzapine, or clozapine is not the most important factor in determining risk of T2DM onset. Rather, body mass and psychiatric diagnosis were the most important determinants in our sample. (Regenold et al, 2000)
It is difficult to determine whether schizophrenia per se has an independent role in the development of abnormal glucose metabolism, as both conventional and atypical neuroleptics have been implicated in the pathogenesis of T2DM and impaired glucose tolerance (Mir and Taylor, 2001; Liebzeit et al, 2001; Lindenmayer et al, 2001). Prior to the

introduction of the first modern antipsychotics in the 1950's, several studies suggested that schizophrenia was associated with an increased risk of diabetes (Lorenz, 1922, Meduna et al., 1942, Braceland et al., 1945, Freeman, 1946, Langfeldt, 1952, Robinson and Shelton, 1940). Unfortunately, those studies did not use explicit diagnostic criteria for schizophrenia, and potentially confounding factors such as body mass index (BMI) and smoking were not considered. Some recent studies of newly diagnosed, antipsychotic-naïve patients with schizophrenia or non affective psychosis have had stronger methods, although problems with potential confounding by hypercortisolemia in the psychosis group, and incomplete matching for key demographic variables, have weakened some of the studies (Ryan et al., 2003, Arranz et al., 2004, Spelman et al., 2007). Despite these reservations, support for the hypothesis that schizophrenia and diabetes may be linked independently of medication comes from the observation that the rate of T2DM in family members of schizophrenic patients is between 18% and 30% (Mukherjee et al, 1989), which is far higher than the rate in the population at large (1.2%-6.3%) (Adams and Marano, 1994). Therefore, patients with schizophrenia and their first-degree relatives appear to be predisposed to developing T2DM.

Leaving aside the issues of medication and age, factors such as ethnicity, physical inactivity, and smoking and diet habits may also play a crucial role in the development of T2DM (Shaten et al, 1993; King and Rewers, 1993). Some researchers have contended that patients with schizophrenia who are severely ill with either negative or positive symptoms may have poorer glycemic control (Brambilla et al, 1976; Brown et al, 1999).

In a study conducted by Kirkpatrick (2008), newly diagnosed, antipsychotic-naïve patients with non affective psychosis and features of deficit schizophrenia were found to differ from other patients without deficit features on the GTT. The non deficit group had significantly higher two-hour glucose concentration than did the deficit group, and both the deficit and non deficit groups had higher two-hour glucose concentrations than did matched control subjects. Because, deficit and non deficit schizophrenia differ with regard to many variables, including those related to etiopathophysiology, the author tested the hypothesis that they would also differ in the results of a GTT. The evidence that diabetes has an increased prevalence in the relatives of people with schizophrenia, and that deficit and non deficit schizophrenia differ with regard to family history (Hong et al., 2003, Kirkpatrick et al., 2000a, Kirkpatrick et al., 2000b and Ross et al., 2000) provided support for this hypothesis. Consistent with other studies, the two groups would not differ at baseline, but would differ on two-hour glucose concentrations.

It was hypothesized that deficit schizophrenia was a separate disease within the syndrome of schizophrenia, based on studies that had shown that deficit and non deficit schizophrenia differed with regard to signs and symptoms, risk factors, course of illness, biological correlates, and treatment response (Kirkpatrick et al., 2001). The alternative interpretation of the many deficit/non deficit differences is that the deficit group simply has a more severe form of the same etiopathophysiology found in the non deficit group. The greater severity interpretation was based on poorer function and outcome, poorer treatment response, and poorer cognitive function, as well as the presence of two forms of serious pathophysiology (positive psychotic symptoms and primary negative symptoms) in the deficit group, compared to one (psychotic symptoms) in the non deficit group. Other studies have supported the separate disease hypothesis: Mucci et al. (2007) found a double dissociation in evoked potential variables; and more normal regional brain volume has been found in deficit compared to non deficit patients by separate groups (Gur et al., 1994, Quarantelli et al., 2002 and Galderisi et al., 2008).

The improved tolerability of AAP compared to typical antipsychotics, and emerging data suggesting improved psychiatric outcomes (Csernansky et al., 2002), has led clinicians to begin prescribing these agents for other disorders such as bipolar disorder, post traumatic stress disorder, personality disorders, dementia with psychosis, conduct disorder and severe aggression in children. Now, 15 years after the first atypical antipsychotic entered the U.S. market, clinicians and researchers have gradually come to realize that while EPS and TD occur less frequently with atypical agents, these medications may present a different set of adverse effects than typical antipsychotics. Of particular concern are the metabolic side effects of excessive weight gain and obesity, glucose intolerance, new-onset T2DM, diabetic ketoacidosis (DKA) and hypertriglyceridemia (Meyer, 2002; Jin et al., 2002 and Meyer and Koro, 2004).

This heightened level of concern is reflected in the actions of various health regulatory authorities throughout the world that have issued warnings and recommend labeling changes for atypical antipsychotic medications (Japan Ministry of Health, Labour and Welfare, 2002; Pierson, 2003; Risperdal Package Insert, 2003; Seroquel Package Insert, 2004; Zyprexa Package Insert, 2003 and Abilify Package Insert, 2004). While regulatory agencies have failed at times to provide specific monitoring recommendations or guidance regarding differential risk for hyperglycemia or DM among various AAP, consensus guidelines are now being published which elaborate on the differences in risk between agents, and provide rational monitoring schemes (American Diabetes Association et al., 2004; and Marder et al., 2004)

Historical evidence of abnormal glucose metabolism in psychiatric patients has been accumulating since the early 20th century (Kooy, 1919). The evidence consists of numerous reports of increased rates of impaired glucose tolerance, insulin resistance, and frank diabetes mellitus among psychiatric patients (Braceland, 1945; Waitzkin, 1966; Mueller, 1969; Keskiner, 1973; Brambilla, 1976 and Winokur, 1988).

Eaton et al. (1996), following up on individuals who had been diagnosed with major depression in 1981, found that major depression was associated with a 2.23 relative risk of diabetes onset over the 13 years since diagnosis. In a study of spouses and first-degree relatives of probands, Moldin et al. (1993) found that individuals diagnosed and treated for major depression had a 1.87 relative odds of also having a diagnosis of diabetes.

Regarding bipolar disorder, there have been two chart review studies reporting an increased prevalence of diabetes in hospitalized patients. Lilliker (1980) found a threefold higher rate of diabetes in 203 "manic-depressive" inpatients compared to other psychiatric inpatients and to the general population. Cassidy et al. (1999) compared the rate of diabetes in 345 hospitalized "manic-depressives" to the expected general population rate weighted for age, race and gender and found a similarly increased rate.

A study by Newcomer et al. (1999) is worth noting, because it compared schizophrenic and bipolar patients to controls on a glucose tolerance test and matched subjects for age and body mass. This study found that schizophrenic patients had significantly higher plasma glucose levels than both bipolar patients and controls 75 min after a 50 g oral dextrose load; however, schizophrenic and bipolar patients were equally insulin resistant with significantly elevated insulin levels compared to controls.

Findings of increased prevalence of diabetes in bipolar I patients relative to the general population is consistent with the aforementioned chart review studies of Lilliker (1980) and

Cassidy et al. (1999) that found rates significantly greater than the general population in their younger patient samples (mean ages of 49 and 40.6 years, respectively). The increased rate of bipolar patients compared to schizophrenic patients and the lack of an increased prevalence in schizophrenic patients are also consistent with the findings of Lilliker (1980), a previously published large-scale study of diabetes prevalence that compared rates among inpatients with a variety of psychiatric diagnoses.

It is important to emphasize that while Newcomer et al (1999) did not find bipolar patients to be glucose intolerant, they did find them to be just as insulin resistant as their schizophrenic subjects, indicating that the glucose metabolism of their bipolar subjects was not normal. Continued and worsening insulin resistance is the typical pattern of disease that eventually results in hyperglycemia and the diagnosis of T2DM. Why the bipolar subjects in their study had not yet manifested plasma glucose levels indicative of frank glucose intolerance is unclear.

In addition to factors that are typically controlled in diabetes prevalence studies, such as age, race, and gender, diabetes prevalence in psychiatric patients can be affected by treatment with psychotropic medications, many of which can cause weight gain and several of which have been associated with new-onset diabetes. Psychotropic medications of a newer (e.g., clozapine and olanzapine) and an older (e.g., phenothiazines) vintage have been reported to be associated with new-onset diabetes (Thonnard-Neumann, 1968; Wirshing et al, 1998 and Goldstein. 1999).

The possibility raised by these studies that schizophrenia may be associated with diabetes independently of poor health habits and medication side effects has received indirect support from family studies. Mukherjee et al. (1989) found an increased prevalence of T2DM among first degree relatives of schizophrenia patients, although that study used norms from population data, rather than a comparison of patients with matched controls. Another study (Spelman et al., 2007) also found an increased prevalence of impaired glucose tolerance in an oral glucose tolerance test (GTT) in both newly diagnosed, antipsychotic-naïve patients with schizophrenia (10.8%) and their first degree relatives (18%) compared to healthy controls (0%). In a study with closer matching and without confounding by hypercortisolemia in the relatives group, increased two-hour glucose concentrations in first degree relatives were also found (Fernandez-Egea et al., 2008).

Shortly after the introduction of chlorpromazine, clinicians noticed that antipsychotics use led to weight gain. It was further noted that lower-potency agents (chlorpromazine and thioridazine) induced greater weight gain than the higher-potency drugs (fluphenazine and haloperidol). Conventional antipsychotics-associated weight gain appears to be comparable for oral and depot formulations of the same drug.

Among the atypical medications, varying degrees of weight gain have been reported. Hummer et al. (1995) reported that after 1 year of treatment, 36% of patients treated with clozapine had gained > 10% of their initial body weight. Seven patients continued to gain weight, reaching a maximum gain of 30% of their initial body weight. Clozapine-induced weight gain does not appear to plateau early in treatment, and it has been shown to continue for 30 weeks. Olanzapine, with a similar chemical structure, has also been associated with significant weight gain. In prospective, double-blind studies, olanzapine has led to nearly twice the weight gain of risperidone. This weight gain is not apparently related to dose and can persist for up to 1 year (Lindenmayer et al, 2003)

Weight gain for risperidone and quetiapine appears to be intermediate among the antipsychotic medications. Weight gain is reported to be lower than that seen with olanzapine and clozapine but greater than that seen with conventional drugs. Weight gain associated with risperidone and quetiapine does appear to correlate with dose. Ziprasidone is associated with little weight gain, even after 1 year of treatment. Average weight gain associated with aripiprazole after 1 year of treatment was 2 kg. Among the atypical antipsychotics, the relative tendency to cause weight gain is as follows: clozapine > olanzapine > risperidone = quetiapine > ziprasidone = aripiprazole. (American Diabetes association, 2004)

Some studies also demonstrated positive correlations between indirect measures of visceral obesity, such as waist-to-hip ratio and waist circumference, and plasma levels of glucose and triglycerides. Although no comprehensive explanation has been put forward to account for the co-occurrence of this group of conditions, it would appear that dysregulation of the hypothalamic-pituitary-adrenal (HPA) axis may play a role. Using a crude indicator of HPA axis activity Ryan et al (2003) have shown that many schizophrenic patients had hypercortisolemia, which in turn may explain why they have excessive visceral fat, hyperglycemia, hyperinsulinemia, and insulin resistance. Alternatively, the stress of hospitalization may lead to impaired fasting glucose tolerance, as in major depression, and the endocrine abnormality may resolve with successful treatment. In conclusion, 15.4% of the drug-naive, first-episode patients with schizophrenia in their study had impaired fasting glucose tolerance, compared to none of the matched healthy subjects. The patients also had higher levels of plasma glucose, insulin, and cortisol and were less insulin sensitive than the comparison subjects.

Increased serum levels of total cholesterol, LDL cholesterol, and triglycerides are all associated with obesity and weight gain. Because several of the newer antipsychotics are associated with significant weight gain, one would expect that hyperlipidemia should also be associated with the use of these medications. Results of database analyses, chart reviews, and clinical trials indicate that clozapine and olanzapine use is associated with increased serum triglyceride levels. This hypertriglyceridemia correlates directly with weight gain. Findings are equivocal regarding changes in cholesterol levels.

The concept of metabolic syndrome (MetS) or Syndrome X as elucidated by Reaven (1988) is a reality today. Originally proposed as a link between insulin resistance and hypertension in the causation of cardiovascular disease (Levitt and Lambert, 2002), it has now been extended to psychiatry and is seen as an adverse effect of psychotropic drugs, especially second-generation antipsychotics. Recent comprehensive reviews have well established thatmetabolic syndrome is indeed the concern of the future, with prevalence ranging between 20%–60%, at least double the prevalence in the general population (Toalson, 2004, Thakore, 2004, Shirzadi and Ghaemi, 2006, De Hert et al, 2006, Haupt, 2006 and Newcomer and Haupt, 2006). Added to this is the increasing recognition that MetS is escalating in economically developing countries (Saw, 1997 and Gu, 2005). On the other hand, several studies have also shown a link between psychiatric illnesses and a vulnerability to developing metabolic syndrome (Thakore, 2004, Thakore et al., 2002, Brugha et al., 1989 and Kendrick, 1996). The picture is therefore far from clear.

Atypical antipsychotic medications have many useful applications for patients other than those with schizophrenia. In our clinical experience, the mood-stabilizing and calming effects are useful in patients with mood disorders, PTSD, and in some patients with unstable personality disorder. Additional research is needed to identify the specific effect of diagnosis on relative risk of diabetes and weight gain with these medications. At the current time, only schizophrenia has been identified as frequently having an independent risk of T2DM (Citrome et al., 2005).

Multiple studies indicate that patients with severe mental illness are not highly motivated to address obesity (Meyer, 2002), and, when motivated to enter a behavioral program for weight loss, experience high drop-out rates with limited success (Loh et al., in press). The outcomes data from CATIE address the medication-related issues in a prospective manner, and thereby provide useful information on the effects of antipsychotic switching on medical comorbidity and associated symptom and quality of life measures. Clinicians are advised to heed the recent expert consensus recommendations on metabolic and general health monitoring for patients with schizophrenia (American Diabetes Association et al., 2004 and Marder et al., 2004), and be attentive to the psychic impact which medical comorbidity may have on their patients with severe mental illness.

Clinicians need to be concerned not only about the development of DM, but also about impaired glucose tolerance in the non diabetic range which represents a source of ongoing cardiovascular risk even if the patient does not develop overt DM. Recently, the ADA reduced the upper limit of fasting normoglycemia from 109 to 99 mg/dl, and thereby increased the range of impaired fasting glucose to 100–125 mg/dl (Expert Panel, 2004).

All clinicians who prescribe AAP must be aware of the additive risk posed by the traditional risk factors for type 2 DM aside from obesity. These are:

1. Age 45 and older,
2. High risk ethnicity (African American, Hispanic, Asian, South Asian, Native American, Pacific Islander),
3. Gestational diabetes, or delivery of infant weighing >9 lbs,
4. Hypertension,
5. Dyslipidemia,
6. Previous history of impaired fasting glucose or impaired glucose tolerance.

The increased obesity, smoking, and unhealthy dietary habits and the inadequate utilization of preventative and primary health care in psychiatric patients underscore the importance of comprehensive medical and behavioral assessments. Patients should have baseline weight and BMI measured, as well as laboratory studies to screen for diabetes, lipid abnormalities, and thyroid disease. In addition, inquiries concerning exercise habits, eating patterns, caffeine usage, and smoking should be included in an initial evaluation. (McIntyre et al, 2005)

Weight loss is a particular challenge for patients with mental illness. (Devlin et al, 2000). Diet and exercise counseling should be provided to all patients, preferably before weight gain, and definitely once weight gain has occurred. (Fagiolini et al, 2003). Behavioral therapies are also effective adjuncts in weight loss treatment. (Devlin et al, 2000; McElroy, 2009) weight gain is clearly related to a specific medication, switching to an alternative agent or lowering the drug dose, if possible, should be considered. (Newcomer, 2009). Pharmacotherapy for obesity may be appropriate for obese patients who have failed to lose weight through diet and exercise alone. Surgical treatment, such as gastric bypass, should be considered in patients with a BMI >40 kg/m^2 who have not responded to other methods of weight reduction and who present with obesity-related comorbid conditions such as hypertension, diabetes, and obstructive sleep apnea. (Snow et al, 2005). Patients who smoke should be provided with smoking cessation support, counseling, and pharmacologic treatment, if appropriate. (Newcomer, 2007)

The National Cholesterol Education Program recommends screening of all adults over age 20 with a fasting lipoprotein profile every 5 years. (NCEP, 2001). Since patients with psychiatric disorders who take atypical antipsychotics associated with weight gain tend to have a greater prevalence of metabolic syndrome, (Fiedorowicz et al, 2008), more frequent metabolic monitoring has been recommended in these patients. Modifiable risk factors should be evaluated at or near baseline and serially after prescription of antipsychotics. Patients should have their weight and BMI evaluated at baseline and assessed at 4, 8, and 12 weeks after initiating or changing an atypical antipsychotic medication (then quarterly thereafter at the time of routine visits). Fasting plasma glucose, lipid levels, and blood pressure also should be assessed 3 months after initiation of antipsychotic medications. Thereafter, blood pressure and plasma glucose values should be obtained annually, or more frequently in those who have a higher baseline risk for the development of diabetes or hypertension. In patients with a normal lipid profile at 3 months, repeat testing should be performed at 5-year intervals, or more frequently if clinically indicated. (American Diabetes Association, 2004)

Results of numerous studies, suggest that physicians should counsel their patients that risk of T2DM can be significantly reduced by lifestyle changes involving diet and exercise. Some studies may also suggest that bipolar I and schizoaffective disorder patients could be inherently prone to T2DM, suggesting that caution is indicated when prescribing potentially hyperglycemic medications, or any medication that might promote weight gain, to patients with these disorders.

5. References

Abilify Package Insert, 2004. Bristol-Myers Squibb, Princeton, NJ.

Adams PF, Marano MA: Current Estimates From the National Health Interview Survey, 1994: Vital and Health Statistics Series 10, Number 193. DHHS Publication PHS 96-1521. Hyattsville, Md, National Center for Health Statistics, 1995

Ali S., Stone M.A., Peters J.L., Davies M.J. and Khunti K., The prevalence of co-morbid depression in adults with type 2 diabetes: a systematic review and meta-analysis, *Diabet Med* 23 (2006), pp. 1165–1173.

American Diabetes Association, American Psychiatric Association, American Association of Clinical Endocrinologists, North American Association for the Study of Obesity. Consensus Development Conference on Antipsychotic Drugs and Obesity and Diabetes. Diabetes Care 2004;27:596-601.

American Diabetes Association, Consensus development conference on antipsychotic drugs, obesity, and diabetes,*Diabetes Care* 27 (2004) (2), pp. 596–601.

American Diabetes Association; American Psychiatric Association; American Association of Clinical Endocrinologists; North American Association for the Study of Obesity. Consensus development conference on antipsychotic drugs and obesity and diabetes. *Diabetes Care*. 2004;27(2):596-601.

Anderson R.J., Freedland K.E., Clouse R.E.and Lustman P.J., The prevalence of comorbid depression in adults with diabetes: a meta-analysis, *Diabetes Care* 24 (2001), pp. 1069–1078.

Andrews R.C., Herlihy O., Livingstone D.E.W., Andrew R.and Walker B.R., Abnormal cortisol metabolism and tissue sensitivity to cortisol in patients with glucose intolerance, *J. Clin. Endocrinol. Metab.* 87 (2002), pp. 5587–5593.

Anisman H. Cascading effects of stressors and inflammatory immune system activation: implications for major depressive disorder. *J Psychiatry Neurosci* 34(1):4-20, 2009.

Arranz B., Rosel P. and Ramirez N. *et al.*, Insulin resistance and increased leptin concentrations in noncompliant schizophrenia patients but not in antipsychotic-naive first-episode schizophrenia patients, *J. Clin. Psychiatry* 65 (10) (2004), pp. 1335–1342.

Arvanitakis Z, Wilson RS, Bienias JL, et al. Diabetes mellitus and risk of Alzheimer disease and decline in cognitive function. Arch Neurol 2004;61(5):661-666.

Bao AM, Meynen G, Swaab DF. The stress system in depression and neurodegeneration: focus on the human hypothalamus. *Brain Res Rev* 57:531-553, 2008.

Beck-Nielsen H, Vaag A, Poulsen P and Gaster M, Metabolic and genetic influence on glucose metabolism in type 2 diabetic subjects—experiences from relatives and twin studies, *Best Pract Res Clin Endocrinol Metab* 17 (2003), pp. 445–467.

Beliard S., Valero R. and Vialettes B., Atypical neuroleptics and diabetes, *Diabetes Metab* 29 (2003) (3), pp. 296–299.

Bergman RN, Lilly lecture 1989. Toward physiological understanding of glucose tolerance. Minimal-model approach, *Diabetes* 38 (1989), pp. 1512–1527.

Biswasl, P.N., Wilton, L.V., Pearcel, G.L., Freemantle, S. and Shakir, S.A., 2001. The pharmacovigilance of olanzapine: results of a post-marketing surveillance study on 8858 patients in England. *J. Pharmacol.* 15, pp. 265–271.

Björntorp P. Do stress reactions cause abdominal obesity and comorbidities? *Obes Rev* 2:73-86, 2001.

Bogner H.R., Morales K.H., Post E.P. and Bruce M.L., Diabetes, depression, and death: a randomized controlled trial of a depression treatment program for older adults based in primary care (PROSPECT), *Diabetes Care* 30 (2007), pp. 3005–3010.

Bonnet F, Irving K, Terra JL, Nony P, Berthezène F, Moulin P. Anxiety and depression are associated with unhealthy lifestyle in patients at risk of cardiovascular disease. *Atherosclerosis* 178(2):339-344, 2005.

Braceland F.J., Meduna L.J.and Vaichulis J.A., Delayed action of insulin in schizophrenia, *Am. J. Psychiatry* 102 (1945), pp. 108–110.

Brambilla F, Guastalla A., Guerrini A., Riggi F., Rovere C., Zanoboni A.and Zanoboni-Muciaccia W., Glucose–insulin metabolism in chronic schizophrenia. *Dis. Nerv. Syst.* 37 (1976), pp. 98–103.

Brownlee M., Biochemistry and molecular cell biology of diabetic complications, *Nature* 414 (2001), pp. 813–820.

Bruehl H., Rueger M., Dziobek I., Sweat V., Tirsi A., Javier E., Arentoft A., Wolf O.T. and Convit A., Hypothalamic–pituitary–adrenal axis dysregulation and memory impairments in type 2 diabetes, *Journal of Clinical Endocrinology Metabolism* 92 (2007), pp. 2439–2445.

Brugha T.S., Wing J.K and Smith B.L., Physical health of the long-term mentally ill in the community: is there unmet need?, *Br. J. Psychiatry* 155 (6) (1989), pp. 777–781.

Buse JB, Cavazzoni P, Hornbuckle K, Hutchins D, Breier A, Jovanovic L: A retrospective cohort study of diabetes mellitus and antipsychotic treatment in the U.S. J Clin Epidemiol 56:164 -170, 2003

Canli T., Desmond J.E., Zhao Z. and Gabrieli J.D.E., Sex differences in the neural basis of emotional memories, *Proceedings of the National Academy of Sciences* 99 (2002), pp. 10789–10794.

Cappuccio FP, D'Elia LD, Strazzullo P, Miller MA. Quantity and quality of sleep and incidence of type 2 diabetes: a systematic review and meta-analysis. *Diabetes Care* 33:414-420, 2010.

Caro J.J., Ward A., Levinton C. and Robinson K., The risk of diabetes during olanzapine use compared with risperidone use: a retrospective database analysis, *J Clin Psychiatry* 63 (2002), pp. 1135–1139.

Caro, J., Ward, A., Levinton, C., Robinson, K. and Kopala, L., 2002. The risk of diabetes during olanzapine use compared with risperidone use: a retrospective database analysis. *J. Clin. Psychiatry* 63, pp. 1135–1139. View Record in Scopus | Cited By in Scopus (103)

Cassidy F., Ahearn E. and Carroll B.J. , Elevated frequency of diabetes mellitus in hospitalized manic-depressive patients. *Am. J. Psychiatry* 156 (1999), pp. 1417–1420.

Cervos-Navarro J. and Diemer N.H., Selective vulnerability in brain hypoxia, *Critical Reviews in Neurobiology* 6 (1991), pp. 149–182.

Citrome L., Blonde L. and Damatarca C., Metabolic issues in patients with severe mental illness, *South Med J* 98 (2005) (7), pp. 714–720.

Cohen S.T., Welch G., Jacobson A.M., de Groot M. and Samson J.A., The association of lifetime psychiatric illness and increased retinopathy in patients with Type I diabetes mellitus. *Psychosomatics* 38 (1997), pp. 98–108.

Cohen, S., Fitzgerald, B., Okos, A., Khan, S. and Khan, A., 2003. Weight, lipids, glucose and behavioral measures with ziprasidone treatment in a population with mental retardation. *J. Clin. Psychiatry* 64, pp. 60–62.

Convit A., Links between cognitive impairment in insulin resistance: an explanatory model, *Neurobiology of Aging* 26 (2005), pp. 31–35.

Convit A., Wolf O.T., Tarshish C. and de Leon M.J., Reduced glucose tolerance is associated with poor memory performance and hippocampal atrophy among normal elderly, *Proceedings of the National Academy of Sciences of the United States of America* 100 (2003), pp. 2019–2022.

Csernansky, J.G., Mahmoud, R. and Brenner, R., 2002. A comparison of risperidone and haloperidol for the prevention of relapse in patients with schizophrenia. *NEJM* 346, pp. 16–22.

Cuijpers P. and Smit F., Subthreshold depression is a risk factor for major depressive disorder. A systematic review of prospective studies, *Acta Psychiatr Scand* 109 (2004), pp. 325–331.

Danese A., Pariante C.M., Caspi A., Taylor A. and Poulton R., Childhood maltreatment predicts adult inflammation in a life-course study, *Proc Natl Acad Sci* 104 (2007), pp. 1319–1324.

Das-Munshi J., Stewart R., Ismail K., Bebbington P.E., Jenkins R. and Prince M.J., Diabetes, common mental disorders, and disability: findings from the UK National Psychiatric Morbidity Survey, *Psychosom Med* 69 (2007), pp. 543–550.

de Groot M., Anderson R., Freedland K.E., Clouse R.E. and Lustman P.J., Association of depression and diabetes complications: a meta-analysis,*Psychosom. Med.* 63 (2001), pp. 619–630.

De Hert M.A. *et al.*, Prevalence of the metabolic syndrome in patients with schizophrenia treated with antipsychotic medication, *Schizophr. Res.*83 (1) (2006), pp. 87–93.

de Kloet E.R., Stress in the brain, *Eur. J. Pharmacol.* 405 (2000), pp. 187–198.

de la Monte SM, Wands JR. Review of insulin and insulin-like growth factor expression, signaling, and malfunction in the central nervous system: Relevance to Alzheimer's disease. J Alzheimers Dis 2005;7(1):45-61.

den Heijer T., Vermeer S.E., van Dijk E.J., Prins N.D, Koudstaal P.J., Hofman A. and Breteler M.M.B., Type 2 diabetes and atrophy of medial temporal lobe structures on brain MRI, *Diabetologia* 46 (2003), pp. 1604–1610

Department of Veterans Affairs, Antipsychotics and metabolic effects: 2002–2003 update. VHA pharmacy benefits management strategic healthcare group and medical advisory panel (2002) Washington DC.

Devlin MJ, Yanovski SZ, Wilson GT. Obesity: what mental health professionals need to know. *Am J Psychiatry*. 2000;157(6);854-866.

Devlin MJ, Yanovski SZ, Wilson GT. Obesity: what mental health professionals need to know. *Am J Psychiatry*. 2000;157(6);854

Eaton WW, Armenian H, Gallo J, et al. Depression and risk for onset of type II diabetes. A prospective population-based study. Diabetes Care 1996;19:1097-1102.

Egede L., Nietert P. and Zheng D., Depression and all-cause and coronary heart disease mortality among adults with and without diabetes, *Diabetes Care*28 (2005), pp. 1339–1345.

Engum A. The role of depression and anxiety in onset of diabetes in a large population-based study.*J Psychosom Res* 62:31-38, 2007.

Expert Panel on Detection, Evaluation, and Treatment of High Blood Cholesterol in Adults. Executive Summary of The Third Report of The National Cholesterol Education Program (NCEP) Expert Panel on Detection, Evaluation, And Treatment of High Blood Cholesterol in Adults (Adult Treatment Panel III). *JAMA*. 2001

Expert Panel on the Diagnosis and Classification of Diabetes Mellitus, 2004. Diagnosis and classification of diabetes mellitus. *Diabetes Care* 27, pp. S5–S10.

Fagiolini A, Kupfer DJ, Houck PR, et al. Obesity as a correlate of outcome in patients with bipolar I disorder. *Am J Psychiatry*. 2003;160(1):112-117.

Fajans SS, Bell GI and Polonsky KS, Molecular mechanisms and clinical pathophysiology of maturity-onset diabetes of the young, *N Engl J Med* 345(2001), pp. 971–980

Farmer A., Korszun A. and Owen M.J. *et al.*, Medical disorders in people with recurrent depression, *Br J Psychiatry* 192 (2008), pp. 351–355.

Fernandez-Egea E., Bernardo M., Parellada E., Justicia A., Garcia-Rizo C., Esmatjes E., Conget I. and Kirkpatrick B., Glucose abnormalities in the siblings of people with schizophrenia, *Schizophr. Res.* 103 (1–3) (2008), pp. 110–113 Aug.

Fiedorowicz JG, Palagummi NM, Forman-Hoffman VL, et al. Elevated prevalence of obesity, metabolic syndrome, and cardiovascular risk factors in bipolar disorder. *Ann Clin Psychiatry*. 2008

Fisher L., Shaf M.M., Mullan J.T., Arean P., Mohr D. and Masharani U. *et al.*, Clinical depression versus distress among patients with type 2 diabetes: Not just a question of semantics, *Diabetes Care* 30 (2007), pp. 542–548.

Freeman H., Resistance to insulin in mentally disturbed soldiers, *Arch. Neurol. Psychiatry* 56 (1946), pp. 74–78.

Fuller MA, Shermock KM, Secic M, Grogg AL: Comparative study of the development of diabetes mellitus in patients taking risperidone and olanzapine. Pharmactherapyl 2:1037 -1043, 2003

Galderisi S., Quarantelli M., Volpe U., Mucci A, Cassano G.B. and Invernizzi G. *et al.*, Patterns of structural MRI abnormalities in deficit and non-deficit schizophrenia, *Schizophr. Bull.* 34 (2008), pp. 393–401.

Gianfrancesco (a), F., Grogg, A., Mahmoud, R., Wang, R.H. and Meletiche, D., 2003. Differential effects of antipsychotic agents on the risk of development of type 2 diabetes mellitus in patients with mood disorders. *Clin. Ther.* 25, pp. 1150–1171.

Gianfrancesco (b), F., White, R., Wang, R.H. and Nasrallah, H.A., 2003. Antipsychotic-induced type 2 diabetes: evidence from a large health plan database. *J. Clin. Psychopharmacol.* 23, pp. 328–335.

Gianfrancesco, F.D., Grogg, A.L., Mahmoud, R.A., Wang, R. and Nasrallah, H.A., 2002. Differential effects of risperidone, olanzapine, clozapine, and conventional antipsychotics on type 2 diabetes: findings from a large health plan database. *J. Clin. Psychiatry* 63, pp. 920–930.

Gold S., Dziobek I., Sweat V., Tirsi A., Rogers K., Bruehl H., Tsui W., Richardson S., Javier E. and Convit A., Hippocampal damage and memory impairments as possible early brain complications of type 2 diabetes, *Diabetologia* 50 (2007), pp. 711–719.

Golden SH, Williams JE, Ford DE, Yeh H-C, Paton-Sanford C, Javier-Nieto F, Brancati FL. Anger temperament is modestly associated with the risk of type 2 diabetes mellitus: The atherosclerosis risk in communities study. *Psychoneuroendocrinology* 31:325-332, 2006.

Goldstein, L.E. , Sporn J., Brown S., Kim H., Finkelstein J., Gaffey G.K., Sachs G. and Stern T.A., New-onset diabetes mellitus and diabetic ketoacidosis associated with olanzapine treatment. *Psychosomatics* 40 (1999), pp. 438–443.

Gonzalez J.S., Safren S.A. and Cagliero E. *et al.*, Depression, self-care, and medication adherence in type 2 diabetes: relationships across the full range of symptom severity, *Diabetes Care* 30 (2007), pp. 2222–2227.

Goodnick, P.J. and Jerry, J.M., 2002. Aripiprazole: profile on efficacy and safety. *Expert Opin. Pharmacother.* 3, pp. 1773–1781.

Goodwin RD, Stein MB. Association between childhood trauma and physical disorders among adults in the United States. *Psychol Med* 34:509-520, 2004.

Grigsby A, Anderson R., Freedland K., Clouse R. and Lustman P., Prevalence of anxiety in adults with diabetes: a systematic review, *J Psychosom Res*53 (2002), pp. 1053–1060.

Grodstein F., Chen J., Wilson R.S. and Manson J.E., Type 2 diabetes and cognitive function in community-dwelling elderly women, *Diabetes Care* 24 (2001), pp. 1060–1065.

Gu *et al.*, Prevalence of the metabolic syndrome and overweight among adults in China, *Lancet* 365 (9468) (2005), pp. 1398–1405.

Gur R.E.,. Mozley P.D and.Shtasel D.L *et al.*, Clinical subtypes of schizophrenia: differences in brain and CSF volume, *Am. J. Psychiatry* 151(1994), pp. 343–350.

Gustafson D, Rothenberg E, Blennow K, et al. An 18-year follow-up of overweight and risk of Alzheimer disease. Arch Intern Med 2003;163:1524-1528.

Hagg, S., Joelsson, L., Mjorndal, T., Spigset, O., Oja, G. and Dahlqvist, R., 1998. Prevalence of diabetes and impaired glucose tolerance in patients treated with clozapine compared with patients treated with conventional depot neuroleptic medications. *J. Clin. Psychiatry* 59, pp. 294–299.

Hales CN and Barker DJ, Type 2 (non-insulin-dependent) diabetes mellitus: the thrifty phenotype hypothesis, *Diabetologia* 35 (1992), pp. 595–601.

Hassing LB, Johansson B, Nilsson SE, et al. Diabetes mellitus is a risk factor for vascular dementia, but not for Alzheimer's disease: A population-based study of the oldest old. Int Psychogeriatr 2002;14(3):239-248.

Hattersley AT and Tooke JE, The fetal insulin hypothesis: an alternative explanation of the association of low birthweight with diabetes and vascular disease, *Lancet* 353(1999), pp. 1789–1792.

Haupt DW, Newcomer JW: Hyperglycemia and antipsychotic medications. J Clin Psychiatry 2001; 62(suppl 27):15-26

Hedenmalm, K., Hagg, S., Stahl, M., Mortimer, O. and Spigset, O., 2002. Glucose intolerance with atypical antipsychotics. *Drug Safety* 25, pp. 1107–1116.

Henkin L, Bergman RN and Bowden DW *et al.*, Genetic epidemiology of insulin resistance and visceral adiposity. The IRAS Family Study design and methods, *Ann Epidemiol* 13 (2003), pp. 211–217.

Heraclides A, Chandola T, Witte DR, Brunner EJ. Psychosocial stress at work doubles the risk of type 2 diabetes in middle-aged women. *Diabetes Care* 32:2230-2235, 2009.

Herman J.P., Ostrander M.M., Mueller N.K. and Figueiredo H., Limbic system mechanisms of stress regulation: hypothalamo-pituitary-adrenocortical axis, *Prog. Neuropsychopharmacol. Biol. Psychiatry* 29 (2005), pp. 1201–1213.

Hermanns N., Kulzer B., Krichbaum M., Kubiak T. and Haak T., How to screen for depression and emotional problems in patients with diabetes: comparison of screening characteristics of depression questionnaires, measurement of diabetes-specific emotional problems and standard clinical assessment, *Diabetologia* 49 (2006), pp. 469–477.

Hong L.E., Avila M.T., Adami H., Elliot A. and Thaker G.K., Components of the smooth pursuit function in deficit and non-deficit schizophrenia, *Schizophr. Res.* 63 (2003), pp. 39–48.

Hummer M, Kemmler G, Kurz M, Kurzthaler I, Oberbauer H, Fleischhacker WW: Weight gain induced by clozapine. Eur Neuropsychopharmacol5 : 437-440,1995

Ismail K, Depression and diabetes, Psychiatry and medicine, Volume 8, Issue 6, June 2009, Pages 203-207, Psychological Medicine Part 2 of 2

Jacobson L. and Sapolsky R.M., The role of the hippocampus in feedback regulation of the hypothalamic–pitutiary–adrenocortical axis, *Endocr. Rev.* 12 (1991), pp. 118–134.

Japan Ministry of Health, Labour and Welfare, Safety Division, Pharmaceutical and Medical Safety Bureau, 2002. "Dear Doctor Letter" Diabetic Ketoacidosis and Diabetic Coma Due to Increased Blood Glucose Level Associated with ZYPREXA (Olanzapine) Tablets, an antipsychotic agent (Emergency Safety Information) released April 16, 2002.

Jin H., Meyer J.M. and Jeste D.V., Phenomenology of and risk factors for new-onset diabetes mellitus and diabetic ketoacidosis associated with atypical antipsychotics: an analysis of 45 published cases, *Ann Clin Psychiatry Mar* (2002) (1), pp. 59–64.

Johnson DE, Yamazaki H, Ward KM, Schmidt AW, Lebel WS, Treadway JL, Gibbs EM, Zawalich WS, Rollema H: Inhibitory effects of antipsychotics on carbachol-enhanced insulin secretion from perfused rat islets: role of muscarinic antagonism in antipsychotic-induced diabetes and hyperglycemia. Diabetes54:1552 -1558, 2005

Jones L.E. and Doebbeling C.C., Depression screening disparities among veterans with diabetes compared with the general veteran population,*Diabetes Care* 30 (2007), pp. 2216–2221.

Kaprio J, Tuomilehto J and Koskenvuo M *et al.*, Concordance for type 1 (insulin-dependent) and type 2 (non-insulin-dependent) diabetes mellitus in a population-based cohort of twins in Finland, *Diabetologia* 35 (1992), pp. 1060–1067.

Kato, M.M. and Goodnick, P.J., 2001. Antipsychotic medication: effects on regulation of glucose and lipids. *Expert Opin. Pharmacother.* 2, pp. 1571–1582.

Katon W., Von Korff M., Lin E.B., Simon G., Ludman E. and Russo J. *et al.*, The Pathways Study: a randomized trial of collaborative care in patients with diabetes and depression, *Arch. Gen. Psychiatry* 61 (2004), pp. 1042–1049.

Kawakami N, Araki S, Takatsuka N, Shimizu H, Ishibashi H. Overtime, psychosocial work conditions, and occurance of non-insulin dependent diabetes mellitus in Japanes men. *J Epidemiol Community Health* 53:359-363, 1999.

Kendrick T., Cardiovascular and respiratory risk factors and symptoms among general practice patients with long-term mental illness, *Br. J. Psychiatry* 169 (6) (1996), pp. 733–739.

Kensinger E.A., Negative emotion enhances memory accuracy: behavioral and neuroimaging evidence, *Current Directions in Psychological Science* 16 (2007), pp. 213–218.

Keskiner A., El Toumi A.and Bousquet T., Psychotropic drugs, diabetes and chronic mental illness. *Psychosomatics* 14 (1973), pp. 176–181.

Khani and J.A. Tayek, Cortisol increases gluconeogenesis in humans: its role in the metabolic syndrome, *Clin. Sci.* 101 (2001), pp. 739–747.

Kinder, L.S., Kamarck, T.W., Baum, A., Orchard, T.J., 2002. Depressive symptomatology and coronary heart disease in Type 2 diabetes mellitus: a study of possible mechanisms. Health Psychol. 21, 542–552.

King H, Rewers M (WHO Ad Hoc Diabetes Reporting Group): Global estimates for prevalence of diabetes mellitus and impaired glucose tolerance in adults. Diabetes Care 1993; 16:157-177

Kingsbury, S.J., Fayek, M., Trufasiu, D., Zada, J. and Simpson, G.M., 2001. The apparent effects of ziprasidone on plasma lipids and glucose. *J. Clin. Psychiatry* 62, pp. 347–349.

Kirkpatrick B, Fernandez-Egea E, Garcia-Rizo C, Bernardo M.

Schizophr Res. 2009 Feb;107(2-3):122-7. Epub 2008 Nov 28. Differences in glucose tolerance between deficit and nondeficit schizophrenia.

Kirkpatrick B., Bucharan R.W., Ross D.E. and Carpenter W.T., A separate disease within the syndrome of schizophrenia, *Arch. Gen. Psychiatry* 58 (2001), pp. 165–171.

Kirkpatrick B., Castle D., Murray R.M. and Carpenter W.T. Jr., Risk factors for the deficit syndrome of schizophrenia, *Schizophr. Bull.*26 (2000), pp. 233–242.

Kirkpatrick B., Ross D.E., Walsh D., Karkowski L. and Kendler K.S., Family characteristics of deficit and nondeficit schizophrenia in the Roscommon Family Study, *Schizophr. Res.* 45 (2000), pp. 57–64.

Knol M, Twisk J, Beekman A, Heine R, Snoek F, Pouwer F. Depression as a risk factor for the onset of type 2 diabetes: a meta-analysis. *Diabetologia* 49:837-845, 2006.

Kokoszka A, Pouwer F, Jodko A, Radzio R, Mućko P, Bieńkowska J, Kuligowska E, Smoczyńska O, Skłodowska Z. Serious diabetes-specific emotional problems in patients with type 2 diabetes who have different levels of comorbid depression: a Polish study from the European Depression in Diabetes (EDID) Research Consortium. *Eur Psychiatry* 24(7):425-430, 2009.

Kooy F.H., Hyperglycemia in mental disorders. *Brain* 42 (1919), pp. 214–289.

Kornegay C.J., Vasilakis-Scarmozza C.and Jick H., Incidence of diabetes associated with antipsychotic use in the United Kingdom general practice research database, *J Clin Psychiatry* 63 (2002), pp. 758–762.

Kornegay, C.J., Vasilakis-Scaramozza, C. and Jick, L., 2002. Incident diabetes associated with antipsychotic use in the United Kingdom general practice research database. *J. Clin. Psychiatry* 63, pp. 758–762.

Koro C.E., Fedder D.O., L'Italien G.J., Weiss S.S., Magder L.S. and Kreyenbuhl D.A.*et al.*, Assessment of independent effect of olanzapine on risk of diabetes among patients with schizophrenia: population-based nested case-control study, *BMJ* (2002), pp. 243–247.

Kumari M, Head J, Marmot M. Prospective Study of Social and other risk factors for incidence of type 2 diabetes in the Whitehall II Study. *Arch Intern Med* 164:1873-1880, 2004.

Lambert MT., Copeland LA., Sampson N and Duffy SA. New-onset type-2 diabetes associated with atypical antipsychotic medications Progress in Neuro-Psychopharmacology and Biological Psychiatry Volume 30, Issue 5, July 2006, Pages 919-923

Langfeldt G., The insulin tolerance test in mental disorders, *Acta. Psychiatr. Scand.* 80 (suppl) (1952), pp. 189–200.

Lee Z.S., Chan J.C., Yeung V.T., Chow C.C., Lau M.S., Ko G.T., Li J.K.,. Cockram C.S and Critchley J.A., Plasma insulin, growth hormone, cortisol, and central obesity among young Chinese type 2 diabetic patients, *Diabetes Care* 22 (1999), pp. 1450–1457.

Leonard BE, Myint A. The psychoneuroimmunology of depression. *Hum Psychopharmaco* 24(3):165-175, 2009.

Leslie D.L. and Rosenheck R.A., Incidence of newly diagnosed diabetes attributable to atypical antipsychotic medications, *Am J Psychiatry* 161 (2004) (9), pp. 1709–1711.

Levitt N.S. and Lambert E.V., The foetal origins of the metabolic syndrome – a South African perspective, *Cardiovasc. J. S. Afr.* 13(4) (2002), pp. 179–180.

Liebzeit KA, Markowitz JS, Caley CF: New onset diabetes and atypical antipsychotics. Eur Neuropsychopharmacol 2001; 11:25-32

Lilliker S.L., Prevalence of diabetes in a manic-depressive population. *Comp. Psychiatry* 21 (1980), pp. 270–275.

Lindenmayer JP, Czobor P, Volavka J, Citrome L, Sheitman B, McEvoy JP, Cooper TB, Chakos M, Lieberman JA: Changes in glucose and cholesterol levels in patients with schizophrenia treated with typical or atypical antipsychotics. Am J Psychiatry 160:290 -296, 2003

Lindenmayer JP, Nathan AM, Smith RC: Hyperglycemia associated with the use of atypical antipsychotics. J Clin Psychiatry 2001; 62(suppl 23):30-38

Liu H., Bravata D.M., Cabaccan J., Raff H. and Ryzen E., Elevated late-night salivary cortisol levels in elderly male type 2 diabetic veterans,*Clin. Endocrinol.* 63 (2005), pp. 642–649

Llorente et al, 2006; Maria D. Llorente, MD, Julie Malphurs, PhD, Susana Prieto, MD, Marilyn SanJuan-Horvath, MD, and Michael A. Silverman, MD, Assessment of Psychiatric Disorders Among Older Adults With Diabetes Mellitus, Clinical Geriatrics, Volume 14 - Issue 8 - August 2006

Loh, C., Meyer, J.M., Leckband, S.G., in press. A comprehensive review of behavioral interventions for weight management in schizophrenia. Ann Clin Psychiatry.

Lorenz W.F., Sugar tolerance in dementia praecox and other mental disorders, *Arch. Neurol. Psychiatry* 8 (1922), pp. 184–196.

Lund, B.C., Perry, P.J., Brooks, J.M. and Arndt, S., 2001. Clozapine use in patients with schizophrenia and the risk of diabetes, hyperlipidemia, and hypertension: a claims-based approach. *Arch. Gen. Psychiatry* 58, pp. 1172–1176.

Lustman P., Clouse R. and Nix B. *et al.*, Sertraline for prevention of depression recurrence in diabetes mellitus. A randomized, double-blind, placebo-controlled trial, *Arch Gen Psychiatry* 63 (2006), pp. 521-529.

Lustman P.J. and Clouse R.E., Depression in diabetic patients. The relationship between mood and glycaemic control, *J Diabetes Complications* 19(2005), pp. 113–122.

Lustman P.J., Freedland K.E., Griffith L.S. and Clouse R.E., Fluoxetine for depression in diabetes: a randomized double-blind placebo-controlled trial,*Diabetes Care* 23 (2000), pp. 618–623.

Lustman P.J., Griffith L.S., Freedland K.E. and Clouse R.E., The course of major depression in diabetes. *Gen Hosp Psychiatry* 19 (1997), pp. 138–143.

Lustman P.J., Griffith L.S., Freedland K.E., Kissel S.S. and Clouse R.E., Cognitive behavior therapy for depression in type 2 diabetes mellitus. A randomized, controlled trial, *Ann. Intern. Med.* 129 (1998), pp. 613–621.

Lustman P.J., Griffith, L.S., Freedland, K.E., Clouse, R.E., 1997b. The course of major depression in diabetes. Gen. Hosp. Psychiatry 19, 138–143.

Maassen JA, Hart LM 't and Van Essen E *et al.*, Mitochondrial diabetes: molecular mechanisms and clinical presentation, *Diabetes* 53 (2004) (suppl 1), pp. S103–S109

Makine C., Karşıdağ Ç and Kadıoğlu P. *et al.*, Symptoms of depression and diabetes-specific emotional distress are associated with a negative appraisal of insulin therapy in insulin-naive patients with type 2 diabetes mellitus. A study from the European Depression in Diabetes [EDID] Research Consortium, *Diabet Med* 26 (2009), pp. 28–33.

Mannucci E., Rotella F., Ricca V., Moretti S., Placidi G. and Rotella C., Eating disorders in patients with type 1 diabetes: a meta-analysis, *J Endocrinol Invest* 28 (2005), pp. 417–419.

Mannucci E., Tesi F. and Ricca V., Eating behavior in obese patients with and without type 2 diabetes mellitus, *Int J Obes Relat Metab Disord* 26 (2002), pp. 848–853.

Manschot S., Biessels G., de Valk H., Algra A., Rutten G., van der Grond J., Kappelle L. and on behalf of the Utrecht Diabetic Encephalopathy Study Group, Metabolic and vascular determinants of impaired cognitive performance and abnormalities on brain magnetic resonance imaging in patients with type 2 diabetes, *Diabetologia* 50 (2007), pp. 2388–2397.

Marder S.R., Essock S.M. and Miller *et al.*, Physical health monitoring of patients with schizophrenia, *Am. J. Psychiatry* 161 (8) (2004), pp. 1334–1349.

Marder, S.R., Essock, S.M., Miller, A.L., Buchanan, R.W., Casey, D.E., Davis, J.M., Kane, J.M., Lieberman, J.A., Schooler, N.R., Covell, N., Stroup, S., Weissman, E.W., Wirshing, D.A., Hall, C.S., Pogach, L., Pi-Sunyer, F.X., Bigger, J.T., Friedman, A., Kleinberg, D., Yevich, S., Davis, B.R. and Shon, S., 2004. Health monitoring of patients with schizophrenia. *Am. J. Psychiatry* (in press) .

McElroy SL. Obesity in patients with severe mental illness: overview and management. *J Clin Psychiatry*. 2009;70(suppl 3):12

McEwen BS. Stress, adaptation, and disease. Allostasis and allostatic load. *Ann NY Acad Sci* 840:33-44, 1998.

McIntyre RS, Konarski JZ, Misener VL, Kennedy SH. Bipolar disorder and diabetes mellitus: epidemiology, etiology, and treatment implications. *Ann Clin Psychiatry*. 2005;17(2):83-93.

McIntyre RS. Overview of managing medical comorbidities in patients with severe mental illness. *J Clin Psychiatry*. 2009

McTigue K., Screening and interventions for overweight and obesity in adults: a summary of the evidence for the U.S. preventive services task force, *Ann Intern Med* 139 (2003) (11), pp. 933–949.

Meduna L.J., Gerty F.J. and Urse V.G., Biochemical disturbances in mental disorders, *Arch. Neurol. Psychiatry* (1942), pp. 4738–4752.

Melkerson K. and Dahl M.L., Adverse metabolic effects associated with atypical antipsychotics: literature review and clinical implications, *Drugs* 64 (2004), pp. 701–723.

Melkersson KI, Hultin A-L, Brismar KE: Different influences of classical antipsychotics and clozapine on glucose-insulin homeostasis in patients with schizophrenia or realted psychoses. J Clin Psychiatry60 : 783-791,1999

Melkersson, K.I. and Hulting, A.L., 2001. Insulin and leptin levels in patients with schizophrenia or related psychoses—a comparison between different antipsychotic agents. *Psychopharmacologia* 154, pp. 205–212.

Menninger WC. Psychological factors in etiology of diabetes. *J Nerv Ment Dis* 81:1-13, 1935.

Meyer, J.M., 2002. A retrospective comparison of weight, lipid, and glucose changes between risperidone- and olanzapine-treated inpatients: metabolic outcomes after 1 year. *J. Clin. Psychiatry* 63, pp. 425–433.

Mezuk B, Eaton WW, Albrecht S, Golden SH. Depression and type 2 diabetes over the lifespan.*Diabetes Care* 31:2383-2390, 2008.

Mir S, Taylor D: Atypical antipsychotics and hyperglycaemia. Int Clin Psychopharmacol 2001; 16:63-73

Moldin S.O.,. Scheftner W.A, Rice J.P., Nelson E.,. Knesevich M.A and Akiskal H., Association between major depressive disorder and physical illness. *Psychol. Med.* 23 (1993), pp. 755–761.

Mooy JM, De Vries H, Grootenhuis PA, Bouter LM, Heine RJ. Major stressful life events in relation to prevalence of undetected type 2 diabetes. The Hoorn Study. *Diabetes Care* 23:197-201, 2000.

Moussavi S., Chatterji S., Verdes E., Tandon A., Patel V. and Ustun B., Depression, chronic diseases, and decrements in health: results from the World Health Surveys, *Lancet* 370 (2007), pp. 851–858.

Mucci A., Galderisi S., Kirkpatrick B., Bucci P., Volpe U., Merlotti E., Centanaro F., Catapano F. and Maj M., Double dissociation of N1 and P3 abnormalities in deficit and nondeficit schizophrenia, *Schizophr. Res.* 92 (1–3) (2007), pp. 252–261.

Mueller P.S., Heninger G.R. and McDonald R.K., Intravenous glucose tolerance test in depression. *Arch. Gen. Psychiatry* 21 (1969), pp. 470–477.

Mukherjee S., Schnur D.B and Reddy R., Family history of type 2 diabetes in schizophrenic patients (letter), *Lancet* 1 (1989), p. 495.

Nasrallah H.A., Pharmacoeconomic implications of adverse effects of antipsychotic therapy, *Am J Health Syst Pharm* 15 (2002) (22 Suppl 8), pp. S16–S21.

Newcomer J.W. and Haupt D.W., The metabolic effects of antipsychotic medications, *Can. J. Psychiatry* 51 (8) (2006), pp. 480–491.

Newcomer J.W., Craft S., Fucetola R., Moldin S.O., Selke G., Paras L.and Miller R., Glucose-induced increase in memory performance in patients with schizophrenia. *Schizophr. Bull.* 25 (1999), pp. 321–335.

Newcomer JW. Comparing the safety and efficacy of atypical antipsychotics in psychiatric patients with comorbid medical illnesses. *J Clin Psychiatry.* 2009;70(suppl 3):30

Newcomer JW. Metabolic syndrome and mental illness. *Am J Manag Care.* 2007;13(7 suppl):S170

Newcomer, J.W., Haupt, D.W. and Fucetola, R., 2002. Abnormalities in glucose regulation during antipsychotic treatment of schizophrenia. *Arch. Gen. Psychiatry* 59, pp. 337–345.

Newman B, Selby JV, King MC, Slemenda C, Fabsitz R and Friedman GD, Concordance for type 2 (non-insulin-dependent) diabetes mellitus in male twins, *Diabetologia* 30 (1987), pp. 763–768

Norberg N, Stenlund H, Lindahl B, Andersson C, Eriksson JW, Weinehall. Work stress and low emotional support is associated with increased risk of future type 2 diabetes in women. *Diabetes Res Clin Pract* 76:368-377, 2007.

Novak V., Last D., Alsop D.C., Abduljalil A.M, Hu K., Lepicovsky L., Cavallerano J. and Lipsitz L.A., Cerebral blood flow velocity and periventricular white matter hyperintensities in type 2 diabetes, *Diabetes Care* 29 (2006), pp. 1529–1534.

Olson, J.C., Edmundowicz, D., Becker, D.J., Kuller, L.H., Orchard, T.J., 2000. Coronary calcium in adults with type 2 diabetes: a stronger correlate of clinical coronary artery disease in men than in women. Diabetes 49, 1571–1578.

Peyrot M, Rubin RR. Levels and risks of depression and anxiety symptomatology among diabetic adults. Diabetes Care 1997;20:585-590.

Pickup JC. Inflammation and activated innate immunity in the pathogenesis of type 2 diabetes.*Diabetes Care* 27(3):813-823, 2004.

Pierce M, Keen H and Bradley C, Risk of diabetes in offspring of parents with non-insulin-dependent diabetes, *Diabet Med* 12 (1995), pp. 6–13.

Pierson, R., 2003. FDA seeks diabetes warning on anti-psychotic drugs. Reuters News web site (reuters.com) accessed September 17, 2003.

Pouwer et al, 2010, F Pouwer, N Kupper, M C Adriaanse, Does Emotional Stress Cause Type 2 Diabetes Mellitus? A Review from the European Depression in Diabetes (EDID) Research Consortium, Discovery Medicine, 9(45):112-118, February 2010

Pouwer F, Skinner TC, Pibernik-Okanovic M, Beekman AT, Cradock S, Szabo S, Metelko Z, Snoek FJ. Serious diabetes-specific emotional problems and depression in a Croatian-Dutch-English Survey from the European Depression in Diabetes [EDID] Research Consortium. *Diabetes Res Clin Pract* 70(2):166-73, 2005.

Pouwer F., Skinner T.C., Pibernik-Okanovic M., Beekman A.T., Cradock S.and Szabo S. *et al.*, Serious diabetes-specific emotional problems and depression in a Croatian–Dutch–English survey from the European Depression in Diabetes [EDID] Research Consortium, *Diabet Res Clin Pract* 70 (2005), pp. 166–173.

Pozzilli P and Di Mario U, Autoimmune diabetes not requiring insulin at diagnosis (latent autoimmune diabetes of the adult): definition, characterization, and potential prevention, *Diabetes Care* 24 (2001), pp. 1460–1467

Pruessner J.C., Baldwin M.W., Dedovic K., Renwick R., Mahani N.K., Lord C., Meaney M. and Lupien S., Self-esteem, locus of control, hippocampal volume, and cortisol regulation in young and old adulthood, *Neuroimage* 28 (2005), pp. 815–826.

Pruessner M., Pruessner J.C., Hellhammer D.H., Bruce Pike G. and Lupien S.J. The associations among hippocampal volume, cortisol reactivity, and memory performance in healthy young men, *Psychiatry Res.: Neuroimag.* 155 (2007), pp. 1–10.

Quarantelli M., Larobina M., Volpe U., Amati G., Tedeschi E. and Ciarmiello A. *et al.*, Stereotaxy-based regional brain volumetry applied to segmented MRI: validation and results in deficit and non-deficit schizophrenia, *Neuroimage* 17 (2002), pp. 373–384.

Räikkönen K, Matthews KA, Kuller LH. Depressive symptoms and stressful life events predict metabolic syndrome among middle-aged women. *Diabetes Care* 30:872-877, 2007.

Reaven GM: Role of insulin resistance in human disease. Diabetes 1988; 37:1595-1607

Regenold et al., 2000. W.T. Regenold, M.A. Kling and P. Hauser , Elevated sorbitol concentration in the cerebrospinal fluid of patients with mood disorders.*Psychoneuroendocrinology* 25 (2000), pp. 593–606.

Risperdal Package Insert, 2003 Janssen Pharmaceutica, Titusville, NJ.

Robinson G.W. and Shelton P., Incidence and interpretation of diabetic-like dextrose tolerance curves in nervous and mental patients, *JAMA* (1940), p. 1142279.

Rod NH, Grønbaek M, Schnohr P, Prescott E, Kristensen TS. Perceived stress as a risk factor for changes in health behaviour and cardiac risk profile: a longitudinal study. *J Intern Med* 266(5):467-475, 2009.

Rojas A. and Morales M.A., Advanced glycation and endothelial functions: a link towards vascular complications in diabetes, *Life Sci.* 76 (2004), pp. 715–730.

Ross D.E., Kirkpatrick B., Karkowski L.M., Straub R.E., MacLean C.J., O'Neill F.A., Compton A.D., Murphy B., Walsh D. and Kendler K.S., Sibling correlation of the deficit syndrome in the Irish study of high-density schizophrenia families, *Am. J. Psychiatr.* 157 (2000), pp. 1071–1076.

Roy, M.S., Roy, A., Affouf, M., 2007. Depression is a risk factor for poor glycemic control and retinopathy in African-Americans with type 2 diabetes. Psychosom. Med. 69, 537–542.

Ryan C.M. and Geckle M.O., Circumscribed cognitive dysfunction in middle-aged adults with type 2 diabetes, *Diabetes Care* 23(2000), pp. 1486–1493.

Ryan M.C., Collins P.and Thakore J.H., Impaired fasting glucose tolerance in first-episode, drug-naive patients with schizophrenia, *Am. J. Psychiatry* 160 (2) (2003), p. 284-269.

Saw S.M., The epidemiology of obesity: a review, *Ann. Acad. Med. Singapore* 26 (4) (1997), pp. 489–493.

Schram MT, Baan CA, Pouwer F. Depression and quality of life in patients with diabetes: a systematic review from the European depression in diabetes (EDID) research consortium. *Curr Diabetes Rev*5(2):112-119, 2009.

Selye H. Stress and the general adaptation syndrome. *Br Med J* 17:1(4667):1383-1392, 1950.

Sernyak MJ, Leslie DL, Alarcon RD, et al. Association of diabetes mellitus with use of atypical neuroleptics in the treatment of schizophrenia. Am J Psychiatry 2002;159:561-566.

Seroquel Package Insert, 2004. AstraZeneca Pharmaceuticals LP, Wilmington, DE.

Shaten BJ, Smith GD, Kuller LH, Neaton JD: Risk factors for the development of type II diabetes among men enrolled in the usual care group of the Multiple Risk Factor Intervention Trial. Diabetes Care 1993; 16:1331-1339

Shehatah A, Rabie M A, Al-Shahry A, Prevalence and correlates of depressive disorders in elderly with type 2 diabetes in primary health care settings, Journal of Affective Disorders 123 (2010) 197–201

Shirzadi A.A. and Ghaemi S.N., Side effects of atypical antipsychotics: extrapyramidal symptoms and the metabolic syndrome,*Harv. Rev. Psychiatr.* 14 (3) (2006), pp. 152–164.

Sinha R, Fisch G and Teague B *et al.*, Prevalence of impaired glucose tolerance among children and adolescents with marked obesity, *N Engl J Med* 346 (2002), pp. 802–810.

Snow V, Barry P, Fitterman N, et al; Clinical Efficacy Assessment Subcommittee of the American College of Physicians. Pharmacologic and surgical management of obesity in primary care: a clinical practice guideline from the American College of Physicians.*Ann Intern Med.* 2005;142(7):525

Spelman L.M., Walsh P.I., Sharifi N., Collins P. and Thakore J.H., Impaired glucose tolerance in first-episode drug-naive patients with schizophrenia, *Diabet. Med.* 24 (5) (2007), pp. 481–485.

Stiefel F., Zdrojewski C. and Bel Hadj F. *et al.*, Effects of a multifaceted psychiatric intervention targeted for the complex medically ill: a randomized controlled trial, *Psychother Psychosom* 77 (2008), pp. 247–256.

Strachan M.W., Deary I.J., Ewing F.M. and Frier B.M., Is type II diabetes associated with an increased risk of cognitive dysfunction? A critical review of published studies, *Diabetes Care* 20 (1997), pp. 438–445.

Stumvoll M., Goldstein B.J. and van Haeften, Type 2 diabetes: principles of pathogenesis and therapy, *The Lancet* 365 (2005), pp. 1333–1346.

Tattersal RB and Fajans SS, Prevalence of diabetes and glucose intolerance in 199 offspring of thirty-seven conjugal diabetic parents, *Diabetes* 24(1975), pp. 452–462.

Thakore J.H., Metabolic disturbance in first-episode schizophrenia, *Br. J. Psychiatry* 184 (S47) (2004), pp. 76–79.

Thakore JH, Mann JN, Vlahos I, Martin A, Reznek R: Increased visceral fat distribution in drug-naive and drug-free patients with schizophrenia. Int J Obes Relat Metab Disord 26:137 -141, 2002

Thonnard-Neumann E., Phenothiazines and diabetes in hospitalized women. *Am. J. Psychiatry* 124 (1968), pp. 978–982.

Toalson P. *et al.*, The metabolic syndrome in patients with severe mental illnesses, *Prim. Care Companion J. Clin. Psychiat.* 6 (4) (2004), pp. 152–158.

Tooke J.E. and Hannemann M.M., Adverse endothelial function and the insulin resistance syndrome, *J. Intern. Med.* 247(2000), pp. 425–431.

Toshihiro M, Saito K, Takikawa S, Takebe N, Onoda T, Satoh J. Psychosocial factors are independent risk factors for the development of Type 2 diabetes in Japanese workers with impaired fasting glucose and/or impaired glucose tolerance. *Diabet Med* 25:1211-1217, 2008.

U.S. Department of Health and Human Services, National Diabetes Fact Sheet: general information and national estimates on diabetes in the United States, 2002, U.S. Department of Health and Human Services, Center for Disease Control, Atlanta, U.S.A. (2002).

van Harten B., de Leeuw F.E., Weinstein H.C., Scheltens P. and Biessels G.J., Brain imaging in patients with diabetes: a systematic review, *Diabetes Care* 29 (2006), pp. 2539–2548.

Van Tilburg, M.A., McCaskill, C.C., Lane, J.D., Edwards, C.L., Bethel, A., Feinglos, M.N., Surwit, R.S., 2001. Depressed mood is a factor in glycemic control in type 2 diabetes. Psychosom. Med. 63, 551–555.

Vogelzangs N, Kritchevsky SB, Beekman AT, Newman AB, Satterfield S, Simonsick EM, Yaffe K, Harris TB, Penninx BW. Depressive symptoms and change in abdominal obesity in older persons.*Arch Gen Psychiatry* 65:1386-1393, 2008.

Waitzkin L. , A survey for unknown diabetics in a mental hospital. II. Men from age fifty. *Diabetes* 15 (1966), pp. 164–172.

Wang G.-J., Volkow N. and Logan J. *et al.*, Brain dopamine and obesity, *Lancet* 357 (2001), pp. 354–357.

Weyer C, Bogardus C, Mott DM and Pratley RE, The natural history of insulin secretory dysfunction and insulin resistance in the pathogenesis of type 2 diabetes mellitus, *J Clin Invest* 104 (1999), pp. 787–794.

Whitmer RA, Gunderson EA, Barrett-Connor E, et al. Obesity in middle age and future risk of dementia: A 27-year longitudinal population based study. BMJ 2005;330:1360.

WHO. WHO Fact Sheet No 312, www.who.int/mediacentre/factsheets/fs312/en, November 2009.

Wild S, Roglic G, Green A, Sicree R, King H. Global prevalence of diabetes: estimates for the year 2000 and projections for 2030. *Diabetes Care* 27:1047-1053, 2004.

Williams J., Katon W. and Lin E.*et al.*, The effectiveness of depression care management on diabetes-related outcomes in older patients, *Ann Intern Med*140 (2004), pp. 1015–1024.

Willis T. Pharmaceutice rationalis sive diatriba de medicamentorum operationibus in humano corpore. [Oxford]: E Theatro Sheldoniano, M.DC.LXXV, 1675.

Winokur A., Maislin G., Phillips J.L. and Amsterdam J.D., Insulin resistance after oral glucose tolerance testing in patients with major depression. *Am. J. Psychiatry* 145 (1988), pp. 325–330.

Wirshing D.A., Boyd J.A. and Meng L.R., The effects of novel antipsychotics on glucose and lipid levels, *J Clin Psychiatry* 63 (2002), pp. 856–865.

Wirshing D.A.,. Spellberg B.J, Erhart S.M., Marder S.R. and. Wirshing W.C, Novel antipsychotics and new onset diabetes. *Biol. Psychiatry* 44 (1998), pp. 778–783.

Wolf A.M. and Colditz G.A., Current estimates of the economic cost of obesity in the United States, *Obes Res* 6 (1998) (2), pp. 97–106.

Zhang J, Niaura R, Dyer JR, Shen BJ, Todaro JF, McCaffery JM, Spiro A 3rd, Ward KD. Hostility and urine norepinephrine interact to predict insulin resistance: the VA normative aging study. *Psychosom Med* 68:718-726, 2006.[Discovery Medicine, 9(45):112-118, February 2010]

Zhang X., Norris S.L., Gregg E.W., Cheng Y.J., Beckles G. and. Kahn H.S, Depressive symptoms and mortality among persons with and without diabetes,*Am. J. Epidemiol.* 161 (2005), pp. 652–660.

Zyprexa Package Insert, 2003. Eli Lilly and Company, Indianapolis, IN.

14

Type 2 Diabetes Mellitus in Family Practice: Prevention and Screening

Philip Evans, Christine Wright, Denis Pereira Gray and Peter Langley
St Leonard's Research Practice, Exeter
United Kingdom

1. Introduction

There is now a worldwide epidemic of Type 2 Diabetes Mellitus. It is a condition associated with numerous complications, which may well be present even at the time of diagnosis. Effective treatments are available but there is no known cure. The focus therefore is on both prevention and early detection by screening, with a view to preventing or delaying complications.

This chapter gives a brief overview of the evidence for prevention of Type 2 Diabetes (behavioural and pharmacological) and describes various approaches to screening, from an international perspective, together with their relative advantages and disadvantages. Clinical opportunistic screening will be discussed and compared with population screening. The international guidance for screening for Type 2 Diabetes will be reviewed and a summary of the evidence relating to the psychological effects of screening, as well as the costs and cost-effectiveness of the various types of screening programmes, will be presented.

2. The rationale for preventing Type 2 Diabetes and its complications

The prevalence of diabetes, particularly Type 2 Diabetes, is increasing on a worldwide scale. The greatest increases are being seen in developing countries such as those in South East Asia (International Diabetes Federation, 2003; Ramachandran et al., 2010). There are many reasons for this increase in prevalence but it is generally thought that increasing rates of obesity and lack of exercise predicated upon a pre-existing genetic tendency towards diabetes are fuelling the epidemic (Stumvoll et al., 2005).

Diabetes is a common condition affecting 5.4% of the UK population (over 2.3 million people) and the vast majority of these have Type 2 Diabetes (The NHS Information Centre, 2010) with a higher prevalence amongst older people. For example between 10% and 20% of patients aged 60 to 79 years in the European prevalence study (DECODE) had diabetes (DECODE Study Group, 2003). In our own study (Evans et al., 2008), over a period of 20 years, there had been a trebling of the prevalence of Type 2 Diabetes in one family practice in the UK (Figure 1).

Type 2 Diabetes has a significant impact on life expectancy. It has been estimated that having diabetes reduces life expectancy by 17 years in males and 20 years in females, who are diagnosed with the condition at the age of 45 years (Yorkshire & Humber Public Health Observatory, 2007). It is also generally acknowledged that a large number of patients with

Type 2 Diabetes remain undiagnosed. For example in the US, one third to one half of people with Type 2 Diabetes are undiagnosed and thus untreated (Engelgau et al., 2000).

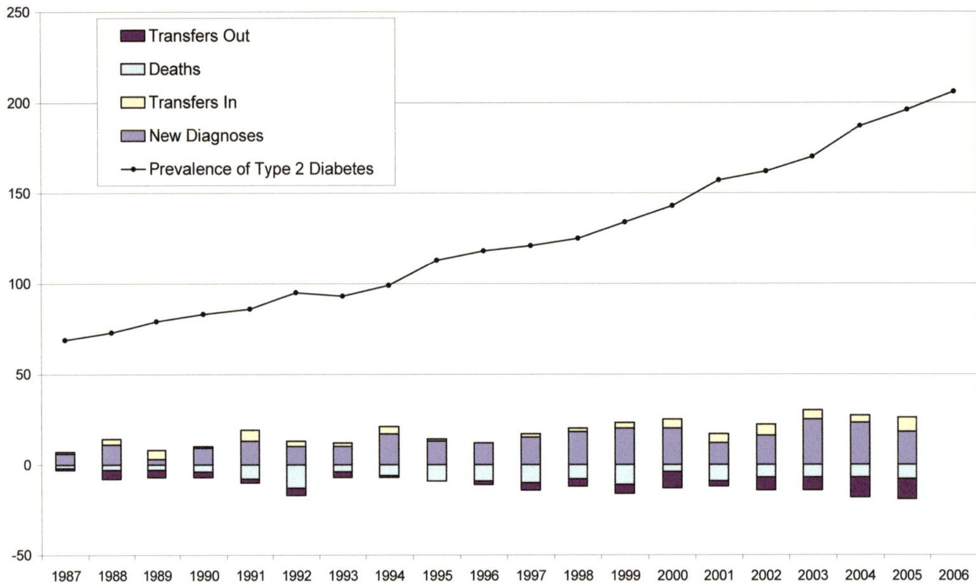

Fig. 1. Increasing prevalence of Type 2 Diabetes in one UK family practice
From: Evans, P., Langley, P., Pereira Gray, D. Diagnosing Type 2 diabetes before patients complain of diabetic symptoms - clinical opportunistic screening in a single general practice. *Family Practice,* 2008; 25(5): 376-381, by permission of Oxford University Press.

Type 2 Diabetes is a relatively unusual chronic disease in that it can have a long latent period prior to clinical diagnosis, perhaps up to 10 years (Harris et al., 1992). Patients who eventually develop Type 2 Diabetes often pass through a phase of intermediate hyperglycaemia when their blood glucose levels are elevated but not above the diagnostic threshold for Type 2 Diabetes. These intermediate states are collectively called Prediabetes and include Impaired Fasting Glucose diagnosed on a fasting plasma glucose test or Impaired Glucose Tolerance diagnosed on an oral glucose tolerance test. More recently the term Impaired Glucose Regulation has been proposed to include these borderline hyperglycaemic states (Diabetes UK, 2009).

Both conditions are increasingly prevalent and it has been estimated that 5.1% of the UK population aged 20 to 79 may have Impaired Glucose Tolerance (International Diabetes Federation, 2003). Prediabetes carries an increased risk of progression to Type 2 Diabetes although this can vary widely, dependent on ethnicity and other factors (Unwin et al., 2002). Nevertheless, it is widely accepted that patients with these conditions are at greater risk of both Type 2 Diabetes and cardiovascular disease (Cautinho et al., 1999), and interventions designed to prevent diabetes have, in the main, been targeted at this group (Tuomilehto et al., 2001).

Type 2 Diabetes is also unusual in that, unlike other conditions such as hypertension, a large proportion of patients have complications at clinical diagnosis. In the Hoorn Study, for example, at entry into the study, 39.5% of patients had ischaemic heart disease (Spijkerman et al., 2004) and 48.1% had impaired foot sensitivity (Spijkerman et al., 2003). In addition, since it is likely that having a high blood glucose for years on end may represent a harmful "legacy effect" (Del Prato, 2009), there is a greater imperative to diagnose early and theoretically reduce diabetic complications in later years.

These characteristics raise the logical possibility of preventing patients progressing to Type 2 Diabetes during this latent phase and hence reducing the complications associated with Type 2 Diabetes, both at diagnosis and afterwards.

2.1 Prevention of Type 2 Diabetes

There is now substantial evidence that progression to Type 2 Diabetes can be prevented or delayed in patients at high risk of Type 2 Diabetes (including those with Impaired Glucose Tolerance or Impaired Fasting Glucose), both by behavioural interventions (Knowler et al., 2002; Ramachandran et al., 2006; Tuomilehto et al., 2001) and by pharmacological interventions (Gillies et al., 2007; Salpeter et al., 2008).

Behavioural interventions included lifestyle interventions promoting weight loss, increased physical activity and dietary modification (Tuomilehto et al., 2001). In the Finnish Diabetes Prevention Study, this was achieved by offering detailed and individualised counselling to achieve set lifestyle goals. Prolonged engagement with a dietary counsellor was needed - for example, the median number of sessions per participant was 20 (Tuomilehto et al., 2001).

Pharmacological interventions have included rosiglitazone (Gerstein et al., 2006), troglitazone (Buchanan et al., 2002), acarbose (Chiasson et al., 2003), metformin (Knowler et al., 2002), and orlistat (Torgerson, 2004). A recent meta-analysis has shown that lifestyle interventions can produce a 50% relative risk reduction in the incidence of Type 2 Diabetes at one year (Yamaoka & Tango, 2005). Typically these interventions are in high-risk individuals such as those with Prediabetes (usually Impaired Glucose Tolerance) and interventions are targeted at halting or slowing β-cell dysfunction and hence incident cases of Type 2 Diabetes.

Our previous work in defining an effective pragmatic strategy for diabetes prevention using general practitioner (GP) databases identified a large proportion of patients with Prediabetes (Greaves et al., 2004). We subsequently developed an educational package for patients with Prediabetes and their healthcare professionals. This package known as WAKEUP (Ways of Addressing Knowledge Education and Understanding in Prediabetes) was found to be acceptable to both patients and health professionals (Evans et al., 2007).

As well as issues relating to clinician education, there are also many practical issues in delivering a national diabetes prevention programme. It is generally acknowledged that the intensity of the lifestyle intervention delivered in these trials is just not feasible in routine practice (Heneghan et al., 2006). A more pragmatic, yet effective, intervention is needed and several research groups in the UK are working on this issue, as are colleagues in Australia (Kilkkinen et al., 2007; Laatikainen et al., 2007).

2.2 Prevention of the complications of Type 2 Diabetes

Once a patient has developed Type 2 Diabetes, the major aim of clinical care is to prevent complications and morbidity related to the disease. The commonest complication of Type 2 Diabetes is cardiovascular disease (American Diabetes Association, 2011) manifested as coronary artery disease, peripheral vascular disease or carotid artery and other cerebrovascular diseases. It is generally acknowledged that patients with Type 2 Diabetes have a raised cardiovascular risk and this may well be present before a clinical diagnosis is made (Hu et al., 2002). Some studies have shown that this risk is equivalent to that of a patient of the same age who does not have diabetes but has already had a coronary event

(Haffner et al., 1998). Hence, Type 2 Diabetes is often termed a "coronary risk equivalent", although this has been contradicted recently in a systematic review and meta-analysis (Bulugahapitiya et al., 2009).

Reducing cardiovascular risk in patients with Type 2 Diabetes is therefore a priority. However, what has yet to be definitively established with regard to screening is whether early diagnosis reduces the risk of complications developing. Our previous work (Evans et al., 2008) showed that patients diagnosed by screening had a significantly lower median HbA1c (1.1% lower) than those presenting with symptoms. As the HbA_{1c} is so closely related to outcomes in Type 2 Diabetes (UK Prospective Diabetes Study (UKPDS) Group, 1998), it is likely that health benefit will ensue for those patients diagnosed by screening - however this is not proven as yet.

2.3 Effectiveness of treatment of Type 2 Diabetes

Effective treatments for the disease are available through lifestyle advice, oral hypoglycaemic drugs, and insulin. Most of the health economic models (e.g. Gillies et al., 2008; Hoerger et al., 2004; Waugh et al., 2007) developed to assess the cost-effectiveness of screening for diabetes include an assessment of the effectiveness of treatment for Type 2 Diabetes, comparing the screened and unscreened groups. As yet, there are no long-term studies of the effectiveness of treatment after diagnosis of Type 2 Diabetes in screened and unscreened groups, so health economic simulations are needed - with their accompanying assumptions.

These models use data from the UK Prospective Diabetes Study (UKPDS, 1998) which showed that intensive treatment of Type 2 Diabetes reduced the risks of microvascular complications but not macrovascular events. However, subsequent follow up after the trial had finished did show a reduction in macrovascular events in the intensive arm (Holman et al., 2008).

National guidance for the effective treatment of Type 2 Diabetes in primary and secondary care exists in the UK (National Collaborating Centre for Chronic Conditions, 2008; National Institute for Health and Clinical Excellence, 2009) and in the US (American Diabetes Association, 2011). These guidelines are evidence-based and should improve outcomes in patients with Type 2 Diabetes. Effective treatments are targeted at optimising cardiovascular risk factors, including serum lipids, HbA_{1c} and blood pressure. In addition, GPs in the UK also receive incentivised payments under the Quality and Outcome Framework when patients with Type 2 Diabetes reach the glycaemic, blood pressure and lipid targets (Roland, 2004).

3. General principles of screening

Screening in medicine is a search process. An examination or a test is offered to asymptomatic people "to classify them as likely or unlikely to have the disease that is the object of screening" (Morrison, 1998). People who are likely to have the disease are then investigated further to arrive at the final diagnosis. The assumption is that an effective intervention is available.

An early diagnosis and treatment activity applied in large groups is often described as 'mass screening' or 'population screening' (Morrison, 1998). Population screening in medicine was introduced in the mid-twentieth century and was applied to a number of diseases including tuberculosis, and more recently to cervical cancer, breast cancer and colon cancer. It was also attempted for diabetes.

There are two inevitable consequences of all screening programmes, namely the occurrence of what are called 'false positive' or 'false negative' results. False positives are people whose test is positive for the disease being sought but who prove not to have the disease. Patients suffer additional investigations and anxiety. People classified as false negative are those who actually have the disease but the test fails to detect it. The patient then suffers the consequences of undiagnosed disease.

3.1 Evaluation of screening programmes

Before any screening programme is introduced, its advantages and disadvantages must be carefully assessed. The general principles of screening were initially set out in the late 1960s (Wilson & Jungner, 1968). Since then, the criteria have been updated (UK National Screening Committee, 1998) and programmes now need to meet a number of criteria. These broadly relate to the health condition, the screening test, the availability of effective treatment, and the screening programme itself. Figure 2 outlines our summary of the criteria currently used by a variety of international health organisations to evaluate population screening. Based on such criteria, there is as yet no justification for population-based screening for Type 2 Diabetes (Borch-Johnsen et al., 2003; Waugh et al., 2007; Wareham & Griffin, 2001), although the case is becoming stronger. Whilst Type 2 Diabetes meets many of the criteria for screening, the main argument against population-based screening is that uncertainty remains about the true benefits arising from the early detection of Type 2 Diabetes through such programmes. In addition, it is unclear whether the economic cost of screening can be justified.

The results of the ADDITION study (Echouffo-Tcheugui et al, 2009 ; Lauritzen et al., 2000; Sandbaek et al., 2008), which will assess the effectiveness of screening for Type 2 Diabetes combined with the provision of intensive treatment to newly-diagnosed patients, will be available soon and will provide much-needed evidence for or against screening.

4. Screening for Type 2 Diabetes

Type 2 Diabetes may well be a suitable disease for screening - it is a serious disease, being associated with many complications, especially in the eyes, heart, kidneys, and limbs and it shortens the expectation of life considerably. Screening tests consist of blood glucose tests and/or oral glucose tolerance tests. These tests are relatively cheap with a blood glucose test costing only £0.48 (US$0.77) in the UK National Health Service. Blood glucose tests and oral glucose tolerance tests have no adverse effects for the patient apart from the inconvenience of having blood tests and the very rare complications of venepuncture.

There are two broad approaches to screening for Type 2 Diabetes - population or opportunistic screening. They have different advantages and disadvantages.

4.1 Population screening

Population screening, as its name implies, is based on a defined population and aims to screen every person in this population (Engelgau et al., 2000). It includes 'universal' screening, which attempts to define the prevalence of diabetes by screening a whole community (Knowler et al., 1978; Sharp, 1964), and 'targeted' or 'selective' screening, which attempts to screen a defined sub-group of the population (Engelgau et al., 2000). In either case, a suitable test such as a screening blood glucose test is offered to a defined population.

The Condition

1. The condition is an important health problem for the individual, and the community or population [a,b,c]
2. The natural history of and risk factor(s) for the condition are understood [a,b,c]
3. There is a recognisable pre-clinical (asymptomatic) stage or an early symptomatic stage in which the condition can be diagnosed [a,b,c]
4. All cost-effective interventions to prevent the condition have been implemented as far as possible [a]

The Test

5. There is a simple, safe, precise and validated screening test [a,b,c]
6. The screening test is acceptable to the population [a,b,c]
7. The distribution of test values in the target population is known and suitable cut-off levels are defined and agreed [a]
8. There is an agreed policy on the further investigation of individuals with a positive screening test result [a]

The Treatment

9. There is an acceptable and effective treatment or intervention for individuals identified through screening [a,c]
10. There is evidence that early treatment leads to better outcomes than late treatment [a,b,c]
11. There are clear, evidence-based policies on which individuals should be offered treatment and the appropriate treatment to be offered [a,c]

The Screening Programme

12. There is evidence from high quality randomised controlled trials that the screening programme is effective in reducing mortality or morbidity [a]
13. The information provided about the test and its outcome must be of value and readily understood by the individual being screened [a]
14. There is evidence that the complete screening programme (test, diagnostic procedures, treatment/intervention) is clinically, socially and ethically acceptable to health professionals and the public [a,c]
15. The benefits from the screening programme outweigh the physical and psychological harm caused by the test, diagnostic procedures and treatment [a,c]
16. The economic costs of the screening programme (including testing, diagnosis, treatment, administration, training, and quality assurance) are balanced in relation to expenditure on medical care as a whole [a,b,c]
17. There is a plan for the organisation, management and monitoring of the screening programme and an agreed set of quality assurance standards [a,c]
18. There are adequate staffing and facilities for testing, diagnosis and treatment [a,b,c]
19. Evidence-based information, explaining the consequences of testing, investigation and treatment, is available to potential participants to help them make an informed choice [a]
20. Screening will be a systematic, ongoing process and not an isolated one-off effort [a,c]

Fig. 2. Criteria for assessing the value of screening programmes
(Criteria adopted by: [a] UK National Screening Committee; [b] American Diabetes Association; [c] World Health Organization).

Historically, screening was offered directly to people in communities and sometimes directly to people in the street – UK examples include surveys undertaken in Bedford (Sharp, 1964), Rotherham (Girt et al., 1969), and Birmingham (Birmingham Diabetes Survey Working Party, 1976). However, the yield was small as many people at low risk were approached and some of those detected failed to consult their GP. Costs per new case detected were therefore high and this approach was abandoned. Community screening could be cost-effective if the prevalence of Type 2 Diabetes in the community was extremely high, although this is rarely the case.

The populations most often identified for screening include people selected because they have one or more risk factors for Type 2 Diabetes. These most commonly include older age, obesity, a family history of diabetes, and hypertension. This approach increases the likelihood of finding new cases and so improves the efficiency of the screening process.

Risk factors are most commonly known to GPs. They are not known to hospitals, as they do not hold the medical records of populations, only those people referred to them. Hence, population screening nowadays is most commonly based on people selected from the population registers of people registered with family practices. This has meant that most of the research reports have come from those countries in which the health system is based on family practices, i.e. Australia, Canada, New Zealand, the Netherlands, the UK, Denmark, and registration-based systems in the USA.

Population screening has several important advantages. It is mathematically precise, readily reproducible, and can operate largely independent of the clinical skills of the doctors and nurses in the family practices. It is easy to transpose arrangements across areas and countries.

Population screening has several important disadvantages. Unless whole community populations are used, various techniques have to be employed to determine potential sub-groups at risk. Selection has to be made on the basis of various clinical risk factors as set out below. This can involve searching of medical records or extraction of risk factors such as age and Body Mass Index (BMI) (Greaves et al., 2004) directly from the GP database or applying external criteria such as those of the American Diabetes Association to the GP's electronic record (Woolthuis et al., 2007). However, there are always people, including those at risk, who decline to accept the offer of screening for a variety of reasons.

The process then involves communication with the people in the target population, usually by writing to them and offering them an appointment. Some people will want to change their appointment and staff of the practice need to accommodate this. Some people will not come and may need to be sent a further appointment. Those who do come need to be recorded. Then, if the screening process is separate from the clinician, the clinician has to be informed and take action. In some US studies, primary care clinicians have not always responded appropriately (Ealovega et al., 2004). There may be a difference in attitude to those tests initiated by clinicians themselves and those tests initiated by others.

It is inevitable that population screening carries administrative costs over and above the cost of the screening investigations. Nevertheless, in the UK, the National Health Service has recently instituted a comprehensive vascular risk assessment programme, known as 'NHS Health Checks' (Department of Health, 2008). These checks are offered to patients aged 40 to 74 years old who do not have existing vascular disease or diabetes. This is a two-step process and diabetes risk is estimated using a self-completed questionnaire, followed by a blood test if appropriate. It is envisaged that the whole of this age group in the population will be screened once every five years. Although it is considered reasonable to include a diabetes assessment within a global cardiovascular risk assessment, there is some current concern about the implementation of this programme (Khunti et al., 2011).

In summary, therefore, population screening, usually of high-risk sub-groups, is the commonest form of screening performed world wide, but in practice is undertaken only in richer and developed countries. Hence, one profound implication is that population screening may well be too costly to be undertaken in developing countries and this is doubly serious as many Asian countries have some of the highest levels of prevalence of Type 2 Diabetes in the world, e.g. 10% in China (Ramachandran et al., 2010).

4.2 Clinical opportunistic screening

Clinical opportunistic screening is quite different from population screening and is a form of clinical case finding. It is essentially an extension of ordinary clinical care in family practice. The key difference from population screening is that the patient, rather than the clinician, makes the appointment. In clinical opportunistic screening, the patient makes the appointment to go to the family practice and then the clinically alert doctor or nurse takes advantage of the patient's presence in the consulting room to offer screening, based on their risk factor profile.

This process has a long tradition in family practice and the whole basis of determining how many people smoke, drink heavily, are overweight or obese, or have raised cholesterol levels has been done in family practices without any national screening programmes. Since more clinical conditions are screened for opportunistically than are screened for by formal population programmes, opportunistic screening can be seen as the usual method of screening. It has just not been recognised as such.

The introduction of computer systems in UK family practices (since the 1980s) has enabled generalist doctors and nurses - for the first time - to organise, handle, and retrieve data live during consultations. Computers have made the family practice consultation much more efficient and opportunistic screening is one aspect of this.

Clinical opportunistic screening has several advantages. Firstly, this process eliminates most of the costly administrative overheads associated with population screening. Secondly, since the offer of screening is made within a therapeutic and trusting patient-doctor relationship, acceptance rates are generally high. An important advantage is that the screening process is offered by the doctor who will care for the patient if the disease is diagnosed, so that, if the test is positive, treatment can start immediately. Thirdly, the relatively high contact rate that people have with their primary health care team underpins clinical opportunistic screening. In the UK, The NHS Information Centre for Health and Social Care (2009) reports that the average contact for adults with their family practice is 5.5 encounters per year of which 3.4 per patient per year are with the doctor. This is important in that the health system offers the doctor repeated opportunities to screen; if a test is missed on one occasion when the patient is distressed or in no state to be screened, or if the doctor simply forgets, then the doctor can be confident that the average patient will be seen again within about four months.

Fourthly, clinical opportunistic screening exploits the key fact that it is family practice, and only family practice, which has the risk factor data and often knows it very well. For example, GPs are spending more and more of their time seeking to alter risk factors for disease. They screen for and increasingly find and then treat hypertension, itself a risk factor for Type 2 Diabetes and also for obesity which is all too obvious to the clinician. Other risk factors such as a positive family history may be very well known too as the family doctor will have often treated the older family members for diabetes and may still be doing so.

Fifthly, this is the only system which can be undertaken in developing countries and is possible wherever there are generalist doctors. Fortunately, family medicine and computerisation of family practice records is spreading steadily around the world, hence the potential for this approach is increasing rapidly worldwide.

In one recent method, university staff determined the risk groups and worked with a group of associated family practices to develop a 'flagging system' which jogged the doctor's memory when at risk patients are seen (Woolthuis et al., 2009). The authors concluded that because it was 'embedded within daily care' and achieved a high uptake rate, this approach was feasible and inexpensive; however, no estimate of the screening costs was reported.

Clinical opportunistic screening has some important disadvantages. Realistically, it cannot be expected to cover the entire at-risk population and it is dependent on the patient consulting for some reason. It also depends on the clinical alertness of the family physicians and practice nurses. This is not standard, and there are inevitable variations in clinical skills, which means variations in the screening process being delivered. The offer of clinical opportunistic screening is a judgement and different clinicians will make different judgements at different times. These types of interventions therefore cannot be completely standardised. Hence, they have been criticised by some as inefficient (Law, 1994) and can be seen as untidy, and potentially unpredictable. Furthermore, patients vary greatly in their emotional state in consultations and, if they are upset with anxiety, depression or having just received bad news, it becomes inappropriate to offer screening.

4.3 International guidelines on screening for Type 2 Diabetes

Whilst there is not yet sufficient evidence to support the introduction of general population screening, there is broad support for screening programmes that focus on defined sub-groups of the population who are at higher risk of developing Type 2 Diabetes. A number of organisations have issued position statements relating to targeted or opportunistic screening for Type 2 Diabetes (e.g. American Diabetes Association, 2011; Diabetes UK, 2006; World Health Organization, 2003). These make recommendations about the patient sub-groups that should be considered for screening, the frequency of screening, where screening should take place, and the preferred screening test.

4.3.1 Who should be offered screening and how frequently?

It is generally accepted (American Diabetes Association, 2011; Diabetes UK, 2006) that clinical judgement and patient preference should guide decisions about screening for Type 2 Diabetes. Several organisations in the UK, Europe and USA (American Diabetes Association, 2011; Diabetes UK, 2006; Paulweber et al., 2010) have made recommendations about the risk factors that might indicate a need for screening and these are summarised in Figure 3.

The optimal frequency of screening is not known. However, Diabetes UK (2006) and the American Diabetes Association (2011) recommend that health professionals should consider proactively screening adults at risk of developing the condition every three years. Both organisations note that it may be necessary to screen more frequently, for example, where individuals are overweight and have one or more of the other risk factors shown in Figure 3.

4.3.2 Where should screening take place?

Currently, the consensus view is that screening should take place in a clinical setting, with testing offered by health care providers, based on an assessment of the individual patient. Diabetes UK argue that "screening is probably most-effective when performed as part of a general health review in primary and community care services, when other cardiovascular risks can be measured … and appropriate advice is immediately available" (Diabetes UK, 2006; p.6).

To achieve screening in 'hard-to-reach' groups, particularly ethnic minorities in developed countries, other locations have been suggested, including religious and community venues or assessments in the workplace (Grant et al., 2004; Oberlinner et al., 2008; Porterfield et al., 2004; Somannavar et al., 2008; Tabaei et al., 2003), although the evidence base for screening in these settings is limited at present.

One potential disadvantage is that community screening of this nature does not reach the groups who are most at risk of developing the condition, and may inappropriately test those who are at low risk or those already diagnosed with diabetes. Diabetes UK (2006) supports community screening for patient groups who do not routinely access family practice services, *provided that* the screening process is guided by clear protocols, staff receive appropriate training, and good medical support is available from local health services. In contrast, the American Diabetes Association (2011) does *not* recommend community screening, even for high-risk populations, because there is a risk that those screened may not seek or be able to access appropriate follow-up and care.

4.3.3 Which screening test should be used?

There is insufficient evidence to identify a single ideal screening test (Waugh et al., 2007). A range of tests exist which might be used for screening purposes and these vary in their sensitivity and specificity, as well as their convenience, acceptability and cost (Cox & Edelman, 2009). Sensitivity is the "proportion of true positives that are correctly identified by the test", while specificity is the "proportion of true negatives that are correctly identified by the test" (Altman & Bland, 1994).

Diabetes UK (2006)

The following people should be offered screening for diabetes every 3 years:

a. White people aged over 40 years and people from Black, Asian and minority ethnic groups aged over 25 years, with one or more of the following risk factors:
   - A first degree family history of diabetes (parents or siblings with diabetes);
   - Overweight, obese or morbidly obese (body mass index of 25-30 kg/m^2 and above) and a sedentary lifestyle;
   - Waist measurement of 94 cm (37 inches) or above for White and Black men, and 80 cm (31.5 inches) or above for White, Black and Asian women, and 90 cm (35 inches) or above for Asian men.

b. People with ischaemic heart disease, cerebrovascular disease, peripheral vascular disease or treated hypertension;

c. Women who have had gestational diabetes who have tested normal following delivery (screen within 6 weeks of delivery, then 1 year post-partum and then three-yearly);

d. Women with polycystic ovary syndrome who have a body mass index of 30 kg/m^2 or more;

e. People who are known to have impaired glucose tolerance or impaired fasting glycaemia;

f. People who have severe mental health problems;

g. People who have hypertriglyceridaemia not due to alcohol excess or renal disease.

IMAGE guidelines (Paulweber et al., 2010)

a. White people aged over 40 years or people from Black, Asian and minority ethnic groups, aged over 25 years with one or more of the following risk factors:
   - A first degree family history of diabetes; and/or
   - Body mass index over 25 kg/m²; and/or
   - Waist measurement of $\geq$ 94 cm for White and Black men and $\geq$ 80 cm for White, Black and Asian women, and $\geq$ 90 cm for Asian men; and/or
   - Systolic blood pressure $\geq$ 140 mm Hg or diastolic blood pressure $\geq$ 90 mm Hg or treated hypertension; and/or
   - HDL-cholesterol $\leq$ 0.35 g/l (0.9 mmol/l) or triglycerides $\geq$ 2g/l (2.2 mmol/l) or treated dyslipidaemia.

b. Women with a history of gestational diabetes or with a child weighing > 4 kg at birth;

c. People with history of temporarily induced diabetes - e.g. steroids;

d. People who have ischaemic heart disease, cerebrovascular disease, peripheral vascular disease;

e. Women with polycystic ovary syndrome who have a body mass index $\geq$ 30 kg/m²;

f. People who have severe mental health problems and/or receiving long term antipsychotic drugs;

g. People with a history of Impaired Glucose Tolerance or Impaired Fasting Glucose.

American Diabetes Association (2011)

Screening for diabetes should be considered every 3 years (with consideration of more frequent testing depending on initial results and risk status):

a. In all adults who are overweight (body mass index $\geq$ 25 kg/m²) and have one or more of the following risk factors:
   - Physical inactivity
   - Family history of diabetes (first-degree relative, i.e. parents or siblings with diabetes);
   - High-risk race/ethnicity (e.g. African-American, Latino, Native American, Asian-American, Pacific Islander);
   - Women who delivered a baby weighing >9lbs or were diagnosed with gestational diabetes mellitus;
   - Hypertension (blood pressure 140/90 mm Hg or higher or on therapy for hypertension);
   - HDL cholesterol of 35 mg/dl (0.90 mmol/l) or less and/or a triglyceride level of 250 mg/dl (2.82 mmol/l) or more;
   - Women with polycystic ovary syndrome;
   - A_{1c} $\geq$ 5.7%, Impaired Glucose Tolerance or Impaired Fasting Glucose on previous testing;
   - Other clinical conditions associated with insulin resistance (e.g. severe obesity, acanthosis nigricans);
   - History of cardiovascular disease.

b. In the absence of the above criteria, screening should begin at age 45 years.

Fig. 3. UK, European and US Guidance on who should be screened for Type 2 Diabetes

Options include the fasting blood glucose test, the oral glucose tolerance test, random (or casual) blood glucose test, or a fasting capillary blood glucose test. More recently, it has been suggested that the glycated haemoglobin (HbA_{1c}) test might also be appropriate for screening, because it does not require fasting and reflects longer-term glycaemia rather than a value at a single time point (American Diabetes Association, 2011; Bennett et al., 2007; Saudek et al., 2008). HbA_{1c} may also have more relevance to clinicians dealing with patients who have diabetes. Urine testing is not strongly recommended for screening purposes, because it is less sensitive than the blood tests.

Currently, a fasting blood glucose test is recommended as the screening test for Type 2 Diabetes in the UK and the USA (American Diabetes Association, 2011; Diabetes UK, 2006). It is easier and faster to perform in clinical settings, more convenient and acceptable to patients, and less expensive than other tests. The latest US guidance (American Diabetes Association, 2011) also states that the HbA_{1c} and 2-hour 75g oral glucose tolerance test are appropriate tests to screen for diabetes. European guidance has tended to encourage the use of the oral glucose tolerance test as the gold standard diagnostic test (Waugh et al., 2007).

Diabetes UK (2006) suggest a fasting capillary blood test can be used for initial screening purposes, although this has lower sensitivity and specificity than venous blood glucose measurement and requires careful interpretation and feedback to the patient. Random (or casual) blood or plasma glucose testing can also be carried out if the patient has taken food or drink prior to the screening test; in this sense, it is practical but the results can be more difficult to interpret than those obtained via fasting tests.

Where a screening test result is suggestive of diabetes, it is recommended that a second, fasting test be repeated on a different day to exclude the possibility of laboratory error, unless the patient has classic symptoms of diabetes. Guidance (American Diabetes Association, 2011; Diabetes UK, 2006) exists for health professionals with regard to the interpretation of test results. This includes the action needed (e.g. further testing, appropriate referrals) as well as the patient education that is required when positive, borderline, or normal test results are received.

4.4 Approaches to screening

A number of targeted screening programmes have been piloted in the UK, Europe and the USA in the last decade (e.g. Echouffo-Tcheugui et al., 2009; Edelman et al., 2002a; Franciosi et al., 2005; Greaves et al., 2004; Goyder et al., 2008; Janssen et al., 2007; O'Connor et al., 2001; Woolthuis et al., 2009).

Many have employed a 'stepwise' approach, whereby participants progress through increasingly invasive screening procedures until they are diagnosed with diabetes or found not to have the condition. The number of steps in the screening process varies across studies.

Typically, in the first step, potential screening participants are identified by:

- their responses on a self-completed questionnaire that assesses their risk of diabetes, such as the FINDRISC (Saaristo et al., 2005), the Symptom Risk Questionnaire (Adriaanse et al., 2002) or the Diabetes Risk Score (Franciosi et al., 2005); or
- using the GP electronic medical records to search for people who match specific risk criteria (e.g. Greaves et al., 2004); or
- using a standardised risk calculator based on clinical data held on the computerised medical record to assess the patient's risk of diabetes, such as the Cambridge Risk Score (Griffin et al., 2000) or QDRISK (Hippisley-Cox et al., 2009).

A recent alternative approach has been the use of online self-completion risk tools to determine a person's risk of diabetes and hence the need for further action. Both the American Diabetes Association and Diabetes UK have online risk calculators available for the public to use (http://www.diabetes.org/diabetes-basics/prevention/diabetes-risk-test/; and http://www.diabetes.org.uk/riskscore respectively).

Individuals who are identified as being 'at risk' of diabetes after the first step are offered (by invitation letter or during a GP consultation) a blood test to directly measure their glucose levels. The initial test tends to be relatively simple and convenient; in some studies, this has been a random blood glucose or HbA_{1c} sample (which do not require prior fasting); in others, a capillary blood sample ('finger prick' test) has been used.

If the results of the initial blood test fall within the normal range, the participant does not progress to the next level, but may receive lifestyle advice. If the results of the initial test reveal glucose levels above a specified threshold, participants are invited back for further testing. At that stage, the screening test may require the patient to fast for a prescribed period prior to the blood sample or undergo a more complex and lengthy screening process, such as the oral glucose tolerance test.

Uptake of screening has varied across the studies and this may be a reflection of the type of test offered, how the invitation is made and where the testing takes place. In one study (O'Connor et al., 2001), the uptake of an initial random blood glucose test (offered via letter) was 44%. Where random capillary blood tests were offered, however, uptake was around 60-70% (Echouffo-Tcheugui et al., 2009). In one study, the reported uptake of a fasting capillary blood glucose test offered directly by the GP was 90% (Woolthuis et al., 2009). Further dropout is evident at the later stages of many of the stepwise screening processes, whereby individuals who have abnormal results in initial tests fail to return for further tests (Woolthuis et al., 2009), particularly where this involves more invasive or complex tests or where the patient is referred to an outpatient clinic (e.g. Franciosi et al., 2005; Janssen et al., 2007; O'Connor et al., 2001).

4.5 The St Leonard's Practice approach to screening for Type 2 Diabetes

The system of screening for Type 2 Diabetes in the St Leonard's Practice, Exeter, UK is one special form of clinical opportunistic screening (Evans et al., 2008). It does not employ any external resources to screen for risk factors. The process relies on the clinical alertness of the GPs and practice nurses, and the efficient protocol-driven screening of patients with chronic conditions known to be associated with Type 2 Diabetes. The doctors and nurses screen adult patients with cardiovascular or cerebrovascular disease, hypertension, hypercholesterolaemia, obesity, recurrent skin infections, or a positive family history of diabetes.

Its advantages are that it eliminates another layer of costs that arise from the involvement of an external agency, such as a university or medical school. It also means that people from external organisations do not see confidential medical records. It fosters professional interest amongst GPs in patients as people with individual risks. It also fosters professional pride in GPs in ultra-early diagnosis. It is possible to maintain the system year after year and it has been so maintained in this practice since 1987 (Evans et al., 2008). Clinical opportunistic screening has the advantage that, since so many blood tests are taken nowadays in family practice, it is often possible to add the blood glucose screening test to samples being taken already, thus saving the patient an additional blood test.

The main advantage of this system is that it can identify, year after year, two-thirds of all new cases of Type 2 Diabetes before a single symptom of diabetes has been reported by a patient (Evans et al., 2008).

Some family practices, including St Leonard's, operate personal lists (Pereira Gray, 1979). When these are in use, it is also possible to compare the performance between doctors. Its main advantage internationally is that the method is more easily reproducible in family practices around the world. All that is needed is an enthusiastic family practitioner or nurse and an efficient computerised medical record system. Both family practice and computer systems are spreading rapidly.

The disadvantages of the St Leonard's system are that the intervention is not standardised and that there are variations between the six doctor partners operating it. It is not yet known how easy it will be to roll it out into other family practices more widely and it may be difficult where morale is low or burnout amongst the doctors is a serious problem (Soler et al., 2008).

4.6 The psychological effects of screening

Marteau (1990) notes that the receipt of an invitation to participate in a cancer or general health screening programme can be enough to evoke anxiety for some patients. As one might expect, receiving a 'positive' result after the screening test can also cause negative emotional reactions. People are not always reassured, even by a 'normal' result, and other adverse psychological effects can occur. For example, a 'normal' result may reinforce an unhealthy lifestyle or perceptions of invulnerability, and make patients less likely to return for future screening (Marteau 1989).

Recently, studies in Europe and the USA have specifically explored the psychological effects of undergoing screening for Type 2 Diabetes and these tend to support the conclusions of Marteau's work. Some studies have assessed the impact of screening by asking patients to complete rating scales that measure their levels of anxiety, depression, and disease-specific worry (Eborall et al., 2007a; Park et al., 2008), or their health-related quality of life (Edelman et al., 2002b). Such studies have generally found no lasting or significant adverse psychological effects in terms of anxiety, depression, worry, or perceived quality of life after screening. However, there is some evidence that simply being invited for screening can increase state anxiety and that, six weeks after attending, anxiety is higher amongst people who have progressed further through the screening process, particularly those who were eventually diagnosed with diabetes (Park et al., 2008).

Other studies have explored patients' experiences of screening in more depth. One study, which interviewed people shortly after they underwent screening tests (Adriaanse et al., 2002), found most participants had positive views of the screening process and had not found it burdensome. Most individuals who had been newly-diagnosed with diabetes did not feel alarmed or concerned about their results. Many appeared to believe they had a 'mild' version of the condition that they could control, although they felt the required lifestyle changes would have a significant impact on their life. People whose test results were normal reported feelings of relief or reassurance but saw no reason to change their lifestyle. Only a quarter of this group intended to have their blood glucose tested in future. Another study, which interviewed participants at different stages of a stepwise screening process (Eborall et al., 2007b), reported similar findings but noted that the stepped nature of the screening process appeared to help participants to adjust psychologically.

The World Health Organization (2003) has cautioned that, as public awareness increases about the significance of a diagnosis of diabetes and its possible complications, the psychological effects of screening may become more marked. Marteau (1990) and Griffin et al. (2000) argue that some of the negative effects of screening can be avoided or reduced, if health professionals attend to the patient's psychological and information needs at each stage of the screening process, including the point of invitation, the test procedure itself, discussing the results, and later follow-up.

4.7 The economic cost of screening for Type 2 Diabetes

Economic modelling studies have been conducted to estimate the cost-effectiveness of screening for Type 2 Diabetes and Impaired Glucose Tolerance. In the UK, decisions about funding of interventions are made by the National Institute for Health and Clinical Excellence (NICE), based on cost-effectiveness. This body considers that interventions below an incremental cost-effectiveness ratio (ICER) threshold of £20,000 to £30,000 per quality-adjusted life-year (QALY) are cost-effective (National Institute for Health and Clinical Excellence, 2004).

One systematic review and economic modelling exercise (Waugh et al., 2007), which included four studies, reached the conclusion that screening for diabetes appeared to be cost-effective for people aged 40-70 years. Whilst screening was more cost-effective for the older age bands (50-69 and 60-69 years), even for people aged 40-49 years, the ICER for screening (when compared to a policy of not screening) was £10,216 per QALY. Screening was found to be more cost-effective for people who were hypertensive and obese and, for many groups, the costs of screening were offset by lower treatment costs in the future. However, because the most comprehensive model in the review came from the USA (Hoerger et al., 2004), the applicability of these findings in the UK was questioned.

A more recent modelling study (Gillies et al., 2008), based on data derived from England and Wales, concluded that screening for Type 2 Diabetes and Impaired Glucose Tolerance - combined with appropriate lifestyle or pharmacological interventions for those found to have Impaired Glucose Tolerance to delay or prevent diabetes - appeared to be cost-effective in a population aged 45 years with 'above-average' risk of developing diabetes. When comparing a policy of *not* screening to one of screening for Type 2 Diabetes *and* Impaired Glucose Tolerance, there were differential costs for each QALY gained, depending on whether diagnosis of Impaired Glucose Tolerance was followed by lifestyle interventions or by pharmaceutical interventions. The costs per QALY gained were £6,242 for screening followed by *lifestyle* interventions, and £7,023 for screening followed by *pharmacological* interventions. In contrast, the cost-effectiveness of a policy of screening for Type 2 Diabetes only was less certain. Here, compared to a policy of not screening, the estimated costs for each QALY gained in respect of screening for Type 2 Diabetes alone were £14,150.

The results of the above studies suggest that it may be more cost-effective to screen for Type 2 Diabetes *and* Prediabetes, rather than Type 2 Diabetes alone. The ADDITION study will also include a cost-effectiveness analysis of screening plus intensive intervention for Type 2 Diabetes and the results of this work are awaited (Lauritzen et al., 2000).

Other studies have attempted to determine the costs of targeted or opportunistic screening, based on the cost of identifying one new case of Type 2 Diabetes. In one US study (O'Connor et al., 2001), which used a two-step screening protocol (random blood glucose followed by oral glucose tolerance test), one new case of diabetes was identified for every 40 high-risk patients screened. The uptake of screening was relatively low (44% of patients who were invited attended) and the screening costs per new case were estimated at $4,064 per new case identified.

More recently, a Danish study (Dalsgaard et al., 2010) has compared three different stepwise screening strategies for Type 2 Diabetes. In the first strategy, diabetes risk questionnaires were sent by the family practice to people aged 40-69 years and those found to be at high risk were asked to contact their GP to arrange a screening test. This strategy detected new cases of Type 2 Diabetes in 0.8% of the target population, at a cost of €1,058 (US$1,535)" per case. Two opportunistic screening programmes were also piloted. In these approaches, people who were consulting their GP were asked to complete the risk questionnaire in the waiting room and were either offered a screening test during the consultation (OP-direct) or asked to return for a fasting screening test at a subsequent consultation (OP-subsequent). The OP-direct strategy detected new cases of Type 2 Diabetes in 0.9% of the target population, at a cost of €707 (US$1,026) per case, while the OP-subsequent strategy detected Type 2 Diabetes in 0.5% of the target population, at a cost of €727 (US£1,055) per new case. The authors concluded that opportunistic screening can identify a similar proportion of new cases as mail-distributed questionnaires, but at lower cost.

5. Conclusions

The worldwide epidemic of diabetes, mainly Type 2 Diabetes, calls for a major response as, in some countries, prevalence now exceeds 10% of the whole adult population. Clinicians are seeking to prevent the condition developing and to screen for undiagnosed cases. Since Type 2 Diabetes is increasingly managed in family practice or primary care, education and support is important.

Prevention of Type 2 Diabetes is now possible through lifestyle alteration but, so far, only after expensive interventions. Drugs can aid prevention but adverse effects are a big issue. Research on simplifying lifestyle interventions is urgent. Once Type 2 Diabetes is diagnosed, health professionals can then intervene as early as possible, before symptoms develop, in order to prevent complications.

In the meanwhile, achieving earlier diagnosis of Type 2 Diabetes depends on screening. Population screening is likely to be introduced in richer countries and has recently started in the UK.

Clinical opportunistic screening in family practice offers an important alternative approach since it may well be more cost-effective, provides the quickest route to treatment, and can detect two-thirds of all new cases of Type 2 Diabetes in a defined population. However, the effectiveness of this type of screening in routine care without extra resources has only been demonstrated in one practice and needs replication. If the early reports are confirmed, then clinical opportunistic screening warrants further consideration as an affordable alternative to population screening, particularly in the developing world.

6. Acknowledgements

We acknowledge with thanks the assistance of Ms Beverley Berry, Information Manager at the Royal College of General Practitioners, London, who provided references for reports relating to early community screening programmes in Rotherham, Bedford and Birmingham. We also acknowledge with thanks the assistance of Dr Maurice Salzmann, Consultant Clinical Biochemist at the Royal Devon and Exeter NHS Foundation Trust, Exeter, who provided details of the local NHS laboratory cost of a blood glucose test.

7. References

Adriaanse, M.C., Snoek, F.J., Dekker, J.M., van der Ploeg, H.M., Heine, R.J. (2002). Screening for type 2 diabetes: an exploration of subjects' perceptions regarding diagnosis and procedure. *Diabetic Medicine,* Vol. 19, pp. 406-411.

Altman, D.G., Bland, J.M. (1994). Diagnostic tests : sensitivity and specificity. *British Medical Journal,* Vol. 308 (11 June 1994), p. 1552.

American Diabetes Association (2011). Standards of medical care in diabetes - 2011. *Diabetes Care,* Vol. 34, Supplement 1 (January 2011), pp. S11-S61.

Bennett, C.M., Guo, M., Dharmage, S.C. (2007). HbA_{1c} as a screening tool for detection of type 2 diabetes : A systematic review. *Diabetic Medicine,* Vol. 24, pp. 333-343.

Birmingham Diabetes Survey Working Party (1976). Ten year follow-up report on Birmingham Diabetes Survey of 1961. *British Medical Journal,* Vol. 2 (3 July 1976), pp. 35-37.

Borch-Johnsen, K., Lauritzen, T., Glumer, C. and Sandbaek, A. (2003). Screening for type 2 diabetes - should it be now ? *Diabetic Medicine,* Vol. 20, pp. 175-181.

Buchanan, T.A., Xiang, A.H., Peters, R.K., Kjos, S.L., Marroquin, A., Goico, J., Ochoa, C., Tan, S., Berkowitz, K., Hodis, H.N., Azen, S.P. (2002). Preservation of pancreatic beta-cell function and prevention of type 2 diabetes by pharmacological treatment of insulin resistance in high-risk hispanic women. *Diabetes,* Vol. 51, pp. 2796–2803.

Bulugahapitya, U., Siyambalapitiya, S., Sithole, J., Idris, I. (2009). Is diabetes a coronary risk equivalent? Systematic review and meta-analysis. *Diabetic Medicine,* Vol. 26, pp. 142-148.

Cautinho, M., Gerstein, H.C., Wang, Y., Yusuf, S. (1999). The relationship between glucose and incident cardiovascular events. A meta-regression analysis of published data from 20 studies of 95,783 individuals followed for 12.4 years. *Diabetes Care,* Vol. 22, Supplement 2, pp. 233–240.

Chiasson, J.L., Josse, R.G., Gomis, R., Hanefeld, M., Karasik, A., Laakso, M. (2003). Acarbose treatment and the risk of cardiovascular disease and hypertension in patients with impaired glucose tolerance: the STOP-NIDDM trial. *The Journal of the American Medical Association,* Vol. 290, pp. 486–494.

Cox, M.E., Edelman, D. (2009). Tests for screening and diagnosis of type 2 diabetes. *Clinical Diabetes,* Vol. 27, No. 4, pp. 132-138.

Dalsgaard, E.M., Christensen, J.O., Skriver, M.V., Borch-Johnsen, K., Lauritzen, T., Sandbaek, A. (2010). Comparison of different stepwise screening strategies for type 2 diabetes : Findings from Danish general practice, ADDITION-DK. *Primary Care Diabetes,* Vol. 4, No. 4 (December 2010), pp. 223-229.

DECODE Study Group (2003). Age- and sex-specific prevalences of diabetes and impaired glucose regulation in 13 European cohorts. *Diabetes Care,* Vol. 26, No. 1 (January 2003), pp. 61-69.

Del Prato, S. (2009). Megatrials in type 2 diabetes. From excitement to frustration? *Diabetologia,* Vol. 52, pp. 1219-1226.

Department of Health (2008). *Putting Prevention First – Vascular checks: Risk assessment and management,* Department of Health, London.

Diabetes UK (2006). *Position Statement : Early identification of people with type 2 diabetes,* Diabetes UK, London.

Diabetes UK (2009). *Position Statement : Impaired glucose regulation (IGR)/Non-diabetic hyperglycaemia (NDH)/Prediabetes,* Diabetes UK, London.

Ealovega, M.W., Tabaei, B.P., Brandle, R., Burke, R., Herman, W.H. (2004). Opportunistic screening for diabetes in routine clinical practice. *Diabetes Care,* Vol. 27, No. 1, pp. 9-12.

Eborall, H.C., Griffin, S.J., Prevost, A.T., Kinmonth, A.L., French, D.P., Sutton, S. (2007a). Psychological impact of screening for type 2 diabetes: controlled trial and comparative study embedded in the ADDITION (Cambridge) randomised controlled trial. *British Medical Journal,* 31 August 2007, doi: 10.1136/bmj.39303.723449.55 (abridged text in print : *British Medical Journal,* Vol. 335, pp. 386-489).

Eborall, H., Davies, R., Kinmonth, A.L., Griffin, S., Lawton, J. (2007b). Patients' experiences of screening for type 2 diabetes: prospective qualitative study embedded in the ADDITION (Cambridge) randomised controlled trial. *British Medical Journal,* 31 August 2007, doi: 10.1136/bmj.39308.392176.BE (abridged text in print : *British Medical Journal,* Vol. 335, pp. 490-493).

Echouffo-Tcheugui, J.B., Simmons, R.K., Williams, K.M., Barling, R.S., Prevost, A.T., Kinmonth, A.L., Wareham, N.J., Griffin, S.J. (2009). The ADDITION-Cambridge trial protocol : a cluster-randomised controlled trial of screening for type 2 diabetes and intensive treatment for screen-detected patients. *BMC Public Health,* Vol. 9, pp. 136.

Edelman, D., Edwards, L.J., Olsen, M.K., Dudley, T.K., Harris, A.C., Blackwell, D.K., Oddone, E.Z. (2002a). Screening for diabetes in an outpatient clinic population. *Journal of General Internal Medicine,* Vol. 17, pp. 23-28.

Edelman, D., Olsen, M.K., Dudley, T.K., Harris, A.C., Oddone, E.Z. (2002b). Impact of diabetes screening on quality of life. *Diabetes Care,* Vol. 25: 1022-1026.

Engelgau, M.M., Narayan, K.M.V., Herman, W.H. (2000). Screening for type 2 diabetes. *Diabetes Care,* Vol. 23, No. 10 (October 2000), pp. 1563-1580.

Evans, P.H., Greaves, C., Winder, R., Fearn-Smith, J., Campbell, J.L. (2007). Development of an educational 'toolkit' for health professionals and their patients with prediabetes : the WAKEUP study (Ways of Addressing Knowledge Education and Understanding in Prediabetes). *Diabetic Medicine,* Vol. 24, No. 7, pp. 770-777.

Evans, P., Langley, P., Pereira Gray, D. (2008). Diagnosing type 2 diabetes before patients complain of diabetic symptoms – clinical opportunistic screening in a single general practice. *Family Practice,* Vol. 25, No. 5, pp. 376-381.

Franciosi, M., De Berardis, G., Rossi, M.C.E., Sacco, M., Belfiglio, M., Pellegrini, F., Tognoni, G., Valentini, M., Nicolucci, A., for The IGLOO Study Group (2005). Use of the

Diabetes Risk Score for opportunistic screening of undiagnosed diabetes and impaired glucose tolerance. *Diabetes Care,* Vol. 28, pp. 1187-1194.

Gerstein, H.C., Yusuf, S., Bosch, J., Pogue, J., Sheridan, P., Dinccag, N., Hanefeld, M., Hoogwerf, B., Laakso, M., Mohan, V., Shaw, J., Zinman, B., Holman, R.R. (2006). Effect of rosiglitazone on the frequency of diabetes in patients with impaired glucose tolerance or impaired fasting glucose: a randomised controlled trial. *Lancet,* Vol. 368, pp. 1096–1105.

Gillies, C.L., Abrams, K.R., Lambert, P.C., Cooper, N.J., Sutton, A.J., Hsu, R.T., Khunti, K. (2007). Pharmacological and lifestyle interventions to prevent or delay type 2 diabetes in people with impaired glucose tolerance: systematic review and meta-analysis. *British Medical Journal,* Vol. 334 (19 January 2007), pp. 299-302.

Gillies, C.L., Lambert, P.C., Abrams, K.R., Sutton, A.J., Cooper, N.J., Hsu, R.T., Davies, M.J., Khunti, K. (2008). Different strategies for screening and prevention of type 2 diabetes in adults: cost effectiveness analysis. *British Medical Journal,* Vol. 336 (21 April 2008), doi: 10.1136/bmj.39545.585289.25.

Girt, J.L., Hooper, L.A., Abel, R.A. (1969). *The multiple health screening clinic, Rotherham 1966: A social and economic assessment. A report prepared by the Social Science Research Unit,* Her Majesty's Stationery Office/Department of Health and Social Security, London.

Goyder, E., Wild, S., Fischbacher, C., Carlisle, J., Peters, J. (2008). Evaluating the impact of a national pilot screening programme for type 2 diabetes in deprived areas of England. *Family Practice,* Vol. 25, pp. 370-375.

Grant, T., Soriano, Y., Marantz, P.R., Nelson, I., Williams, E., Ramirez, D., Burg, J., Nordin, C. (2004). Community-based screening for cardiovascular disease and diabetes using HbA_{1c}. *American Journal of Preventive Medicine,* Vol. 26, No. 4 (May 2004), pp. 271-275.

Greaves, C.J., Stead, J.W., Hattersley, A.T., Ewings, P., Brown, P., Evans, P.H. (2004). A simple pragmatic system for detecting new cases of type 2 diabetes and impaired fasting glycaemia in primary care. *Family Practice,* Vol. 21, pp. 57-62.

Griffin, S.J., Little, P.S., Hales, C.N., Kinmonth, A.L., Wareham, N.J. (2000). Diabetes risk score: towards earlier detection of type 2 diabetes in general practice. *Diabetes / Metabolism Research and Reviews,* Vol. 16, pp. 164-171.

Haffner, S.M., Lehto, S., Ronnemaa, T., Pyorala, K., Laakso, M. (1998). Mortality from coronary heart disease in subjects with type 2 diabetes and in nondiabetic subjects with and without prior myocardial infarction. *The New England Journal of Medicine,* Vol. 339, No. 4, pp. 229-234.

Harris, M.I., Klein, R., Welborn, T.A., Knuiman, M.W. (1992). Onset of NIDDM occurs at least 4-7 yr before clinical diagnosis. *Diabetes Care,* Vol. 15, No. 7, pp. 815-819.

Heneghan, C., Thompson, M., Perera, R. (2006). Prevention of diabetes. *British Medical Journal,* Vol. 333 (14 October 2006), pp. 764-765.

Hippisley-Cox, J., Coupland, C., Robson, J., Sheikh, A., Brindle, P. (2009). Predicting risk of type 2 diabetes in England and Wales: prospective derivation and validation of QDScore. *British Medical Journal,* Vol. 338: b880.

Hoerger, T.J., Harris, R., Hicks, K.A., Donahue, K., Sorensen, S., Engelgau, M. (2004). Screening for Type 2 Diabetes Mellitus: A cost-effectiveness analysis. *Annals of Internal Medicine,* Vol. 140, No. 9 (4 May 2004), pp. 689-699.

Holman, R.R., Paul, S.K., Bethel, M.A., Matthews, D.R., Neil, H.A.W. (2008). 10-year follow-up of intensive glucose control in type 2 diabetes. *The New England Journal of Medicine,* Vol. 359, No. 15 (9 October 2008), pp. 1577-1589.

Hu, F.B., Stampfer, M.J., Haffner, S.M., Solomon, C.G., Willett, W.C., Manson, J.E. (2002). Elevated risk of cardiovascular disease prior to clinical diagnosis of type 2 diabetes. *Diabetes Care,* Vol. 25, No. 7 (July 2002), pp. 1129-1134.

International Diabetes Federation (2003). *Diabetes Atlas (Second Edition).* International Diabetes Federation, Brussels.

Janssen, P.G.H., Gorter, K.J., Stolk, R.P., Rutten, G.E.H.M. (2007). Low yield of population-based screening for type 2 diabetes in the Netherlands: the ADDITION Netherlands study. *Family Practice,* Vol. 24, pp. 555-561.

Khunti, K., Walker, N., Sattar, N., Davies, M. (2011). Unanswered questions over NHS health checks. *British Medical Journal,* Vol. 342 (5 February 2011), pp. 316-318.

Kilkkinen, A., Heistaro, S., Laatikainen, T., Janus, E., Chapman, A., Absetz, P., Dunbar, J. (2007). Prevention of type 2 diabetes in a primary health care setting : interim results from the Greater Green Triangle (GTT) Diabetes Prevention Project. *Diabetes Research and Clinical Practice,* Vol. 76, pp. 460-462.

Knowler, W.C., Bennett, P.H., Hamman, R.F., Miller, M. (1978). Diabetes incidence and prevalence in Pima Indians : A 19-fold greater incidence than in Rochester, Minnesota. *American Journal of Epidemiology,* Vol. 108, No. 6, pp. 497-505.

Knowler, W.C., Barrett-Connor, E., Fowler, S.E., Hamman, R.F., Lachin, J.M., Walker, E.A., Nathan, D.M. (2002). Reduction in the incidence of type 2 diabetes with lifestyle intervention or metformin. *The New England Journal of Medicine,* Vol. 346, pp. 393-403.

Laatikainen, T., Dunbar, J.A., Chapman, A., Kilkkinen, A., Vartiainen, E., Heistaro, S., Philpot, B., Absetz, P., Bunker, S., O'Neil, A., Reddy, P., Best, J.D., Janus, E.D. (2007). Prevention of type 2 diabetes by lifestyle intervention in an Australian primary health care setting : Greater Green Triangle (GGT) Diabetes Prevention Project. *BMC Public Health,* Vol. 7, p. 249.

Lauritzen, T., Griffin, S., Borch-Johnsen, K., Wareham, N.J., Wolffenbuttel, B.H., Rutten, G. (2000). The ADDITION study : proposed trial of the cost-effectiveness of an intensive multifactorial intervention on morbidity and mortality among people with type 2 diabetes detected by screening. *International Journal of Obesity and Related Metabolic Disorders,* Vol. 24 (September 2000), Supplement 3, pp. S6-S11.

Law, M. (1994). 'Opportunistic' screening. *Journal of Medical Screening,* Vol. 1, No. 4 (October 1994), p. 208.

Marteau, T.M. (1989). Psychological costs of screening. *British Medical Journal,* Vol. 229 (26 August 1989), p. 527.

Marteau, T.M. (1990). Screening in practice : Reducing the psychological costs. *British Medical Journal,* Vol. 301 (7 July 1990), pp. 26-28.

Morrison, A.S. (1998). Screening. In: *Modern Epidemiology (Second Edition),* K.J. Rothman and S. Greenland (Editors), pp. 499-518, Lippincott Williams & Wilkins, ISBN 0-316-75780-2, Philadelphia, USA.

National Collaborating Centre for Chronic Conditions (2008). *Type 2 diabetes: National clinical guideline for management in primary and secondary care (update),* The Royal College of Physicians, London.

National Institute for Health and Clinical Excellence (2004). *Guide to the methods of technology appraisal,* National Institute for Health and Clinical Excellence, London.

National Institute for Health and Clinical Excellence (2009). *Type 2 diabetes: The management of type 2 diabetes (NICE Clinical Guideline 87),* National Institute for Health and Clinical Excellence, London.

NHS Information Centre for Health and Social Care (2009). *Trends in consultation rates in general practice 1995/1996 to 2008/2009 : Analysis of the QResearch® database,* The Health and Social Care Information Centre, London.

NHS Information Centre for Health and Social Care (2010). *Prevalence: Quality and Outcomes Framework (QOF) for April 2009 - March 2010, England - Numbers on QOF disease registers and raw prevalence rates, England,* accessed 12 April 2010, available from: http://www.ic.nhs.uk/webfiles/QOF/2009-10/Prevalence%20tables/QOF0910_National_Prevalence.xls

O'Connor, P.J., Rush, W.A., Cherney, L.M., Pronk, N.P. (2001). Screening for diabetes mellitus in high-risk patients : Cost, yield and acceptability. *Effective Clinical Practice,* Vol. 4, pp. 271-277.

Oberlinner, C., Neumann, S.M., Ott, M.G., Zober, A. (2008). Screening for pre-diabetes and diabetes in the workplace. *Occupational Medicine,* Vol. 58, No. 1 (January 2008), pp. 41-45.

Park, P., Simmons, R.K., Prevost, A.T., Griffin, S.J. (2008). Screening for type 2 diabetes is feasible, acceptable but associated with increased short-term anxiety : A randomised controlled trial in British general practice. *BMC Public Health,* Vol. 8, (October 2008), p. 350.

Paulweber, B., Valensi, P., Lindstrom, J., Lalic, N.M., Greaves, C.J., McKee, M., Kissimova-Skarbek, K., Liatis, S., Cosson, E., Szendroedi, J., Sheppard, K.E., Charlesworth, K., Felton, A.M., Hall, M., Rissannen, A, Tuomilehto, J, Schwarz, PE, Roden, M, on behalf of the IMAGE Study Group (2010). A European evidence-based guideline for the prevention of type 2 diabetes. *Hormone and Metabolic Research,* Vol. 42, Supplement 1, pp. S3-S36.

Pereira Gray, D.J. (1979). The key to personal care. *Journal of the Royal College of General Practitioners,* Vol. 29, pp.666-678.

Porterfield, D.S., Din, R., Burroughs, A., Burrus, B., Petteway, R., Treiber, L., Lamb, B., Engelgau, M. (2004). Screening for diabetes in an African-American community: The Project DIRECT experience. *Journal of the National Medical Association,* Vol. 96, No. 10 (October 2004), pp. 1325-1331.

Ramachandran, A., Snehalatha, C., Mary, S., Mukesh, B., Bhaskar, A.D., Vijay, V. (2006). The Indian Diabetes Prevention Programme shows that lifestyle modification and metformin prevent type 2 diabetes in Asian Indian subjects with impaired glucose tolerance (IDPP-1). *Diabetologia,* Vol. 49, pp. 289–297.

Ramachandran, A., Ma, R.C.W., Snehalatha, C. (2010). Diabetes in Asia. *Lancet;* Vol. 375, pp. 408-418.

Roland, M. (2004). Linking physicians' pay to the quality of care - a major experiment in the United Kingdom. *The New England Journal of Medicine,* Vol. 351 (30 September 2004), pp. 1448-1454.

Saaristo, T., Peltonen, M., Lindstrom, J., Saarikoski, L., Sundvall, J., Eriksson, J.G., Tuomilehto, J. (2005). Cross-sectional evaluation of the Finnish Diabetes Risk Score: a tool to identify undetected type 2 diabetes, abnormal glucose tolerance and metabolic syndrome. *Diabetes and Vascular Disease Research,* Vol. 2, No. 2 (May 2005), pp. 67-72.

Salpeter, S.R., Buckley, N.S., Kahn, J.A., Salpeter, E.E. (2008). Meta-analysis: Metformin treatment in persons at risk for diabetes mellitus. *The American Journal of Medicine,* Vol. 121, Issue 2 (February 2008), pp. 149-157.

Sandbaek, A., Griffin, S.J., Rutten, G., Davies, M., Stolk, R., Khunti, K., Borch-Johnsen, K., Wareham, N.J., Lauritzen, T. (2008). Stepwise screening for diabetes identifies people with high but modifiable coronary heart disease risk: The ADDITION study. *Diabetologia,* Vol. 51 (29 April 2008), pp. 1127-1134.

Saudek, C.D., Herman, W.H., Sacks, D.B., Bergenstal, R.M., Edelman, D., Davidson, M.B. (2008). A new look at screening and diagnosing diabetes mellitus. *Journal of Clinical Endocrinology and Metabolism,* Vol. 93, No. 7 (July 2008), pp. 2447-2453.

Sharp, C.L. (1964). Diabetes survey in Bedford 1962. *Proceedings of the Royal Society of Medicine,* Vol. 57, No. 3 (March 1964), pp. 193-195.

Soler, J.K., Yaman, H., Esteva, M., Dobbs, F., Asenova, R.S., Katic, M., Ozvacic, Z., Desgranges, J.P., Moreau, A., Lionis, C., Kotanyi, P., Carelli, F., Nowak, P.R., de Aguiar Sa Azeredo, Z., Marklund, E., Churchill, D., Ungan, M. (European General Practice Research Network Burnout Study Group) (2008). Burnout in European family doctors: the EGPRN study. *Family Practice,* Vol. 25, No. 4, pp. 245-265.

Somannavar, S., Lanthorn, H., Pradeepa, R., Narayanan, V., Rema, M., Mohan, V. (2008). Prevention Awareness Counselling and Evaluation (PACE) Diabetes Project: A mega multi-pronged program for diabetes awareness and prevention in South India (PACE-5). *Journal of the Association of Physicians of India,* Vol. 56 (June 2008), pp. 429-435.

Spijkerman, A.M.W., Dekker, J.M., Nijpels, G., Adriaanse, M.C., Kostense, P.J., Ruwaard, D., Stehouwer, C.D.A., Bouter, L.M., Heine, R.J. (2003). Microvascular complications at time of diagnosis of type 2 diabetes are similar among diabetic patients detected by targeted screening and patients newly diagnosed in general practice: The Hoorn Screening Study. *Diabetes Care,* Vol. 26, No. 9, pp. 2604-2608.

Spijkerman, A.M.W., Henry, R.M.A., Dekker, J.M., Nijpels, G., Kostense, P.J., Kors, JA., Ruwaard, D., Stehouwer, C.D.A., Bouter, L.M., Heine, R.J. (2004). Prevalence of macrovascular disease amongst type 2 diabetic patients detected by targeted screening and patients newly diagnosed in general practice: the Hoorn Screening Study. *Journal of Internal Medicine,* Vol. 256, pp. 429-436.

Stumvoll, M., Goldstein, B.J., van Haeften, T.W. (2005). Type 2 diabetes: principles of pathogenesis and therapy. *The Lancet*, Vol. 365 (9 April 2005), pp. 1333-1346.

Tabaei, B.P., Burke, R., Constance, A., Hare, J., May-Aldrich, G., Parker, S.A., Scott, A., Stys, A., Chickering, J., Herman, W.H. (2003). Community-based screening for diabetes in Michigan. *Diabetes Care*, Vol. 6, No. 3, pp. 668-670.

Torgerson, J.S., Hauptman, J., Boldrin, M.N., Sjostrom, L. (2004). XENical in the prevention of diabetes in obese subjects (XENDOS) study: a randomized study of orlistat as an adjunct to lifestyle changes for the prevention of type 2 diabetes in obese patients. *Diabetes Care*, Vol. 27, pp. 155–161.

Tuomilehto, J., Lindstrom, J., Eriksson, J.G., Valle, T.T., Hamalainen, H., Ilanne-Parikka, P., Keinanen-Kiukaanniemi, S., Laakso, M., Louheranta, A., Rastas, M., Salminen, V., Uusitupa, M., for the Finnish Diabetes Prevention Study Group (2001). Prevention of type 2 diabetes mellitus by changes in lifestyle among subjects with impaired glucose tolerance. *The New England Journal of Medicine*, Vol. 344, No. 18, pp. 1343-1350.

UK National Screening Committee (1998). *First report of the National Screening Committee*, Health Departments of the United Kingdom, London.

UK Prospective Diabetes Study (UKPDS) Group (1998). Intensive blood-glucose control with sulphonylureas or insulin compared with conventional treatment and risk of complications in patients with type 2 diabetes (UKPDS 33). *The Lancet*, Vol. 352 (12 September 1998), pp. 837-853.

Unwin, N., Shaw, J., Zimmet, P., Alberti, K.G.M.M. (2002). Impaired glucose tolerance and impaired fasting glycaemia : the current status on definition and intervention. *Diabetic Medicine*, Vol. 19, pp. 708-723.

Wareham, N.J. & Griffin, S.J. (2001). Should we screen for type 2 diabetes ? Evaluation against National Screening Committee criteria. *British Medical Journal*, Vol. 332 (21 April 2001), pp. 986-988.

Waugh, N., Scotland, G., McNamee, P., Gillett, M., Brennan, A., Goyder, E., Williams, R., John, A. (2007). Screening for type 2 diabetes: literature review and economic modelling. *Health Technology Assessment*, Vol. 11, No. 17, pp. 1-144.

Wilson, J.M.G., Jungner, G. (1968). *Principles and practice of screening for disease*, World Health Organization, Geneva.

Woolthuis, E.P.K., de Grauw, W.J.C., van Gerwen, W.H.E.M., van den Hoogen, H.J.M., van de Lisdonk, E.H., Metsemakers, J.F.M., van Weel, C. (2007). Identifying people at risk for undiagnosed type 2 diabetes using the GP's electronic medical record. *Family Practice*, Vol. 24, pp. 230-236.

Woolthuis, E.P.K., de Grauw, W.J.C., van Gerwen, W.H.E.M, van den Hoogen, H.J.M., van de Lisdonk, E.H., Metsemakers, J.F.M., van Weel, C. (2009). Yield of opportunistic targeted screening for type 2 diabetes in primary care : The Diabscreen Study. *Annals of Family Medicine*, Vol. 7, No. 5, pp. 422-430.

World Health Organization (2003). *Screening for type 2 diabetes : Report of a World Health Organization and International Diabetes Federation meeting*, World Health Organization, Geneva.

Yamaoka K, Tango T. (2005). Efficacy of lifestyle education to prevent type 2 diabetes: a meta-analysis of randomized controlled trials. *Diabetes Care,* Vol. 28, pp. 2780-2786.

Yorkshire and Humber Public Health Observatory (2007). *Diabetes key facts : Supplement 2007,* Yorkshire and Humber Public Health Observatory, York.

15

Community Participation Model for Prevention and Control of Diabetes Mellitus

Víctor Manuel Mendoza-Núñez, María de la Luz Martínez-Maldonado and Elsa Correa-Muñoz
Unidad de Investigación en Gerontología, Facultad de Estudios Superiores Zaragoza, Universidad Nacional Autónoma de México (UNAM), México D.F., México

1. Introduction

The health of the population is a product of the society and at the same time an indispensable contribution to economic growth and political stability. The degree of health of the population is a very important indicator of human development. In this regard, it is necessary for the Ministry of Health to forge alliances with other public and private actors, including organizations of the civil society, because it has been shown recently that one of the key elements that contribute to maintenance of health is the support that is received from interpersonal interaction.

At present, there has been a significant increase worldwide of chronic degenerative diseases, among which Diabetes mellitus (DM) is prominent.

Diabetes mellitus constitutes a public health problem worldwide. In this respect, the International Diabetes Federation estimates that 285 million people around the world suffer from DM. This total is expected to rise to 438 million within 20 years. Each year, an additional seven million persons develop diabetes (International Diabetes Foundation [IDF], 2011). This disease is the leading cause of death in Mexican population and is the most cost-intensive item for the nation's health care system. The majority of patients with diabetes in Mexico are in poor metabolic control (Villalpando et al., 2010a). In this respect, the current care model has not been effective for the prevention and control of DM. Thus, it is necessary to develop feasible strategies for adapting the current care model into a context of shared responsibility between the community and the health-team system (Villalpando et al., 2010b).

In this chapter, we present a community participation model for the prevention and control of diabetes mellitus. This model establishes as its fundamental strategy the implementation of a formal health-promoters training program so that program participants will achieve empowerment and constitute a social capital of benefit to themselves through active participation in the community with the practice of self-care, mutual aid, and self-promotion in an organized and systematic social network (Mendoza-Núñez et al., 2009a). For management of diabetes mellitus in the community, the following are established as key elements: (i) adoption of healthy lifestyles; (ii) treatment individualization and health promotion strategies, (iii) aggressive prevention and management of risk factors, and (iv) rigorous glycemic control as an element of prevention and management (Mendoza-Núñez & Rosado-Pérez, 2010).

2. Health concepts

Health is a fundamental quality of the human being, who is a biological, living, dynamic, and unique being; a social being who is in permanent interaction with other human beings, situated in a time and space that depend on their environment and that act on it; a being of emotions, of sensations, of desires, of intentions; a spiritual being; a being of knowledge, of rationality, of reflection. Therefore, health will be expressed in each of these dimensions (Contandriopoulos, 2006).

On the other hand, in order to understand the determinants of the wellness-sickness of individuals and populations, it is necessary to explore the biological, social, and psychic spaces of humans. Each of these dimensions constitutes a viewpoint on wellness-sickness and on the factors affecting this. None of these dimensions is independent of the others, nor is any sufficient for summarizing the significance of health and what the determinants of the latter are.

It is also important to recognize that the protection or promotion of the population in the broadest sense cannot constitute a responsibility that the society delegates to one institution in particular (a health system, or a private group: physicians; social workers; community groups, etc.). This should be assumed by the entire society and depends on the capacity of the State to guarantee access to education, health services, safety, and a healthy environment. In these terms, health is the concern of each of the citizens (Contandriopoulos, 2006).

The manner of conceptualizing health and disease should evolve so that it is not only the result of consensuses of normality and abnormality, of statistical tables or measurements by techno-scientific apparatuses, but rather, the result of a dialog in which the scientific, subjective, and contextual aspects of biopsychosocial humans participate (Caponi, 1997).

On the other hand, it is important to recognize that the human, as are all living beings, is an integrated whole that constitutes a dynamic suprasystem, which is in turn comprises the following many perfectly coordinated subsystems: the physical subsystem; the chemical; the biological; the psychological; the social; the cultural; the ethico-moral, and the spiritual. All of these, together and integrated, constitute the personality, and their lack of integration or coordination unleashes pathological processes of different natures: organic; psychological; social, or several together.

Within this context, the definitions of health, as with other human qualities, are generated at specific historical moments and are linked with the social and economic circumstance under which the spaces for application of this definition gain in practice, signify the way to obtain power to overcome this particular circumstance; thus, these definitions cannot be more than historically perishable. Notwithstanding its transitory situation, the way of looking at health by those wielding power over more or less extensive population groups defines the way of acting in relation to their health and the purposes and forms of utilizing their resources (Chapela, 2008a).

In this work, we understand health as "the capacity of the human corporeal nature to decide and contract viable futures and of reaching these". This definition of health, on the one hand, conceives of the subject as body-subjectivity, that is, as only one thing, and on the other, sets forth a cross-disciplinary and multi-conceptual position on health and ponders the subject in collective fashion (Chapela, 2008a).

This definition allows us to disassociate health from sickness, to understand that the former is an essential part of the subject and not solely a state or a moment in life. The latter term shows us that the subject has a great deal to do with the construction of health at the individual as well as at the collective level, without forgetting that the human corporeal-nature capacity of deciding and constructing futures is mediated not only by the individual's world vision, by history, that is, by past, present, and future happenings that have permeated the person's being and the individual's being in the world, but also by the social guidelines that structure the ways that subjects proceed, without forgetting the psychobiological dimension in which aspirations, wishes, sensations, and emotions, and, of course, actions take place, having the political and economic dimensions as a framework (Chapela, 2008a).

3. Health Promotion (HP)

The notion of HP is also complex and controversial, and to date, a consensus has not been reached with regard to its significance. HP is a relatively recent notion and acquired importance during the mid-XX Century. However, throughout history we are able to find practices and conceptions directed toward improving the conditions of life of the people that, in the light of present-day conceptions and values, could be recognized as antecedents of HP, although with significant differences (Restrepo, 2001; Gómez-Arias and González, 2004; Eslava- Castañeda, 2006; Chapela, 2008b).

According to the Ottawa Charter, HP is a process that permits people to increase control over their health to improve it. It constitutes a political, social, and global progression that encompasses not only actions directed precisely toward strengthening the abilities and capacities of individuals, but one that is also directed toward modifying social, environmental, and economic conditions with the aim of mitigating their impact on public and individual health. HP is the process that allows people to increase their control over the determinants of health and, consequently, to improve it. Participation is essential to sustain action in matters of health promotion (Ottawa Charter for the Promotion of Health, World Health Organization [WHO] Geneva, Switzerland 1986).

However, after Ottawa, multiple health promotions may be found in distinct countries and practiced by distinct international organizations, although these affirm that they have adopted the Ottawa Charter as their directorate. The original concept that is planned in the document involves conducting changes in many structural instances; however, not all of the organisms that have understood the document are disposed to change; thus, the actions in many cases have been very restricted (Chapela 2008b).

4. Community models for the prevention and control of diabetes mellitus

In the past decades, the implementation of community programs for the prevention and control of DM has been a priority worldwide (Shephard et al., 2005; Castillo, 2010; Ciccone et al., 2010). In this regard, the study published by Wagner et al. in 1996 permitted determination of the common elements of community programs for chronic disease control with the participation of the community, which allowed for developing the so-called "The Chronic Care Model (CCM)". The CCM focuses on improving and optimizing six key elements of the health care system: i) health care organization; ii) delivery system design; iii) clinical information systems; iv) decision support; v) self-management support, and vi) community resource linkages. The usefulness of this model has been widely demonstrated for the prevention and control of DM (Wagner et al., 1996; Wagner et al., 1999; Glasgow et al., 2001 Parchman et al., 2007; Piatt et al., 2006; Battersby et al., 2010; Strickland et al., 2010).

Although the usefulness of the CCM is widely recognized for the prevention and control of chronic diseases, the need has been recognized to broaden, modify, or adapt it, taking into consideration the specific needs of the population; therefore, some options, one denominated the Expanded Chronic Care Model (ECCM), have been proposed (Barr et al., 2003). Among the best known proposals, we are able to cite Racial and Ethnic Approaches to Community Health (REACH) (Giachello et al., 2003; Jenkins et al., 2010) and Community-based Participatory Research (CBPR) (Savage et al., 2006; Horowitz et al., 2009).

In Latin America, the Program for Education of Non-insulin-dependent Diabetics-Latin America (PEDNID-LA) was proposed, which was implemented simultaneously in Argentina, Bolivia, Brazil, Chile, Colombia, Costa Rica, Cuba, Mexico, Paraguay, and Uruguay, demonstrating satisfactory results for the adoption of healthy lifestyles (Gagliardino & Etchegoyen, 2001).

In Mexico, the Ministry of Health's General Directorate of Health Promotion developed the Health Promotion Operational Model in 2006. Based on Ottawa Charter functions, the model integrates health promotion activities within the overall health care system (Santos-Burgoa et al., 2009). However, the results relative to the implementation and effectiveness of the model have not been reported.

The National Autonomous University of Mexico (UNAM, FES-Zaragoza Campus) has developed a model for the prevention and control of chronic diseases that is directed toward older adults (Mendoza-Núñez et al., 1996; Martínez-Maldonado et al., 2007, Mendoza-Núñez et al., 2009a); notwithstanding this, its application is not limited to this age group, but rather, can be useful for the adult population in general.

The model is based fundamentally on the integral development of the person, understood as a process that is carried out throughout and until the end of the person's lifetime. It implies becoming active in many ways, making use of and potentiating the resources possessed. It is a process of transformation and continuous growth in which the social capital is fundamental. Integral development involves the following elements: citizenship; social capital; potentialities; social networks, and empowerment.

a. The concept of citizenship, which makes relevant the fact of "being subject to" with rights (rights to life, freedom, dignity, health, well-being, etc.) and of being able to make use of these.
b. Social capital, which permits the potential exchange of the opportunities of a social support network.
c. The concept of potentialities, which all of us human beings possess physically (functional efficiency, muscular force, and motor skills), psychologically (sensitivity, affect, knowledge acquisition, creativity, etc.), and socially (links, productivity, social participation, the creation of culture and values, etc.).
d. Social support networks, by means of which, through personal, community, and institutional contacts, the individual maintains his/her identity and his social development.
e. Empowerment, the process of participative development through which individuals, communities, and organizations achieve greater control over their lives and environment.

5. Social support networks and health

The study of social support and its repercussions on the state of health, well-being, and Quality of life (QOL) has experienced significant development dating from the last three decades of the XX Century, above all in some related disciplines, such as preventive medicine, public health, community psychology, social work, anthropology, and sociology. Notwithstanding this, self-help groups, as they are now known, arose in the 1930s in the U.S. with the foundation of Alcoholics Anonymous (AA) (Llopis, 2005).

Social networks refer to the personal, community, and institutional contacts through which the individual maintains his/her social identity and receive material, instrumental, emotional, and informative support. The basic elements of social support networks comprise social capital, which is defined as the potential exchange of opportunities of a social network. Therefore, social capital depends in large measure on the social contacts possessed by the individual (Burt, 1997). Likewise, social support represents the tangible element of social capital, which is represented by the material, instrumental, affective, and informative contributions, real or perceived, provided by family, friends, the community, and formal institutions (Fernández, 2005; Guzmán et al., 2002) (Figure 1).

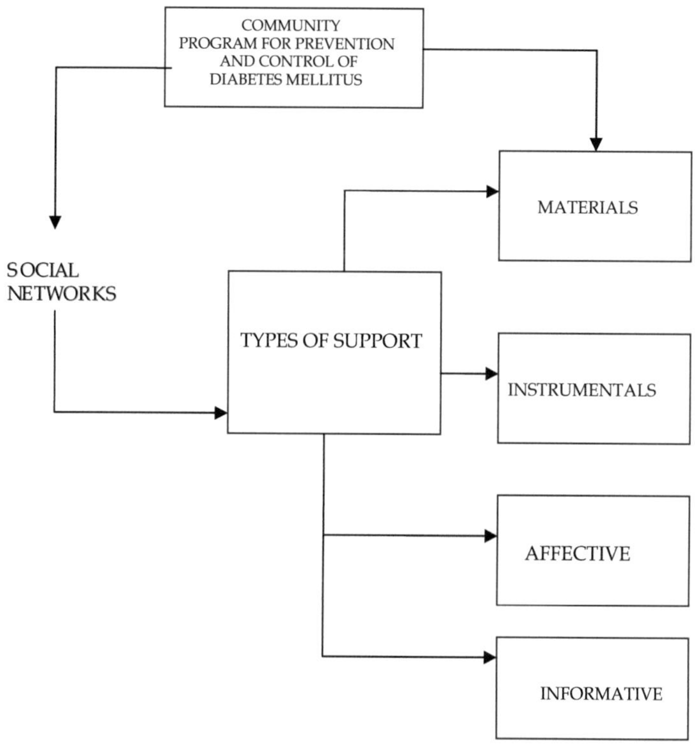

Fig. 1. Types of support that individuals can offer through social networks of social support in Community Programs for prevention and control of Diabetes Mellitus..

Program

Among elements to measure social networks, we find size, density, reciprocity, family relationship, homogeneity, type of support received, and social network analysis is approached through individualized description and the application of standardized instruments (Kloseck, 2007; Mendoza-Núñez & Martínez-Maldonado, 2009b).

Reciprocity is the key element of social networks and assumes that when support is requested from the social support network, the individual is aware that he/she, too, is a potential element of support for the group (Dabas & Perrone, 1999). Likewise, it is proposed that the social network wields an influence on health-related habits, because the individual is more likely to adopt healthy lifestyles if he/she has someone to share these with, and, on the other hand, internalization of the norms of behavior that the family, friends, and the community group offer can be of significant influence. In addition, the social control that is exercised by means of regulations, sanctions, or interventions can also exert an influence on attitudes and changes in conduct (Arechabala & Miranda, 2002). Therefore, a suitable social network is considered as an open, multicenter system made up of informal (family, friends, community) and formal components (professional and institutional), with defined objectives and goals framed within a program that, through the empowerment of individuals, achieves maximal health and well-being according to their sociocultural context. At present, it is recognized that one of the basic strategies for the prevention and control of diabetes mellitus is the establishment, coordination, and monitoring of social support networks as part of public policy (Mendoza-Núñez et al., 2009b).

Social support networks are a potential source of well-being and health, because health can be transmissible and the vehicle is the social support network.

6. Empowerment and health

Empowerment is defined as a process of participative development by means of which individuals, communities, and organizations achieve greater control over their lives and environment, acquiring rights and new life goals, in addition to a reduction of social marginalization (Kar, 1999; Anderson & Funnell, 2005; Maton, 2008). Empowerment involves self-strengthening, control, self-power, self-confidence, making decisions of one's own accord, a fitting life according to one's values, the capacity to fight for one's rights, independence, to the right to make one's own decisions. It is noteworthy that empowerment is relevant at the individual as well at the collective level (Ho et al., 2010).. In this regard, in order to exercise empowerment in an efficient and efficacious manner, it is indispensible to consider four key elements (Narayan, 2002):

i. Access to information. Information is power; it is in this way that informed citizens have more opportunities to access to services, to exercise their rights, and to ensure that non-governmental as well as governmental actors respond to their needs;
ii. Inclusion and participation. Individuals should be included in decision-making to ensure that the use of public and private resources responds to the real needs of the population.
iii. Responsibility or rendering of accounts. Public servants and those responsible for Non-governmental organizations (NGOs) should respond for their policies, actions, and the use of funds.
iv. Local organizational capacity. The population should possess the ability to organize itself and to work in a group, with the goal of participating actively in the community intervention programs that are developed in its milieu.

On the other hand, the importance has been highlighted of empowerment for the detection of chronic diseases according to the biopsychosocial model and patient-centered care, demonstrating that active participation of the individual is fundamental for to achieving maximum well-being and QOL at different ages and within different contexts (Salmon, 2003; Savage et al., 2006).

The main methods employed at the community level to achieve empowerment are the following (Kar, 1999): a) training for empowerment and the development of leadership; b) support for the establishment of policies and aid programs; c) public education and opinion for sources of support; d) the organization of associations; e) cooperative unions for the creation of empowerment collectives; f) empowerment for work and microentrepreneurs to achieve autonomy and control of their situation, and h) the protection of rights and social action for legislation to benefit specific groups.

Empowerment within the framework of health promotion considers motivation for action, empowerment-oriented support, individual participative actions, and an empowerment program for its institutionalization and replication (Maton, 2008). Likewise, it has been recognized that education is basic for achieving empowerment (Aujoulat et al., 2007). It has also been cited that social and educational activity in community interventions avoids isolation (Cattan, 2005).

The model contemplates a Community United for Human Growth (CUHG), whose purpose is to coordinate the large net of social networks of mutual-aid groups, in which self-care is a daily practice for the prevention and control of diabetes mellitus, as well as for achieving maximal well-being and health as components of one's human development (Figure 2).

Participation of the population aged 45 years and over (diabetics and non-diabetics) is considered, in that the common objective is to establish strategies for the individual to continue his/her integral human development. One of the determining factors for lack of control of chronic diseases, and especially for diabetes mellitus, comprises the prejudices and stereotypes that deriving form lack of information, which leads to negation of the disease and abandonment of treatment, or resorting to "miraculous or cure-all" treatments.

On the other hand, it has been demonstrated that apathy is one of the principal difficulties for the population in its adoption of healthy lifestyles for chronic disease prevention and control (Padala et al., 2008).

Thus, our proposal establishes the elimination of the stigma of the disease and proposes a model of community intervention for integral human development in which maintenance of health constitutes the key factor. This model avoids the social prejudices that label "groups of diabetics as sick people who do not follow the rules", which generates social rejection and abandonment of the group in many participants, who "seek at all times the cure for their incurable disease" in order to "stop being part of the group of diabetics".

In 1996, our research group proposed a community care model, considering the active participation of the individual in order to achieve maximum QOL in their social milieu (Mendoza-Núñez et al., 1996). In this respect, although the results have been satisfactory, we adapted the model in 2004 according to the paradigm of active aging and subsequently submitted this to a process of investigation to determine its feasibility and pertinence (Martínez-Maldonado et al., 2007). As previously mentioned, our proposal is not limited to older adults, because the principles and strategies can be applied to adult population in general.

The model establishes as the key element the formation of promoters of integral human development. In this regard, promoters function as mutual aid-group coordinators, establishing self-care and self-management actions for their members' well-being and social development, in which health maintenance is fundamental.

Self-care, mutual aid, and self-management constitute the basic strategic elements for the model proposed, and the former are closely linked; thus, we are unable to propose these in

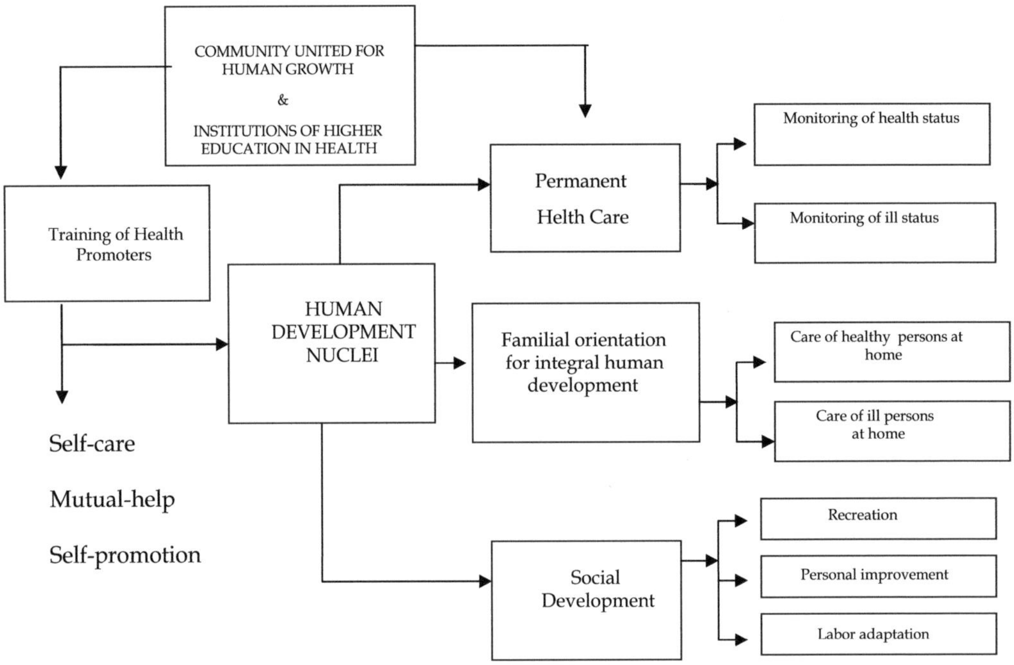

Fig. 2. Community Participation Model for Prevention and Control of Diabetes Mellitus. Community United for Human Growth linked to Institutions of Higher Education in Health is responsible for the design and implementation of educational programs and guides the training of the health promoters for the development of mutual-help groups (human development nucleus). A human development nuclei is a group integrated by 10 to 15 adults of nearby communities with similar interests. They are mainly involved in the practice of self-care, mutal-help, and self-promotion guidelines established by the program. The model is addressed toward the following objectives: (i) the supervision of the health status of participants in the program; (ii) the training of qualified health care promoters, certified on the basis of a formal continuous education program offered by a renowned academic institution; (iii) to provide orientation and guidance to families with regard to basic care practices with both healthy and sick adults; (iv) to promote the social and human development of the populations in Mexico.

isolated fashion. Therefore, any community program directed toward human development in which maintenance of health and improving QOL are considered should establish the mechanisms that allow for its harmonic and complementary execution. In this sense, knowledge, attitudes, and behaviors required for adequately exercising self-care, mutual aid, and self-management require the formal training of the persons who function as leaders and who promote the active participation of the members of mutual-aid groups (Song, 2010).

Self-care refers to the reasoned behavior of the individual with a theoretical basis that allows him/her to decide on and act upon the prevention, diagnosis, and treatment of acute and chronic diseases, as well as in maintenance of health and maximum enjoyment of their QOL, according to their sociocultural context, utilizing formal and informal social support networks in optimal fashion. Similarly, mutual aid includes the reasoned and requisite behavior that a group of individuals who share similar problems and who are aware of the advantages and commitments acquired adopts on voluntarily accepting to be part of the group. With regard to self-management, this involves the actions that an individual or self-help group performs in an autonomous manner, in an expected and optimal way, taking into consideration the elements and mechanisms of formal and informal social support networks.

The CUHG is one of the elements of the social support network, responsible for training Human Development Promoters (HDP), who are in turn responsible for coordinating mutual-aid groups denominated Human Development Nuclei (HDN), which are made up of 10 to 15 adults groups according to their affinities and the geographical closeness to their domiciles. HDN function under the directorates of self-care, -help, and -management.

The model's established pillars are:

- Permanent monitoring of the health state: The fundamental objective of this is to maintain, prolong, and recover health, as well as to improve the individual's self-perception of psychosocial well-being, according to his/her physical condition and sociocultural milieu. For this, self-care programs should be implemented for the healthy and sick individual, with pre-established evaluation, surveillance, and primary care-action protocols.
- Formation of Human Development Promoters: The CUHG, supported by an educative institution, is responsible for the formation of HDP, following a formal academic program, considering continuous education and a certification of the topicality and pertinence of the knowledge imparted.
- Familial orientation for integral human development: HDP possess sufficient knowledge to orient and train the individual's relatives to provide support for the psychosocial development of their family members, considering the basic skills for the care of the healthy and sick individual in the home.
- Adaptation and social development: The model took into consideration among its goals that adults would enjoy their situation to the maximum, taking into consideration their human life-cycle stage and sociocultural conditions. Thus, we recommend the implantation of programs of recreation, adaptation, and psychosocial and occupational self-improvement under an anthropological focus, according to the individual's interests, age, schooling, gender, health state, socioeconomic situation, etc.

The model establishes flexible general guidelines that could be adopted for rural and urban population, as well as for groups of adults of different sociocultural and economic conditions.

As an integral part of the model, the implementation has been established of a "Healthy Life" Program in which, under a constructivist focus, participants establish the strategies for adopting healthy lifestyles, utilizing a self-efficacy instrument to maintain and strengthen behavioral changes.

7. Model viability

The model has been implemented in Mexico with an older adult population from rural and urban areas. Notwithstanding this, as mentioned previously, its application is not limited to this age group (Mendoza-Núñez et al., 2009b).

Among the most relevant aspects of the model, we find that community groups are not labeled with "groups of diabetics" stigma. In this regard, it has been proposed that

unfundamented social representations of diabetes leads to prejudices on and negative stereotypes of the disease (Torres-López et al., 2005) that affect self-esteem, causing apathy, rejection, and abandonment of the "groups of diabetics" (Padala et al., 2008).
On the other hand, the anthropological aspects associated with the disease should be considered in community interventions, because cultural aspects determine negative lifestyles (sedentary life style and inadequate nutrition), which raises the risk of diabetes mellitus (Martorell, 2005).
For this reason, the purpose of our model is the conformation and integration of a "great network of networks" of mutual-aid groups who practice scientifically founded principles of daily self-care and self-management for their human development. In this light, the prevention of chronic diseases, and especially diabetes mellitus, constitutes one of the basic objectives.
Our experience in the application of the model demonstrates that it is viable in the technical and operative ambits at the community level; notwithstanding this, the most important weakness of the model lies in the discrepancy of its participative focus with State Social Development and Health Programs, in which neither empowerment nor the active participation of the population are considered, which generates frustration and, occasionally, program abandonment.

8. Healthy lifestyles and diabetes mellitus

Healthy lifestyles constitute key elements for preventing and controling DM. In this regard, it has been amply demonstrated that the periodic practice of physical exercise together with a healthy diet for a minimum of 2 years significantly diminishes the blood concentration of glucose, triglycerides, and cholesterol, and body weight, and increase the levels of High density lipoprotein (HDL) cholesterol, significantly diminishing the risk for metabolic syndrome, diabetes mellitus, and their complications (Steyn et al., 2004; Schulze & Hu, 2005; Barclay et al., 2008; Brown et al., 2009). Although the effectiveness of healthy lifestyles is known for the prevention and control of DM, the problematic resides in achieving the adoption and maintenance of the population of compliance with these lifestyles, In this respect, it has been cited that to maintain healthy lifestyles, the strategies should not be limited to the individual, but instead, should involve the family, the workplace, and community networks, in addition to the establishment of social reinforcement programs (Bazzano, 2005; Teufel-Shone et al., 2005; Toft et al., 2007; Marrero, 2009).
Among the factors linked with compliance with healthy lifestyles, we are able to highlight self-efficacy and self-esteem. In this regard, self-efficacy is a determining factor for self-care for DM (Johnston-Brooks et al., 2002; Hankonen et al., 2009). Similarly, low self-esteem and depression are factors related with low community participation for DM self-care (Fortmann et al., 2010).
In general, a healthy diet that is recommended comprises consuming three to five servings of fruits and vegetables daily and decreasing the consumption of foods rich in saturated fats and refined sugars. Nonetheless, it is important to cite that these recommendations should be adapted to age, gender, occupation, health state, socioeconomic level, food preferences, and food availability. In this respect, one of the errors observed in our environment in community programs for the prevention and control of DM is the recommendation of diets that are not accessible to the economic situation or that have discrepancies with food preferences, which occasions the non-compliance of persons with the program or program abandonment soon after beginning it (Mendoza-Núñez et al., 2008)

On the other hand, the practice of moderate physical exercise with a duration of 50 min daily for a minimum of 5 days weekly has biochemical, psychological, and social benefits (Caspersen et al., 1985; Laitakari, 1996); notwithstanding this, some cultural aspects that are linked with incorrect beliefs determine to a great extent the resistance of the population to adopting and maintaining this lifestyle, thus the need to establish strategies that respond to the sociocultural context (Marcus et al., 2000; Di Loreto et al., 2003).

9. Conclusion

The proposed model of community participation for the prevention and control of diabetes mellitus establishes as fundamental elements a broad concept of health, the concepts of citizenship and empowerment, and as self-care strategies, mutual aid and self-management with the support of social networks. Similarly, the model possesses several characteristics that distinguish it. In the first place is its versatility, because it can be adapted to different populations; in second place, its inclusion for the functioning of a program that is based on the recovery of the daily knowledge of persons with the aim of constructing new knowledge from these; the inclusion of subprograms of relevant aspects for achieving empowerment and disease control, while the integral development of persons is another characteristic that makes the model different from others and that eliminates the disease stigma, another of its benefits.

This model represents important savings of economic resources for the State.

Finally, to strengthen the viability of the model, it is indispensable that the State establish public policies that permit the development of this type of model.

10. Acknowledgments

This work was supported by Consejo Nacional de Ciencia y Tecnología FONSEC SSA/IMSS/ISSSTE S0008-2008-1, Grant 87139, and Instituto para la Atención de los Adultos Mayores del Estado de Hidalgo (IAAMEH), México.

11. References

Anderson, R.M., Funnell, M.M. (2005). Patient empowerment: reflections on the challenge of fostering the adoption of a new paradigm. *Patient Education and Counseling;* 57(2):153-157.

Arechabala, M. M. C. & Miranda, C. C. (2002). Validación de una escala de apoyo social percibido en un grupo de adultos mayores adscritos a un programa de hipertensión de la región metropolitana. *Ciencia y Enfermería;* 8: 49-55.

Aujoulat, I., d'Hoore. W. & Deccache, A. (2007). Patient empowerment in theory and practice: polysemy or cacophony?. *Patient Education and Counseling;* 66(1):13-20.

Barclay, C., Procter, K.L., Glendenning, R., Marsh, P., Freeman, J. & Mathers, N. (2008). Can type 2 diabetes be prevented in UK general practice? A lifestyle-change feasibility study (ISAIAH). *British Journal of General Practice;* 58(553):541-547.

Barr, V.J., Robinson, S., Marin-Link, B., Underhill, L., Dotts, A., Ravensdale, D. & Salivaras, S. (2003). The expanded Chronic Care Model: an integration of concepts and strategies from population health promotion and the Chronic Care Model. Hospital Quarterly;7(1):73-82.

Battersby, M., Von Korff, M., Schaefer, J., Davis, C., Ludman, E., Greene, S.M., Parkerton, M. & Wagner, E.H. (2010). Twelve evidence-based principles for implementing self-management support in primary care. *Joint Commission Journal on Quality and Patient Safety*; 36(12):561-570.

Bazzano, L.A., Serdula, M. & Liu, S. (2005). Prevention of type 2 diabetes by diet and lifestyle modification. *Journal of the American College of Nutrition*; 24(5):310-319.

Brown, T., Avenell, A., Edmunds, L.D., Moore, H., Whittaker, V., Avery, L. & Summerbell, C. (2009). Systematic review of long-term lifestyle interventions to prevent weight gain and morbidity in adults. *Obesity Reviews*; 10(6):627-638.

Burt, R. S. (1997). A note on social capital and network content. *Social Networks*; 19: 355-373.

Caponi, S. (1997). Georges Canguilhem y el estatuto epistemológico del concepto de salud. *História, Ciências, Saúde – Manguinhos*; IV (2):287-307.

Caspersen, C.J., Powell, K.E. & Christenson, G.M. (1985). Physical activity, exercise, and physical fitness: definitions and distinctions for health-related research. *Public Health Reports*;100(2):126-131.

Castillo, A., Giachello, A., Bates, R., Concha, J., Ramirez, V., Sanchez, C., Pinsker, E. & Arrom, J.(2010). Community-based diabetes education for Latinos: The Diabetes Empowerment Education Program. *Diabetes Educator*;36(4):586-594.

Cattan, M., White, M., Bond, J. & Learmouth, A. (2005) Preventing social isolation and loneliness among older people: a systematic review of health promotion interventions. *Ageing & Society; 25: 41–67.*

Ciccone, M.M., Aquilino, A., Cortese, F., Scicchitano, P., Sassara, M., Mola, E., Rollo, R., Caldarola, P., Giorgino, F., Pomo, V. & Bux, F. (2010). Feasibility and effectiveness of a disease and care management model in the primary health care system for patients with heart failure and diabetes (Project Leonardo). *Vascular Health and Risk Management*; 6:297-305.

Contandriopoulos, *A.-P. (2006).* Elementos para una "topografía" de concepto de la Salud. *Ruptures, Revista Interdisciplinaria de la Salud*; 11 (1): 86-99.

Chapela, M. C. (2008a). Promoción de la salud para la disminución del riesgo y el cuidado de las enfermedades crónicas. En: Mendoza-Núñez, V., Sánchez-Rodríguez y Correa-Muñoz, E. Estrategias para el Control de enfermedades crónico-degenerativas a nivel comunitario: México: FES Zaragoza, UNAM. p. 23-45.

Chapela, M.C. (2008b). Una definición de salud para promover la salud. En: Martínez (coord.) Seis miradas sobre la salud y sus relaciones con el mundo social. México: Universidad Autónoma Metropolitana. p. 13-33.

Dabas, E. & Perrone, N. (1999). Redes en salud. FUNCER. Disponible en: http://www.pasteur.secyt.gov.ar/formadores/RedSal-Dabas-Perrone.pdf

Di Loreto, C., Fanelli, C., Lucidi, P., Murdolo, G., De Cicco, A., Parlanti, N., Santeusanio, F., Brunetti, P. & De Feo, P. (2003). Validation of a counseling strategy to promote the adoption and the maintenance of physical activity by type 2 diabetic subjects. *Diabetes Care*;26(2):404-408.

Eslava-Castañeda, J.C. (2006). Repensando la promoción de la salud en el sistema general de seguridad social en salud. *Revista de Salud pública*; 8 (Sup. 2): 106-115.

Fernandez, P. R. (2005) Redes sociales, apoyo social y salud. *Periferia*, 3. Disponible en: www.periferia.name

Fortmann, A.L., Gallo, L.C., Walker ,C. & Philis-Tsimikas, A. (2010). Support for disease management, depression, self-care, and clinical indicators among Hispanics with type 2 diabetes in San Diego County, United States of America. *Revista Panamericana de Salud Pública*; 28(3):230-234.

Gagliardino, J.J. & Etchegoyen, G. (2001). A model educational program for people with type 2 diabetes. *Diabetes Care*; 24:1001-1007.

Giachello, A.L., Arrom, J.O., Davis, M., Sayad, J.V., Ramirez, D., Nandi, C., Ramos, C. & Chicago Southeast Diabetes Community Action Coalition. (2003). Reducing diabetes health disparities through community-based participatory action research: the Chicago Southeast Diabetes Community Action Coalition. *Public Health Reports*;118(4):309-323.

Glasgow, R.E., Orleans, C.T. & Wagner, E.H. (2001). Does the chronic care model serve also as a template for improving prevention?. *Milbank Quarterly*;79(4):579-612,.

Gómez-Arias, R. D., González, E. (2004). Evaluación de la prevención de la enfermedad y la promoción de la salud: Factores que deben considerarse. Revista Facultad Nacional de Salud Pública 20; 22 (1):87-106.

Guzmán, J. M., Huenchuan, S. & Montes de Oca, V. (2002). Redes de apoyo social de las personas mayores: marco conceptual. Santiago de Chile: CEPAL. Disponible en: http://www.eclac.cl/publicaciones/xml/0/14200/lclg2213_p2.pdf

Hankonen, N., Absetz, P., Haukkala, A. & Uutela, A. (2009). Socioeconomic status and psychosocial mechanisms of lifestyle change in a type 2 diabetes prevention trial. *Annals of Behavioral Medicine*;38(2):160-165.

Ho, A.Y., Berggren, I. & Dahlborg-Lyckhage, E. (2010). Diabetes empowerment related to Pender's Health Promotion Model: a meta-synthesis. *Nursing & Health Sciences*;12(2):259-267.

Horowitz, C.R., Robinson, M. & Seifer, S. (2009). Community-based participatory research from the margin to the mainstream: are researchers prepared?. *Circulation*; 19;119:2633-2642.

International Diabetes Federation (2011). Prevalence of diabetes mellitus in the world. *Diabetes Facts*. http://www.idf.org/

Jenkins, C., Pope, C., Magwood, G., Vandemark, L., Thomas, V., Hill, K., Linnen, F., Beck, L.S. & Zapka, J. (2010). Expanding the chronic care framework to improve diabetes management: the REACH case study. *Progress in community health partnerships*; 4(1):65-79.

Johnston-Brooks, C.H., Lewis, M.A. & Garg, S. (2002). Self-efficacy impacts self-care and HbA1c in young adults with Type I diabetes. *Psychosomatic Medicine*;64(1):43-51.

Kar, S.B., Pascual, C.A. & Chickering, K.L. (1999). Empowerment of women for health promotion: a meta-analysis. *Social Science & Medicine; 49: 1431-1460.*

Kloseck, M. (2007). The use of Goal Attainment Scaling in a community health promotion initiative with seniors. *BMC Geriatrics*, 7:16. Available from: http://www.biomedcentral.com/1471-2318/7/16

Laitakari, J., Vuori, I. & Oja, P. (1996). Is long-term maintenance of health-related physical activity possible? An analysis of concepts and evidence. *Health education research*;11(4):463-477.

Llopis, C. J. (2005). Redes sociales y apoyo social. Una aproximación a los grupos de autoayuda.*Periferia;* 3. Disponible en: www.periferia.name

Marcus, B.H., Dubbert, P.M., Forsyth, L.H., McKenzie, T.L., Stone, E.J., Dunn, A.L. & Blair, S.N. (2000) Physical activity behavior change: issues in adoption and maintenance. *Health Psychology* 19(1 Suppl):32-41.

Marrero, D.G. (2009). The prevention of type 2 diabetes: an overview. *Journal of Diabetes Science and Technology;*3(4):756-760.

Martínez-Maldonado, M.L., Correa-Muñoz, E. & Mendoza-Núñez, V.M. (2007). Program of active aging in a rural Mexican community: a qualitative approach. *BMC Public Health; 7:276.*

Martorell, R. (2005). Diabetes and Mexicans: why the two are linked. *Preventing Chronic Disease.* Available from: URL: http://www.cdc.gov/pcd/issues/2005/jan/pdf/04_0100.pdf

Maton, K.I. (2008). Empowering community settings: agents of individual development, community betterment, and positive social change. *American Journal of Community Psychology;* doi 10.1007/s10464-007-9148-6.

Mendoza-Núñez, V.M., Correa-Muñoz, E., Sánchez-Rodríguez, M. & Retana-Ugalde, R. (1996). Modelo de atención de núcleos gerontológicos. *Geriatrika;* 12: 15-21.

Mendoza-Núñez, V.M., Sánchez-Rodríguez, M.A. & Correa-Muñoz, E. (2008). Estrategias para el control de enfermedades crónico-degenerativas a nivel comunitario. México: FES "ZARAGOZA", UNAM.

Mendoza-Núñez, V.M., Martínez-Maldonado, M.de L. & Correa-Muñoz, E. (2009a). Implementation of an active aging model in Mexico for prevention and control of chronic diseases in the elderly.*BMC Geriatrics;* 26;9:40.

Mendoza-Núñez, V.M. & Martínez-Maldonado, M. (2009b). Escala de Redes de Apoyo Social para Adultos Mayores (ERASAM). En: A. L. González-Celis, R. [Coord.]. Evaluación en Psicogerontología. México: Editorial Manual Moderno. p. 95-112.

Mendoza-Núñez, V.M., & Rosado-Pérez, J. (2010). Aging, diabetes mellitus and overweight. In: Hiriart-Urdanivia, M. & Mas-Oliva, J. Advances in obesity-diabetes research at UNAM. México: Manual Moderno/PUIS, UNAM. p. 79-102.

Narayan, D. (2002) Empoderamiento y reducción de la pobreza. México: Banco Mundial /Alfaomega Grupo Editor. p. 1-13.

Parchman, M.L., Pugh, J.A., Wang, C.P. & Romero, R.L. (2007). Glucose control, self-care behaviors, and the presence of the chronic care model in primary care clinics. Diabetes Care 30:2849–2854.

Padala, P.R., Desouza, C.V., Almeida, S., Shivaswamy, V., Ariyarathna, K., Rouse, L., Burke, W.J. & Petty, F. (2008). The impact of apathy on glycemic control in diabetes: a cross-sectional study. *Diabetes Research and Clinical Practice* ;79(1):37-41.

Piatt, G.A., Orchard, T.J., Emerson, S., Simmons, D., Songer, T.J., Brooks, M.M., Korytkowski, M., Siminerio, L.M., Ahmad, U. & Zgibor, J.C. (2006). Translating the chronic care model into the community: results from a randomized controlled trial of a multifaceted diabetes care intervention. *Diabetes Care;* 29(4):811-7.

Restrepo, H. (2001). Conceptos y definiciones. En: Restrepo H. y Málaga, H. Promoción de la Salud: Cómo construir vida saludable. Bogotá: Editorial Médica Panamericana.p.24-33.

Salmon, P. & Hall, G.M. (2003). Patient empowerment and control: a psychological discourse in the service of medicine. *Social Science & Medicine*; 57: 1969-1980.

Santos-Burgoa, C., Rodríguez-Cabrera, L., Rivero, L., Ochoa, J., Stanford, A., Latinovic, L. & Rueda, G. (2009). Implementation of Mexico's Health Promotion Operational Model. Preventing chronic disease; 6(1). Available from: URL http://www.cdc.gov/pcd/issues/2009/jan/pdf/08_0085.pdf

Savage, C.L., Xu, Y., Lee, R., Rose, B.L., Kappesser, M. & Anthony, J.S. (2006). A case study in the use of community-based participatory research in public health nursing. *Public Health Nursing*;23(5):472-478.

Schulze, M.B. & Hu, F.B. (2005). Primary prevention of diabetes: what can be done and how much can be prevented?. *Annual Review of Public Health*; 26:445-467.

Shephard, M.D., Mazzachi, B.C., Shephard, A.K., McLaughlin, K.J., Denner, B. & Barnes, G. (2005). The impact of point of care testing on diabetes services along Victoria's Mallee Track: results of a community-based diabetes risk assessment and management program. *Rural Remote Health*; 5(3):371.

Song, M. (2010). Diabetes mellitus and the importance of self-care. *Journal of Cardiovascular Nursing*; 25(2):93-8.

Steyn, N.P., Mann, J., Bennett, P.H., Temple, N., Zimmet, P., Tuomilehto, J., Lindström, J. & Louheranta, A. (2004). Diet, nutrition and the prevention of type 2 diabetes. *Public Health Nutrition*;7(1A):147-165.

Strickland, P.A., Hudson, S.V., Piasecki, A., Hahn, K., Cohen, D., Orzano, A.J., Parchman, M.L. & Crabtree, B.F. (2010). Features of the Chronic Care Model (CCM) associated with behavioral counseling and diabetes care in community primary care. *Journal of the American Board of Family Medicine*; 23: 295–305.

Teufel-Shone, N.I., Drummond, R., Rawiel, U. (2005). Developing and adapting a family-based diabetes program at the U.S.-Mexico border. Prev Chronic Dis [serial online]. Available from: URL: http://www.cdc.gov/pcd/issues/2005/jan/04_0083.htm

Toft, U.N., Kristoffersen, L.H., Aadahl, M., von Huth Smith, L., Pisinger, C. & Jørgensen, T. (2007). Diet and exercise intervention in a general population--mediators of participation and adherence: the Inter99 study. *European Journal of Public Health*; 17(5):455-463.

Torres-López, T.M., Sandoval-Díaz, M. & Pando-Moreno, M. (2005). "Blood and sugar": social representations of diabetes mellitus by chronic patients in Guadalajara, Mexico. *Cadernos de Saúde Pública*;21(1):101-110.

Villalpando, S., Rojas, R., Shamah-Levy, T., Ávila, M.A., Gaona, B., De la Cruz, V., Rebollar, R. & Hernández, L.. (2010a). Prevalence and distribution of type 2 Diabetes mellitus in Mexican adult population. A probabilistic survey. *Salud Pública de México*;52 (suppl 1):S19-S26.

Villalpando, C.G., Ridaura, R.L., Ponce, E.L. & Villalpando, M.E. (2010b). And now what? Time for daring innovation. Salud Pública de México.;52 (Suppl 1):S80-83.

Wagner, E.H., Austin, B.T. & Von Korff, M. (1996). Organizing care for patients with chronic illness. *Milbank Quarterly*; 74(4):511-544.

Wagner, E.H., Davis, C., Schaefer, J., Von Korff, M. & Austin, B. (1999). A survey of leading chronic disease management programs: are they consistent with the literature?. *Managed Care Quarterly*; 7(3):56-66.

World Health Organization. (1986). Ottawa Charter for Health Promotion. Geneva: WHO/HPR/HEP/95.1.WHQ.

16

A Novel Approach to Adolescent Obesity in Rural Appalachia of West Virginia: Educating Adolescents as Family Health Coaches and Research Investigators

Robert A. Branch et al.,*
University of Pittsburgh, Pittsburgh PA USA

1. Introduction

"Transformation happens less by arguing cogently for something new than by generating active ongoing practices that shift culture's experience of the basis of reality." – R.S. Zander (a psychologist) B. Zander (a conductor, in the Art of Possibility). (Zander & Zander, 2002)

The pandemic of obesity, with its attendant downstream complications of Type II, Diabetes (DM) and Cardiovascular disease (CD) is emerging as an international challenge to public health. (Adams et al., 2007; Grubb, 2002) Despite increased understanding of the complexity of the biology of energy balance, and evidence of how to maintain sustained weight reduction in the context of a randomized clinical trial, (Knowler et al., 2002) the actual epidemic is still inexorably increasing. (USBRFSS, 2002)

Each advance in our understanding of the biology of energy balance provides further evidence for the complexity of multiple interactive processes, and the amazing ability of the human body to auto regulate to counter external interventions and maintain what the body perceives as the ideal basis for competing in its environment. Thus, our perception of the dangers of obesity, based on future predictions of adverse events run counter to biological self-perception of the immediate present.

We have, however, found that perfection is not required to ameliorate an adverse future, as relatively modest reductions in weight, when sustained, provide disproportionate reduction in the risk of DM and CD. (Knowler et al., 2002) This perspective provides the basis for the belief that we can reverse the epidemic.

The authors' opinion, mirrored by others, is that the primary root cause for the current dilemma of, 'knowing what to do, but not doing it' is a clash of biological and cultural

---

*Ann Chester[2], Cathy Morton-McSwain[2], Soleh Udin Al Ayubi[1], Kavitha Bhat Schelbert[1], Philip Brimson[4], Shama Buch[1], Yvonne Cannon[3], Steve Groark[1], Sara Hanks[2], Tomoko Nukui[1], Petr Pancoska[1], Bambang Parmanto[1], Stephanie Paulsen[1] and Elaine Wahl[3]
[1]*University of Pittsburgh, Pittsburgh PA USA*
[2]*West Virginia University, Morgantown WV USA*
[3]*University of Pittsburgh Medical Center, Pittsburgh PA USA*
[4]*University of Surrey, Guildford Surrey UK*

perception. (Patton, 1990) Our tenant is that evolutionary adaptation faced with cycles of feast and famine has led to multiple, often subtle biological mechanisms for energy conservation, that are strengthened by social cultural behaviors of nurturing, sharing and preparing for future fasts. With the 21st century advances of food distribution and refinement, the continuous availability of high energy foods and more sedentary lifestyles now render us maladapted to this new environment.

We propose that this clash of perception is best addressed by enhancing learning skills in the community to consider each approach, and develop a new way forward. (Ausubel, 1962) Applying these learning skills to focus on a dialogue, between biological and cultural urges and knowledge of future risk, is required to create sustained changes in behavior that we know can work. From this prospective, success or failure of any obesity intervention in the long haul will be require to 'shift in cultures experience as the basis of reality' (referred to by the Zanders' quotation above) (Zander & Zander, 2002) as the essential ingredient for transformational change.

We describe an innovative strategy to create such a transformational change by directly addressing this primary root cause. We provide an educational forum through family-oriented learning rather than health care teaching. This strategy is being tested in a rural Appalachian community in the US that is stable, but geographically and economically isolated. It is at the epicenter of the US epidemic, with some of the highest obesity rates yet recorded. (Pancoska et al., 2009) Within this community, the primary target chosen for intervention is the adolescent with a secondary beneficiary being the adolescents' family. The benefits for this concept extend beyond the question of obesity alone, and offer a transformational model for community self-help and self improvement.

Our belief is that even though the infrastructure support for our new paradigm is substantial, it addresses the depth of sophistication needed to create sustained change. Elements of the program are generalizable and could be augmented by changes in local and national policies to improve for the interface between education and health care that could benefit affected communities.

In this chapter, we described the evolution and goals of the CAIRN program for rural Appalachia, (*Figure 1*) and point out the role of some of the multiple key players involved. For any program of this level of sophistication, the individual development will be different, and the key players to influence development will vary in the resources and ideas they contribute; however, it will be the key players who will influence the details of what is developed. We suggest that the common critical elements are community willingness to actively participate, the extensive need for voluntary input from as varied a resource base as possible, the need for help from academia and building a multisource funding base for organization and infrastructure.

2. The Setting: A community network of science clubs for adolescents in rural Appalachia

Rural Appalachia, although one of the most scenically beautiful regions of the US with its extended mountain range, is also one of the poorest in the country. The only state entirely in Appalachia, West Virginia (WV), the Mountain State, was initially settled by a wave of Scottish-Irish early immigrants looking for homestead farming. Its later wave of African-American and Caucasian migration came with the railroads to work coal mines. Those who remained despite the later depression are the communities for this sparsely populated countryside. Even though poverty stricken and unsystematically educated, they are fiercely independent, proud and self-reliant, with a strong culture that centers on cohesive families. (Knowler et al., 2002)

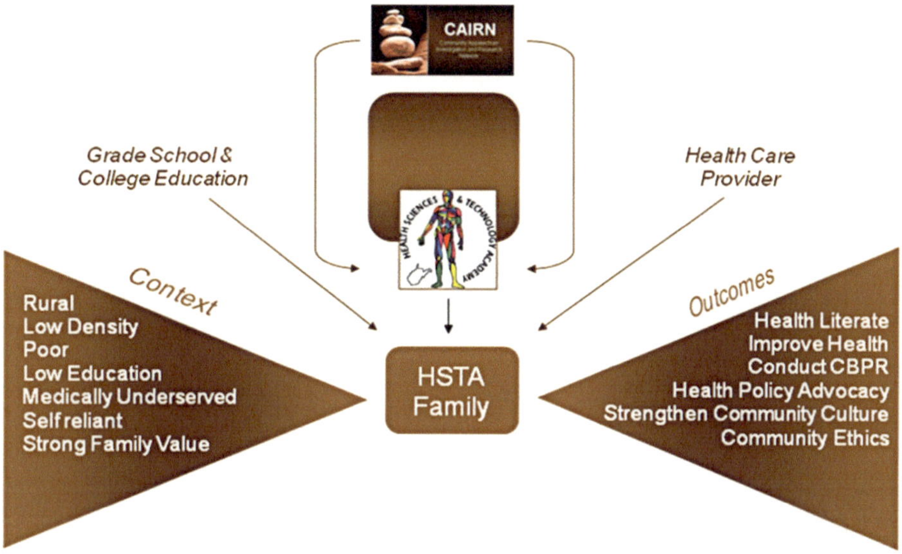

Fig. 1. The vision for the CAIRN collaboration between Pitt and HSTA is to learn how best to enhance cultural values, health related knowledge and life style behavior in rural Appalachian families to improve community health.

Two decades ago, there was a realization that the cycle of poverty could only be broken by a radical change from within the community itself. The initial response from community and academic leaders was to form a cohesive organization, Health, Science and Technology Academy (HSTA), led by the botanist Ann Chester PhD, to focus on education of high school students to limit high school dropout rates and encourage adolescents from families without a history of college education to be successful college graduates in disciplines of value to the community.

Dr. A. Chester, PhD: When I was in the 7th grade, in a new school, my achievement scores were accidently misread, and I was placed in a tract for non-college bound students. From birth, my family told me I was smart and could do anything I wanted to do. Everybody, even my great grandmother, went to college in my family and I was expected to too. Up until that point, I was at the top of my classes. I was always "the good kid" and landing in a class of 'no expectations' was eye opening. To be told by teachers that I was not college material and that I was limited to being a seamstress or a secretary was news to me. My response was to quit trying. I began to get bad grades. I even cut up in class, and got sent to the corner. This went on for 6-weeks before my mother could unravel the situation and get me in the right tract. By that point, the damage to my self-esteem was huge and the 6 weeks of lost work in my new, fast paced classes seemed insurmountable. It took me years to get over what happened in just 6 short weeks. I did recover and went on to college and graduate school and on to obtain a Ph.D. Somewhere along the line, I realized that the potential of many of those other students in that non-college bound tract was no less than mine. The difference: they never got that chance I had. I kept imagining what the effect of a life-time of low expectations can do.

I began to work on this passion in 1985 when I joined the West Virginia University Health Careers Opportunity Program to help under-represented college students be successful in medical school, dental school and pharmacy school. In early 1990's the American Association of Medical Colleges posed a goal to every medical school to collectively get 3000 under-represented students into Medical School by 2000. WVU School of Medicine Dean, Dr. Robert D'Alessandri, asked me what WVU should do for the effort. By this point, after 7 years of trying to recruit under-represented students into a free program offered at WVU, and having trouble finding students that fit the description in the freshman applicants, the obvious solution was to reach into the high schools to capture and nurture them before they were weeded out of college tracts. Dr. D'Alessandri and I, along with others, conceived of HSTA, and got funding from Howard Hughes Medical Institute to start it with 44 kids and 9 teachers in 1994. The HSTA community-campus partnership infrastructure with its community-majority was developed and expanded with funding from the W. K. Kellogg foundation in 1996. It has since expanded to 800 students and 80 teachers with funding from many sources including the WV State Legislature and the Claude Worthington Benedum Foundation and National Institute of Health. HSTA still thrives today – 17 years later with community in the leadership role.

The infrastructure of HSTA is truly just beginning to be tapped as a change agent for bettering the education status, the economic status and health of West Virginians. As intended, HSTA has become a successful pipeline program for recruiting under-represented students to college and STEM careers. (Branch & Chester, 2009) What we never expected was how powerful the community leadership in this community-campus partnership is in changing lives. HSTA also persuaded the WV legislature to provide tuition and fee waivers to any successful HSTA graduate to any WV state college or university all the way through health professions school. HSTA persuaded the WV legislature to fund HSTA with a line item in the state budget. They have supported the students so that 97% of them go to college and 92% stay in WV to work and 73% are in STEM and health fields when they graduate from college to earn on average $26,000 more than their highest earning parent. With community backing, the students are giving back to their communities immediately in the 9th-12th grades through improving health literacy in their families and applying science into everyday lives.

HSTA is a community based participatory learning model that is outside, but complementary to the State school system. Now present in 26 counties in WV, approximately eight hundred (800) 9th-12th grade underrepresented students per year are participating, in an after-school science club network of 79 science clubs. (Bardwell et al., 2009) It focuses on preparing students for the health sciences, and bringing healthcare information and healthcare professionals to the medically underserved communities of West Virginia. Student selection is based on local community nomination. Prioritization is given to poor families, minorities and families with no prior college experience. HSTA then provides the infrastructure and support for community-based science projects and community service in the students' individual communities. HSTA uses an interesting combination of mix and match of its students to encourage interactions. The summer science enrichment week long workshops are separated by grade while community based immersion science projects during the year include all club members across the four grades. Students are mentored by scientists, teachers, and community leaders during the school year. Here, the "learning experience" is translated to "a doing experience" with sharing of their new found knowledge back to their families and communities. With goals to improve science and health education, but self-empowers communities through leadership development of their youth, and ultimately will increase the number of health care providers, scientists, and science educators in West Virginia's currently under-served communities.

The success of this program rests in the community's feelings of ownership and control, and long-term partnerships among higher education, public education at the state and local level, and rural communities. HSTA is governed by a state-wide Joint Governing Board with volunteer representation from 14 Local Governing Boards leading each region. HSTA's governing boards represent all partners: the parents, the students, the schools, communities, and higher education. The majority of the board members represent the local communities with the minority being representatives from institutions of higher education and health professions. This strategy reinforces the role of parents and community in the science education of the youth.

The initial education focus was any topic in the fields of mathematics, science, biology, ecology and technology. It has been amazingly successful. Over 1267 HSTA students enrolled at eighth grade have successfully graduated from high school. Ninety-six percent enter college in comparison to the 56% of the general WV population who attend college. Of these, 89% finish college, relative to 72% in the general WV population and 83% of HSTA African American students are attaining bachelor degrees or higher, compared to only 23% of African Americans of the general WV population. HSTA students earn post graduate degrees 23% of the time and they choose Science, Technology, Engineering and Mathematics majors (STEM) 51% of the time, 4 times more often than the general population of 16% of WV college graduates. Of the greatest importance to the community, 92% stay in WV and have more attractive career opportunities than their parents.

These advances in education of adolescents have not been mirrored by advances in health care in this community. In part as a consequence of the confluence of its geography and economy, rural Appalachia is one of the most medically underserved regions within the US, with all the rural counties in WV being classified as medically underserved. In 2008, the organization "West Virginians for Affordable Health Care" (WVAHC) issued a policy statement entitled '"Early deaths: West Virginians have some of the shortest life expectancies in the United States." (Ezzati et al., 2008) Drawing on a wide variety of resources, this document drew attention by three counties in WV (all with HSTA clubs) that have a life expectancy within the lowest 1% of all counties in the US. For the first time in US history, life expectancy in seven counties actually decreased in the decade of the 1990s. The reason for these changes were largely attributed to poor diet, inadequate exercise and resulting obesity. A plea for policy changes went to what were considered primary stakeholders. These included: local and regional Health Departments, the Bureau of Public Health, the Superintendent of Public Schools, the Secretary of Transportation, the County Commissioners, the West Virginia Department of Agriculture, the Governor's Office of Economic Opportunity, the State Board of Education, the Department of Health and Human Resources, the West Virginia Health Information Network and the State Legislature. The silence in response to this plea has been deafening! There is, therefore, an unmet community need to address this problem.

3. Education and Community Based Participatory Research (CBPR): Health as a focus for HSTA science projects

In 2007, as part of its mission, HSTA saw a need for more direct interaction with clinical scientists working side by side with HSTA students to dissolve barriers for pursuing science and health care careers. The community itself identified obesity as a major health care concern. Encouraged by the prior success of HSTA initiatives (learning), leading to positive community projects (doing), HSTA's community-based joint governing board asked for the same principles to be applied to CBPR in obesity. They encouraged the HSTA students to go beyond baseline data gathering into a new phase of putting into practice the principles of clinical translational science and evidence based medicine, with the community itself playing the leadership role. They encouraged the CAIRN partnership with Clinical Translational Scientists from University of Pittsburgh.

The cross-state collaboration between West Virginia and Western Pennsylvania in the acronym CAIRN also alludes to the Celtic symbol of a beacon to direct a stranger within their country. In this instance, and by analogy, CAIRN is ideally positioned to provide a beacon or direction for self-help in health care behavior in rural Appalachia and to conduct investigational research into whether the strategies used are working. If they are, they have potential to expand and be relevant to Appalachian communities other than in West Virginia, and to be relevant for other diseases relevant to the community.

Initially, Robert A. Branch MD, Clinical Translational Research Scientist and Director of the Center for Clinical Pharmacology at the University of Pittsburgh (Pitt) was invited by HSTA to teach concepts about clinical trials to HSTA club members.

Dr. R. A. Branch, MD: My interest in this interaction was piqued by my own experience in entering an academic career. In this instance, I was a product of a highly regimented, dictatorial, conservative, English, private boarding school developed for military families which I found highly oppressive. I was told early on that the only 'escape' from this environment was to qualify for University in four years, instead of five, and told by my teachers that I would not qualify at all. Motivated by rebellion for learning by rote I developed my own approach to learning without guidance. By happenstance, I used concept mapping for problem solving. This allowed me not only to enter Medical School at 17 years, but obtain a distinction at the head of my medical class in obtaining a MD before the age of 21. The approach of concept mapping is readily adapted to problem based learning which I formally applied to the teaching of advanced therapeutics to medical students at the University of Pittsburgh. (Tofovic et al., 1998) This grounding in educational practice made immediately attractive the challenge of interesting bright adolescents, with essentially no health care background, to become health advocates and educators to their own families. The questions of: Is it feasible? How can it be done? What is its potential? These all became potential hurdles to overcome. The experience of conducting Community Research has proved to be substantially different from Clinical Translational research from three perspectives; firstly to gain trust, there has to be a long term commitment; secondly, the rewards are for an increase in community self-esteem, not the investigators ego and thirdly, the component of providing community feed back to participants at all steps in the process requires a major reorientation and effort. With these cautions, the rewards from the investigator come more from the community than peer group recognition from other scientists.

The first few minutes of the first day of the first summer week long workshop in 2007, organized by Cathy Morton-McSwain and run by Bob Branch, were pivotal to the subsequent program. A group of 22 HSTA students from 18 HSTA clubs had been assembled to teach principles of clinical trials, with a focus on obesity complications. In these first few minutes, the responses to three questions set the stage.

1. How many of you are or have family members who are obese?

   Half of the students were obese, and all had at least one member of the family who was obese.

2. How many of you have a family member with diabetes?
   18 of 22 hands went up. When teachers from those clubs were asked in a later meeting and a quarter were already diabetic themselves.
3. Rather than be taught a topic are you prepared to learn how to conduct CBPR and do something about your problem?

All 22 were enthusiastic.

These three questions provided a basis for the week long, total immersion into the problem of ethics, research and obesity. (Bardwell et al., 2009) Problem based small group learning experiences covered:

- Principles of ethics (Belmont Report, Helsinki Declaration), regulation of confidentiality used in research (HIPAA regulations)
- Principles of CBPR
- Domain specific information obtained from internet searches included
  - Energy Balance
  - Obesity
  - Diabetes Mellitus, Type II
  - Diabetes Prevention
  - Diabetes Management

It was also the basis of their formulation of a pilot prevalence study designed to establish the relevance of this problem in their own community. The students named their study "Diabetes Education to Protect and Defend our Families (DPD)" and participated in designing the written consent form.

4. Adolescents as investigators of obesity and diabetes

Having formulated ideas of what HSTA students could attempt to do as community projects in the following year, the challenge was to put together the logistics to allow the study to take place. With minimal editing and formatting, the protocol and consent from the DPD Study was formulated into a formal proposal to the WVU Institutional Review Board. This included written informed consent for adults, assent for minors and a HIPAA consent (this was for educational purposes, as the data to be collected was self reported and not the property of a covered entity).

Cathy Morton-McSwain: As one of two Education Coordinators responsible for the HSTA student and teacher programs and projects, and a teacher with 25 years experience in the classroom, I quickly realized this project was a learning curve of epic proportions. It was really important that I am a West Virginia girl. I could be trusted to ensure this project was for the good of all and would not in any way lead to making those involved look foolish or be ridiculed. I was born and raised here and I knew that any challenge put to our clubs would be tackled with a fierce determination to succeed. It is just the nature of, and explanation for, why we in WV so often overcome, what to others are insurmountable odds, made even worse by a daunting terrain and infrastructure that is not in any way conducive to success. I knew that to succeed we needed to challenge each hurdle, one by one and have the sass to just show the world we could make this a howling success. I also drew on the knowledge that humor and fun make every task or lesson more memorable. I developed guides and lessons including scripts to follow which allowed for role playing. Drawing from a cast of characters modeled after real, albeit exaggerated family members, I designed skits and scenarios that were funny, silly, but within the range of possible, to mimic what might or could happen and how to handle such situations. Students were introduced to and role played such characters as Amiable Aunt Agnes, who never let you finish a sentence but would agree and sign anything if she thought it would make you happy. Paranoid Patty, who knew for a fact that the government had placed robot bugs in everybody's house so they could spy on all of us cause she saw it on "60 Minutes", Uncle Mo who rode his lawnmower to the corner liquor store and always had a snoot full, Granddaddy Don who wouldn't agree with anyone much less to anything, Brother Joe who would participate if you promised to clean his room for a month, and Momma, who kept everyone out of trouble and under control.

I became a 'mad scientist' researcher and gave all the students terrible diseases to test my newly developed drug, which caused some to have crippling side effects. Students were wearing swimming goggles to mimic eye damage, rubber gloves to mimic neuropathy, slings to mimic strokes and loss of the use of a limb. I withheld information, broke every ethics rule and violated every right, and then made them use their skills and knowledge of ethics to help build a case to bring charges against me and my Pharmaceutical company, while identifying what principles were violated.

But no matter what crazy way we presented and practiced each new concept and process of implementing this program, it was all designed to follow the same format which was a designed step by step checklist that students used to make sure no procedure or process was overlooked. This transformed what was a rote process to something that was memorable because students had practiced it as various crazy characters while learning how to deal with awkward situations that could present certain barriers.

The reasons for my passion to see this program be successful were many but centered in that I knew there was so much untapped potential in our communities, and I love to teach, be creative and have fun. It was the excitement and pride I witnessed in the faces of students, when they rose to the occasion and excelled at something most believed they could not do. They understood research and more importantly how to use it to bring about change. They were health advocates in their families and vectors of change.

The energy was contagious and it spread through all of us including the family members. When they realized that together they could address issues they had researched and were important to them, their loved ones, and their communities the projects took on a life of their own. It suddenly was as if they found a key to open the door and had a way to make a difference. This ownership was empowerment and a gateway to get others involved. My role evolved and changed to that of the coach and mentor. I brought together community resources and groups. I reassured, encouraged and was a sounding board and guide for proposed interventions and projects. Sometimes I nudged, but rarely because for so many of those participating, it was if they were finally able to 'get in the game' and were not just sidelined waiting for that unknown someone or something to get things started and done. It is how the role of Community Research Associate began, and is still evolving.

In addition to preparing the young investigators and their club teachers, the essential infrastructure for the study conduct had to be provided. This included developing standard operating procedures (SOP) so that each club would perform the study with the same quality. In order to ensure integration of activities between clubs, we were fortunate in the existing HSTA regional, county and club levels of structure and prior experience in conducting community projects. We did have to formulate the structure of the questionnaire and ensure its easy conversion from paper to electronic format, centralize flow of data and provide appropriate management of identified (kept in West Virginia) and de-identified information (organized and curated in Pittsburgh). The resource base and information technology capability at the University of Pittsburgh were essential in planning, design and execution, but the activities provided a tremendous opportunity for the community to achieve more than they believed possible. It is worth emphasizing that these behind the scenes activities were vital to a successful outcome and could not have been done at the community level within a short time without the outside expertise available from Pitt.

5. The magnitude of the problem of obesity and diabetes in individuals in rural Appalachia

Our experience provided proof of principle that education can be extended to action to conduct CBPR in the community. It also provided an opportunity to the students to give back the information to the community. In the first year of this initiative, we trained and certified 210 HSTA club teachers and club members in the ethics and principles of clinical research. We developed a paper based questionnaire with the students transferring paper data to an electronic format. The DPD study used appropriate assent/consent and achieved HIPAA compliance in use of identified and de-identified data. Over a 6 month period, 989 subjects were recruited to a baseline evaluation of the extent of the problem by responding to this obesity, diabetes-based questionnaire. The cohort in HSTA-linked family members was enriched in poor and minority participants that reflected outreach into the community, and covered a wide age-range. Enrollment of subjects across the state reflected the distribution of 18 clubs participating in this survey (*Figure 2*). It shows a rural distribution that represented the poorest communities targeted by the HSTA Program.

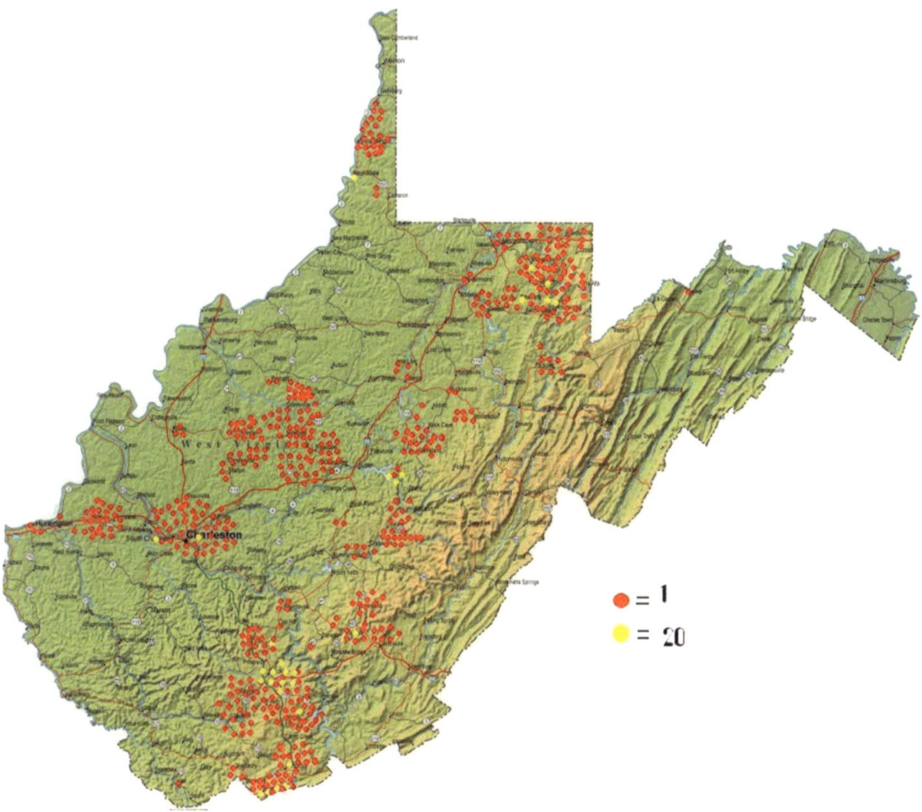

Fig. 2. Geographic location of study participants. (Bardwell et al., 2009)

The students have been successful in enrolling an even distribution of family members over a wide range of 8-80 years old. (Pancoska et al., 2009) The results were appalling and worse than anticipated from other studies. In subjects over 20 years, the mean was at a BMI of 30 (i.e. over

50% were already obese. (*Figure 3*) In subjects under 20 years, there was the expected relationship of age with BMI. Using the regression of this relationship to identify its mean as a correction factor, and linking the two age groups, the age corrected BMI had a similar distribution about the mean in all age groups. Thus, the problem of obesity being shown equally prevalent at all ages. The adolescents already had as much of a problem as their elders.

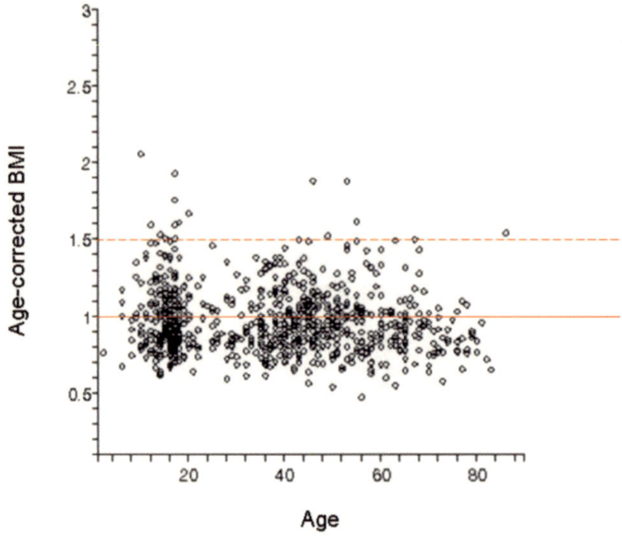

Fig. 3. Age-corrected BMI normalized for mean of BMI which is 30 in subjects> 20 years. (Pancoska et al., 2009)

When all subjects were considered together, the prevalence of diabetics was 10.6%. When only adults were considered, it rose to 16%, and when BMI was subdivided into cohorts of 5 BMI units, there was an exponential relationship of BMI to diabetic frequency, approach 50% with BMIs over 55. (*Figure 4*)

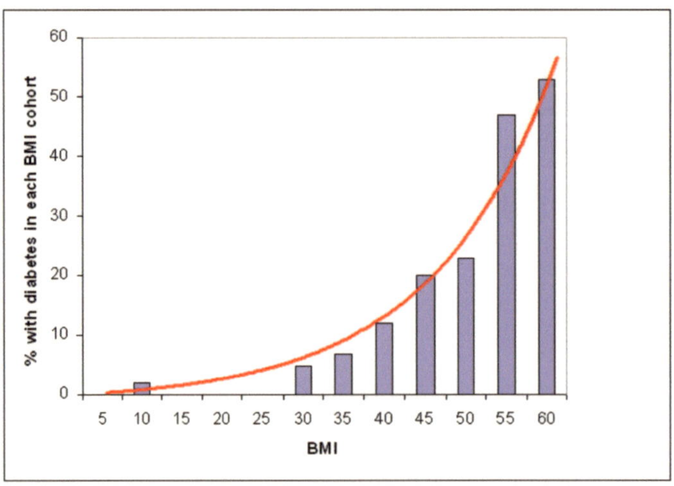

Fig. 4. The change in frequency of diabetes with increasing BMI in rural Appalachia in 2008. (Pancoska et al., 2009)

6. The HSTA cohort in context of obesity: Diabetes epidemic

This region is known to be at the epicenter of an evolving epidemic where the prevalence of obesity has increased by 61% in the last decade in the US, and is mirrored by the prevalence of diabetes, which has increased by 50% within the same period.

Childhood and adolescent obesity has more than doubled in the last decade. In West Virginia, over 43% of children had been classified as at-risk of becoming overweight, or are overweight. Unless these trends are reversed, it has been suggested that a third of all children today will develop Type II diabetes during their lifetime. The impact of this impending epidemic is not only a community health care burden but a financial disaster for an already overstretched, undermanned and under-funded local healthcare system.

The major complications of obesity in adults are DM and CD in mid-life. In the last decade, West Virginia has reported the highest premature death rate in the nation. (WVFAHC, 2008) These diseases also contribute immensely to morbidity, mortality, and health care costs. An illustration of the magnitude of this impact is the recent report that when 2% of counties with the lowest life expectancy are compared with the 2% of counties with the highest life expectancy in Appalachia, the difference in life expectancy for men is 10 years and in women 7.5 years. The counties with the lowest life expectancy are the rural West Virginia communities of the HSTA families.

The 1998-2009 Behavioral Risk Surveillance System (BRFSS) files compiled annually by the Center of Disease Control provides the most detailed information of rate of change. (USBRFSS, 2002) The objectives, design and structure of this report are different from the CAIRN study, but does provide interesting complementary information. This organization uses random digit phone calls for 1000 subjects who respond per state to collect self reported data including height and weight used to calculate BMI, the index of obesity. This system is known to reflect an approximate 10% underreporting, but is considered to yield comparative data between years to look a trends. Using this conservative approach between 1989 and 2008 the national prevalence of obesity has risen from 12% to 27% (with West Virginia being 10 points higher in 2008).

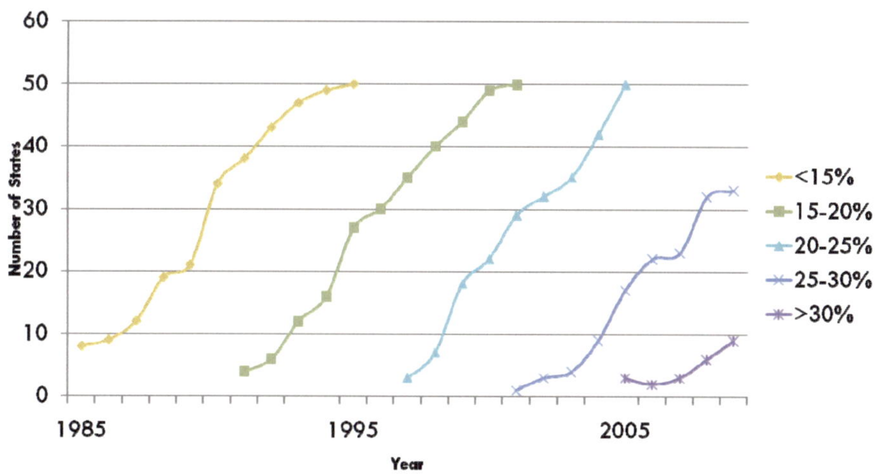

Fig. 5. The number of states in the US that have achieved a prevalence of obesity (BMI>30). Adapted from BRFSS report.

We have adapted the detailed CDC presentation of individual states obesity prevalence rate to illustrate the number of states that achieves an obesity prevalence threshold rate in increments of 5% from 15-35% over the years. This format of presentation reinforces the CDC year by year mapped prevalence to emphasize the problem is national and not local, with all 50 states participating in the epidemic. (*Figure 5*) (USBRFSS, 2002) It is mirrored by similar trends in Europe, the Middle East, India and more recently China. *Figure 5* also emphasizes that the rate of new states reaching the next threshold has been linear over the years of monitoring, with only a possible slowing down in the last 5 years. The state of West Virginia has been at the forefront of States reaching each threshold (*Figure 6*). When the date that each threshold for obesity prevalence in WV is plotted against the year the threshold was exceeded, the result can be fitted equally well to a linear regression, or a more recent exponential increase. (*Figure 6*) If the >50% results of HSTA survey are added, the last data point can be considered as either a part of the exponential increase, or a high outlier to the linear increase. In either case, the implications for the future are ominous.

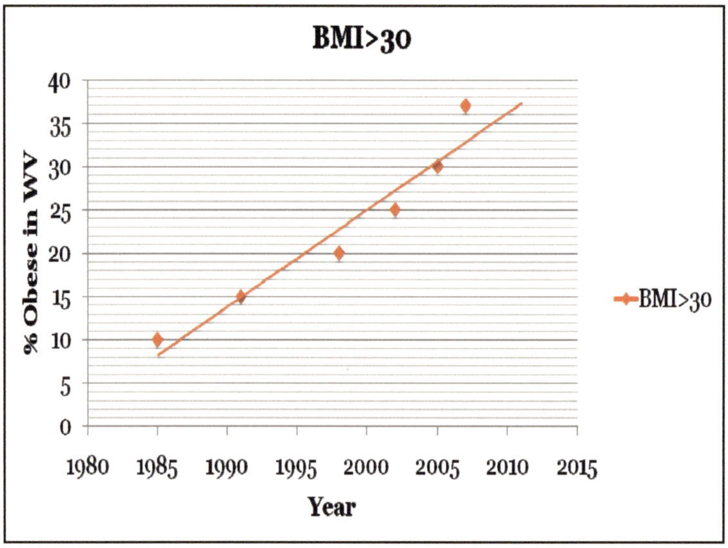

Fig. 6. Linear progression of obesity incidence in West Virginia based on BRFFS data.

At the present time, we favor the idea that the differences in subject selection identify different subsets of the population with the BRFSS random digit dialing in WV favoring population centers, and our study, the more dispersed rural population (*Figure 2*). Longitudinal follow up from both sources will allow us to discriminate based on the slopes of rate of change from each source in the future.

We are aware that in the majority of longitudinal studies of individual subjects, BMI tends to increase with aging. We were, therefore, surprised that age-corrected BMI had no change with aging (*Figure 3*). We reason that if we consider the older cohort in *Figure 3*, that it is likely, based on the BRFFS trend (*Figure 6*) that when this cohort was in their adolescence, that their mean BMI was substantially lower than the mean of today's adolescents. We have modeled this slope (*Figure 7*), and projected the same slope to the future projections of change in BMI based in the assumption that the rate of increase in BMI in these adolescents continues to be linear (*Figure 6*). The results are truly frightening in that in 20 years the mean BMI in adults will be 42 unless we change this rate of progression. (*Figure 7*)

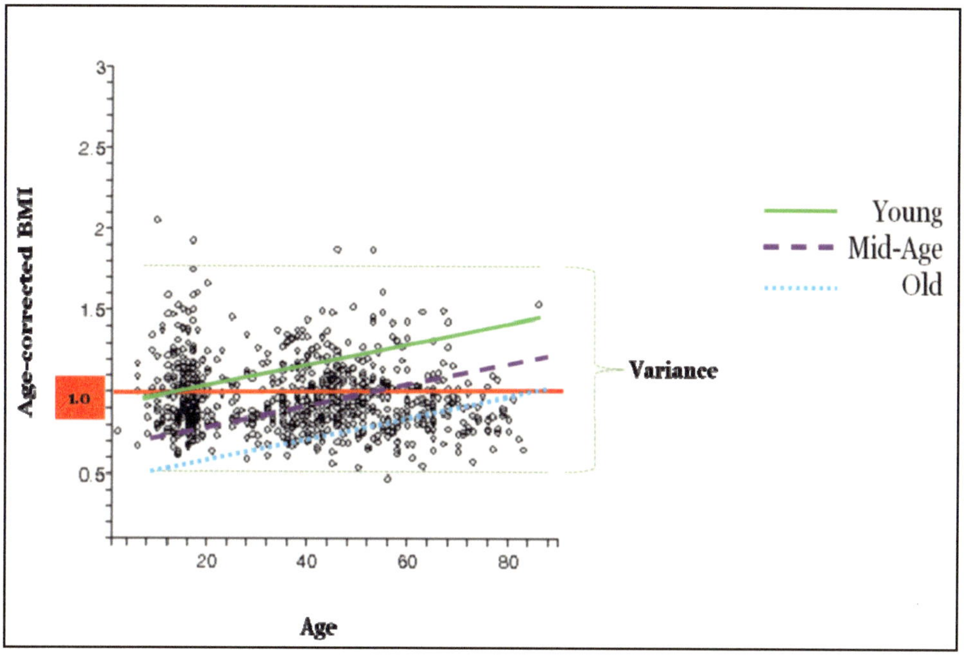

Fig. 7. Projected changes of BMI in HSTA family sample populations of West Virginia in subjects as they age from the present time.

We have, therefore, identified a community at the center of the US Obesity epidemic, and have further identified that the apex and most at risk is in the adolescent within this community. We consider that this is the most vulnerable group to target our interventions.

7. The family as the target for intervention within the HSTA community

We suggest that the primary goal of the HSTA organization has been successful because a subsection of the community has recognized that escape from a cycle of poverty is through education. These adult family members have nominated their children to participate in science club activities. They drive them to activities, provide computers, laptops and smart phones to help their self-confidence and aspiration to seek college education. These families are open to change and to exposure of new ideas. They, by choice, have become part of a HSTA community in which their adolescent family member has become a point person in the inclusion of the whole family.

This position has been strongly reinforced in local discussion and focus groups; it reinforces central themes of West Virginia culture of self reliance and strong family closeness.

Dr. K. Bhat-Schelbert, MD: In 2009, I joined the team as a family physician and researcher with expertise in obesity management, in adolescents, and qualitative methods. I was fascinated by the great potential of this program in motivating activated adolescents to become health advocates for their families and communities. I realized that as adolescents develop their position in the family shifts. They learn a great amount from their peers and teachers, and are personally invested in the welfare of their families. Soon after joining the team, I helped devise focus group discussions to guide the direction of the project and evaluate how teenagers can learn best, then transfer what they have learned on to their families. In 2010, a set of informal groups were conducted when parents and children were present. These groups helped us realize the true potential and value of the club structure, and the level of commitment these teenagers bring to improve their families' lifestyles. Moreover, we came to find that most of these teenagers had access to internet, and that their parents were committed to promoting the education of their children. These statements helped guide our decision to develop a web-based portal as a viable tool for education delivery. The focus groups also helped to assess the level of commitment and involvement of both HSTA students and parents in attempting behavior change in their diet and exercise habits. Recently, a set of formal focus groups were conducted to understand how teenagers communicate with their families, help them change behavior, and tell us how receptive families are to receive this communication. As part of the group HSTA project, they asked their families to perform one simple behavior change, which was decided by the students (reduce soda consumption, monitor pedometer steps or eat wheat rather than white bread). How they promoted and sustained change was decided by the student. Preliminary results of the focus groups suggest that a significant portion of the interviewed families were successful in implementing and sustaining behavior change although little guidance was given as to how to do this. Parents almost unanimously stated that they attempted the behavior change to support their children's desires and education, even when they would not do so by recommendation of their physician. And as a bonus, participation in the behavior change became a venue for adolescents to spend time with their families. These results strongly suggest that and that adolescents can be trusted to translate their knowledge of health-related behaviors, and family members can support one another in their pursuit of a healthy lifestyle.

These focus groups have been of great value because it has led us to identify a central theme of our program. This is for the whole family to be involved in family self-help rather than the isolated family member with the disease entity, in this instance obesity, DM and CD. In this model, all members have value in participating in whole family involvement of lifestyle choices, supporting health care/patient interactions and enhancing patient compliance with health care recommendations as the healthcare consequences of obesity, diabetes and cardiovascular disease, are in practice carried by the whole family, not just the target member. This is of major relevance in these disadvantaged, isolated, rural families.

7.1 Family network analysis

In order to obtain baseline information about family structure, and also to appeal to the curiosity of HSTA club members in their individual heritage in conducting this project, we structured our survey to have the student initially identify a family tree, and then request the family members to complete the individual questionnaire.

The family tree was restricted to living members within a family unit, i.e. those who could be expected to influence each other's behavior. This included only siblings in their own generation (not cousins), parents, uncles, and aunts in the parental generation and only grandparents in the generation above. This information included position in the family, age, gender, and zip code, but did not include any confidential health care information. Consenting individuals in the family tree were then individually approached to request their assent/consent, depending on age, to respond to confidential health care-related questions that enquired about self-reported height and weight, in order to compute Body Mass Index (BMI) and self-reported history of known DM or CD.

A family group was defined as a group in which complete data were available that comprised at least a boy or girl, their mother and their father. All additional members of the family with complete reported data were included in the analysis of that family. Our approach in using graph-based network analysis was made possible by Petr Pancoska PhD, a mathematician in our team.

Dr. P. Pancoska, PhD: I am a mathematician in the Center for Clinical Pharmacology at the University of Pittsburgh. I originally received my Ph.D. in experimental physics at Charles University, Prague. I spent twelve years intensely involved in conducting and teaching mathematical modeling and simulations in chemical physics in Prague. I then spent the next 10 years working in the Department of Chemistry at the University of Illinois, Chicago, where I focused on discrete mathematics. In 2003, I made a major career decision to move from fundamental mathematics as it relates to physical applications in chemistry, to biological applications. I moved and worked at Stony Brook University; trained myself in biology, and became deeply involved in using physicochemical modeling of DNA, using Eulerian graph representation to develop algorithms that predict functional consequences of single nucleotide polymorphisms of allelic gene variants and k-partite graph theory to analyze complex phenotype data sets and disease states. My familiarity in mathematical modeling and network analysis is well illustrated by the innovation applied to the preliminary data in formulating the family diabetes risk potential as a novel single family based metric. I have been instrumental in study design and will be responsible for the analysis of data acquired by the HSTA network and have developed the modeling algorithms.

The family-based approach brought several challenges to the data collection and processing together with development of data-driven descriptors of features we needed to capture, analyze and interpret. Families are social units with different sizes. Our family descriptor has to be therefore designed with ability to compare quantitatively different size families. Our next challenge was to extend from prior approaches characterize the family social structure using only topological indices of the family network graph. (Knowler et al., 2002) We realized that by annotating the family structure graphs by quantitative vertex potentials and edge weights, derived from the family member's clinico-demographic data, the rigorous mathematical tools of extremal graph theory can be used to find a family diabetes risk descriptor with the properties we were seeking. (Pancoska et al., 2009) Another challenge was how to deal with trends in the collected data, which were related to disease and clinical heterogeneity in the population from those that were normal consequences of an age range in the population (from young to elderly). While finding the tool for age correction was a matter of proper data visualization, the identification of heterogeneity required a combination of several complex algorithms, brought from different disciplines. With experience gathered in spectral data processing, we chose to extract and evaluate the information about the structure of data about obesity in our population in rational and efficient way using minimal number of variable parameters. This approach increases the power of the derived conclusions, as well as optimizes the data-driven intervals of age-corrected BMI used for classification of family members. These are used to derive vertex potentials and edge weights in the double-weighted family graphs. While non-linear transformation of newly derived obesity categories into disease risk potentials followed conventional practice, the conversion of them into family risk potential is novel. A deterministic algorithm was used for finding the maximal flow sub graph in the double-weighted graph, representing the obesity and key features of social relationships in every participating family. This approach allows a single value, "obesity-related diabetes risk flow" per family as the final analytical tool. This integration of tools, algorithms, facts and approaches from different disciplines, that are not normally used together providing an intellectually satisfying motivation for me. This approach has the additional appeal in that it can be applied to other diseases.

We based the selection of mathematical tools for quantitative characterization of the family group as a basic, single informational unit upon the following requirements: (1) the ability to quantitatively capture both the network of social relations in the family, the age-corrected BMI and presence or absence of diabetes for individual subjects. (2) Provide a mathematically rigorous way of combining the age-corrected BMI information for individual family members into a (single) numerical family-based descriptor, without losing network information, while capturing individual information explicably and quantitatively in a full family context. (3) Define a quantitative descriptor for comparisons of families or larger social units with diverse sizes and social structures. The quantitative mathematical tool, which satisfies the above criteria, recruits from discrete mathematics and is the weighted graph for the family. (*Figure 8*) In this graph, each vertex represents one family member weighted (in diameter) for age corrected BMI and the edge connecting two vertices, represents the edge as the social relationship between the two subjects. Each edge has been assigned as the mean of the age-corrected BMI-derived number of the two vertices for that edge. The methods have been described in full in Pancoska et al., 2009.

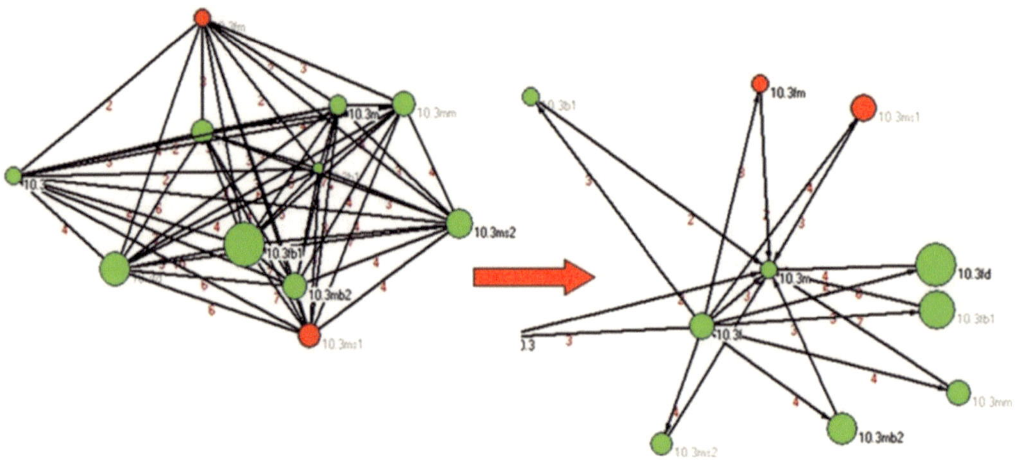

Fig. 8. Examples of (A) full family tree represented as weighted un-oriented graph for family with two incidences of diabetes (red vertices) and (B) corresponding maximal flow oriented sub graph. The size of each vertex is proportional to age-corrected. (Pancoska et al., 2009)

7.2 Family Diabetes Risk Potential (FDRP)

Having analyzed the cohort of participants in this study as individuals, we next proceeded to an analysis of the family as the unit of interest. Within this cohort, there were 142 families with at least an adolescent, a mother, and a father. The majority of families had one or more additional members of their families (average 6.5 members per family). *Figure 8, Left Panel*, illustrates a representative example of a full weighted for a family with two members having diabetes. The complexity of this network is substantially simplified by using an oriented, maximal flow sub-graph. (*Figure 8, Right Panel*) In the family diabetes risk potential (FDRP) analysis, we identified 53 families with at least one report of diabetes.

When the family diabetes risk potential was compared between families with and without diabetes, there was a clear difference between diabetic and non-diabetic containing families (Figure 9). The frequency distribution profile fell into three clusters. In the lowest and most common family cluster the proportion of families with diabetes was less than those without diabetes (43%). In the second cluster the proportion of diabetic families was 69% while in the highest cluster, 100% of families were diabetic.

Using a simpler topographic approach, evidence has been recently been presented to indicate that there is a communicable component to the prevalence of obesity. (Krummel et al., 2001) In the Framingham Heart Study, network analysis suggested that chance of becoming obese increased if an individual had a friend who had previously become obese. We reasoned that in the context of rural Appalachia, the strength and importance of the family as a unit would be equally or more important. It is reasonable to suggest that if the communicable component is perception, then modification of this perception through interactive feedback communication that takes these networks of relationships into account could slow the spread of obesity, and thereby reduce the prevalence of diabetes. We suggest that the FDRP provides a new tool to use in intervention studies that target families at greater risk. This approach has the advantage it frames the starting point for optimizing an intervention in a resource efficient way.

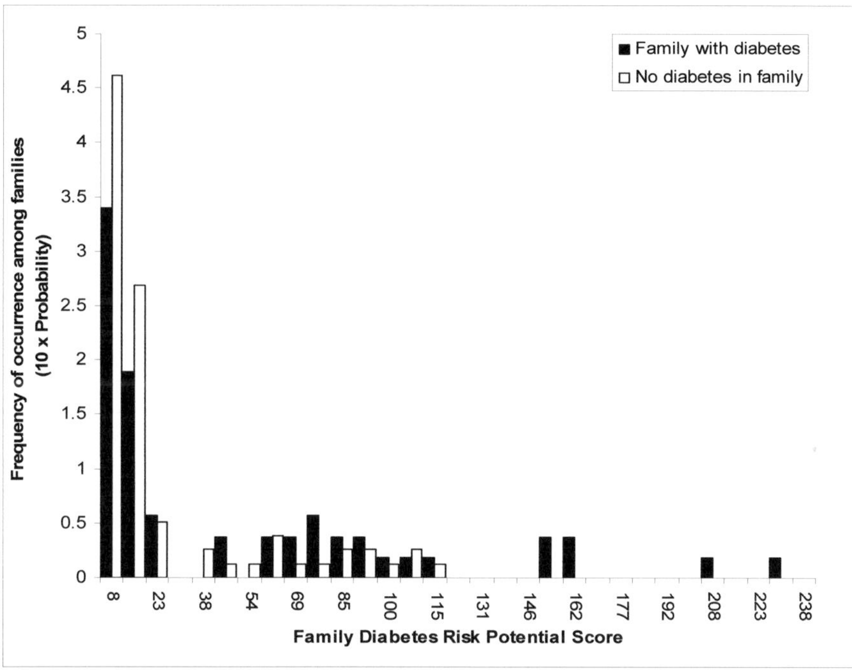

Fig. 9. The frequency distribution of family diabetes risk potential in 55 non diabetic families (open bars) or 87 families (solid bars) with diabetic members. Occurrence frequency of each group has been normalized within rural Appalachia. (Pancoska et al., 2009)

8. The value of decentralized community networking: The spring HSTA symposium

A further major learning experience in our early experience was best illustrated by the symposium in Spring of 2008 when all 800 HSTA club members, and their club teachers assembled for a one day session in which each club community project was presented by the responsible group in a series of parallel group sessions at a centrally located high school. One objective was for every student to have to stand before an audience and publicly speak, even if for a short time. A second objective was to share ideas, and the third was for the students to take ownership and pride in their own clubs' achievements.

As in prior years, the enthusiasm, ingenuity in presenting styles, and use of audio-visual aids was outstanding. What was particularly impressive was that a CBPR activity on obesity that started from 22 students attending the summer course extended to 18 clubs for club projects and resulted in 40 individual group presentations at the symposium that shared an innovative range of ideas that extended from one subject who generated the Google map shown in *Figure 2* to an intervention in which the local high school agreed to modify the lunch program for all students at that school for a semester. In the following year, 30 clubs made the effort to join the CBPR activity and over 300 students were trained in CBPR. In 2011, this is extending further to all 79 clubs with approximately 800 students.

9. Building the Infrastructure: The CAIRN model

The mission of the CAIRN partnership interaction is to increase health knowledge in a culturally sensitive way that lifestyle choices, expectations in health care needs and choices in disease management result in improved community and family family health. (*Figure 1*)
We are well aware that in the instance of obesity, knowing what to do is insufficient to change behavior patterns in a sustainable way. Conventional paternalistic health care teaching has repeatedly led to un-sustained change in weight. (*Figure 10*) The prototypic model of the 'Diabetes Prevention Program' that did reduce new onset of diabetes (Orchard et al., 2005; Lachin et al., 2007; DPP Research Group, 2006; DPP, 2000) and influence other components of the metabolic syndrome in high risk subjects (Knowler et al, 2002) has proved hard to replicate in a cost effective way. Two of its core elements, a modest diet reduction and modest increase in exercise are easy to say but hard to sustain. It appears that the other two key components of the program, a personal health coach and a tool kit for maintaining compliance and introducing new interests over time, are also essential. (Brimson, 2009)

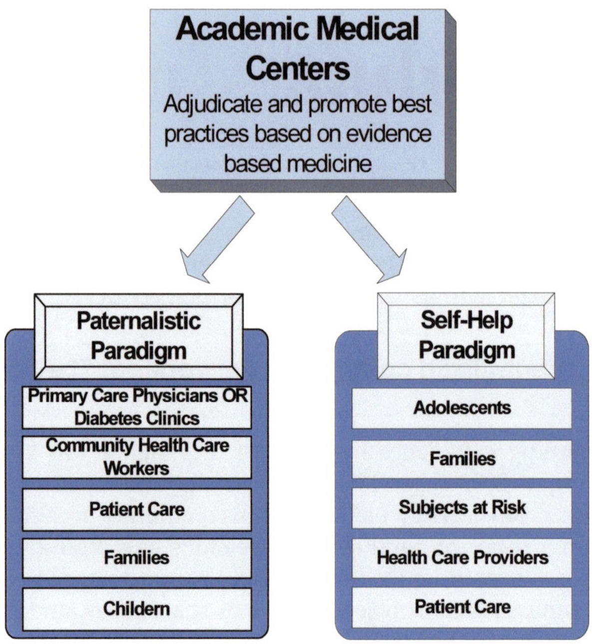

Fig. 10. A changing paradigm of information flow for obesity and diabetes prevention and management.

Our contention is that we can address each of these requirements within the CAIRN partnership by creating a community self-help paradigm in which trained adolescents play a pivotal role in family education to focus on learning (*Figure 10*) and an educated patient presents to health care providers at a time when prevention and early care can be better managed:

- Diet Modification
  - Dietary education
  - Food label reading competitions
  - Club cook off's
- Exercise Modification
  - Individual activities
  - Group activities
  - Electronic games like Wii
- Health coaching
  - Trained HSTA club member as the coach
- Tool Kit
  - Weight monitoring
  - Diet and exercise diaries
  - Movement monitors (arm bands)
  - Knowledge based games and quizzes competition
- Support Groups
  - HSTA family and community
  - HSTA family
  - HSTA club

We also recognize that we do not know what works best or how best to sustain activity within this community. Thus, Investigation and Research (components in the acronym CAIRN) are essential elements to be built into the program to critically assess progress.

In an ongoing dialogue, we have carefully considered the additional elements that would help us create an effective, cost efficient and sustainable program and apply this in a pilot model as an overlay to an existing learning program. Our underlying assumptions in our model are:

1. It builds on community based self-reliance, in which educational information and health care services are external inputs, but the program itself is community driven and not school or health provider driven. The goal is to learn why and how to change behavior. This requires a changing paradigm of paternalistic advocacy to the self-help active paradigm of assuming responsibility. (*Figure 10*) We have found the community is willing and eager to take on this challenge if provided the tools in an organized way.
2. The community itself is geographically dispersed, uniformly poor and medically underserved. This implies that a network of communication has to be provided as a resource base.

Three major new innovative features to promote change have been identified, that with the help of an infrastructure grant from the National Institute of Health are now in place within CAIRN and being further developed. These are:

- Community Research Associates (CRA) as a community education and research leaders.
- Learning Paradigm as contrasted to a teaching program.
- Communication Network for coordination.

9.1 CAIRN Community Research Associate (CRA) Network

In our preliminary experience over three years, the essential ingredient for success has been the willingness of the two experienced educators in high school science for HSTA to assume a double work role and invest their time and energy in developing the prototype of the CRA as a new community career track. (Bardwell et al., 2009) These individuals have responded extremely quickly and effectively to mentoring and training in CBPR from the University of Pittsburgh team and defining the potential in the community for this new career track. Our CRA network consists of a veteran leader, and the three CRAs, who report to her, live in the community and act as science educator liaisons between the clubs and scientists. Our model for this new career track is for senior science teachers to become full time committed individuals. They already have the skills of a science educator, and need to express a willingness to learn the principles of CBPR, disease domain specific medical information and background related science fields for the disease topic. They communicate and teach these ideas to club mentors and science teachers who have no training in these fields, who manage club students, who in turn educate HSTA-related families. We have elected to recruit senior educators rather than health care providers or citizen activists without teaching experience as their orientation to the program is more in line with the mission of the program. They also are ideally situated to know and be able to direct the resource capacity of CAIRN program, to where it can be used most efficiently in the community. Each position is embedded in the local community, so that they play a critical liaison role in interactions with the community. They are also ideally situated to play a mentoring role in college interactions for HSTA club teachers and the placement of HSTA graduates into WV colleges after HSTA matriculation.

In our opinion this CRA network provides the vital integrating element within the community that is enhancing the dynamics and excitement created by self-empowerment across this broadly dispersed region.

9.2 CAIRN Learning Paradigm

Our experience in the 2007-08 year provided us clear evidence that enthusiasm and access to tools for research is not sufficient to effect sustained change in culture. The symposium at the end of the year, and interactions throughout the year indicated the need for a theoretical frame work or pedagogy to build upon.

The CAIRN learning paradigm that we have elected to build has been based on 40 years of science teaching by our education collaborator, P. Brimson PhD.

Dr. P. Brimson PhD: I am an unusual educator in that I acquired my PhD only after retiring from a 40 year teaching career. The motivation to pursue this late dissertation arose from an academic frustration over contemporary methods being applied in adult science education in England, and my interest in enhancing the pedagogical approach of my colleagues. After 20 years of teaching science in the English equivalent of high school, I spent 20 years in adult science education in which I was faced with the challenge of mature students with limited, often misinformed conceptual understanding on the topics of interest. Based on the work arising in psychology, educational theory and science, my approach focused on the root cause of confusion, a clash of community and science cultures. (Patton, 1990; Ausubel, 1962; Novak et al., 1984) In my opinion this conceptual framework provides a sound basis for the CAIRN learning paradigm.

Our assumption is that learning (as opposed to teaching) involves a complex sequential process by which each individual acquires new information, integrates it with prior knowledge and builds a conceptual baseline framework by assimilation. There is a reorganization of understood information and concepts built into revised comprehension and understanding. This consolidated base is a spring board for abstract conceptual expansion. It provides a platform for action and is the motivation for behavior. In this process health learning requires a process of individual discovery and construction that can be sustained by motivation if relevant to the individual.

We also assume that knowledge is being sought as a way of finding novel and productive ways of interacting with a complex world. Thus, simple concepts need to evolve into more complex concepts. We recognize that a challenge arises when new and more complex information is presented to an individual. When the new information is consistent with a preconceived concept, then concept building is emotionally acceptable. In contrast, if a preconceived model is misconceived or incorrect, when new valid, but more complex information is provided, the emotive response is either outright rejection or early 'forgotten learning'. This conflict is fundamental to Patton's 'mutually exclusive competing paradigms of enquiry' and a root cause for the clash between science and culture. Our approach is to adopt methods to bridge the divide that have been proposed by David Ausubel in his cognitive model of the assimilation theory of meaningful learning, (Ausubel, 1962; Novak et al., 1984) and extended into the practical use of concept mapping which in essence asks the learner to examine their prior concepts and evaluate them in the context of the new information. (Branch et al., 2009)

These theoretical constructs are relevant to our program in three major ways. We consider poorly formally educated adults in rural Appalachia have highly developed cultural explanations for their world. However, many such explanations are built on misconception or oversimplification. They are, therefore, predisposed to be resistant to new more complex ideas. In contrast, adolescents are less 'imprinted' with culture and from their concurrent exposure to new ideas in high school, are more open to scientific enquiry and more complex conceptualization. The second implication is that new information is less emotionally challenged if the information is provided by members of that culture even if they happen to be adolescents. The third implication is that learning and assimilation are active process that requires extensive discussion and dialogue in which the learner has to have time and feel comfortable to ask their own questions. This opportunity is available in a family setting. The CAIRN learning paradigm applies this philosophy of learning to the Appalachian community.

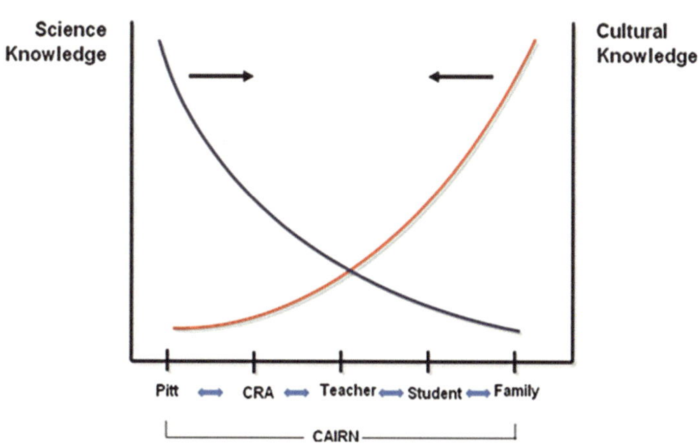

Fig. 11. A schematic representation of the CAIRN tiered, diffusion model of science and cultural learning.

The learning paradigm involves a tiered diffusion structure. It is designed with the premise that transfer of new knowledge embedded in complex concepts is difficult. It involves the sharing of preconceptions, an understanding of the implications of these 'perception of reality' when presented with new information and the willingness to change perception. However, once managed, the changes have the potential to result in a new set of perspectives to influence behavior that if reinforced can be permanently sustained. The tiers of levels of knowledge and of prevailing culture and the diffusion are via the intermediary steps in the exchange of concepts and information. (*Figure 11*) At each level of bi-directional information transfer, the amount of meaningful learning is a fraction of the information provided, and the barrier to learning is dependent on extent of cultural resistance to the new information. The expectation is that the level of sophistication of and differences between perception of conflicts of concepts on science and culture will be more similar between each step of the interactive transition process. Our goal in having a tiered structure is two-fold. The first is to move the shape of the science and cultural curves in *Figure 11* to become more congruent, the second is to construct a logistically feasible model in which amplification from a few with initial knowledge can influence the many who potentially can benefit from it.

Scientific Disciplines	**Physiology**	**Disease Understanding**	**Disease Intervention**
• Clinical Translational Research • Epidemiology • Sociology • Psychology • Medicine • Economics	• Energy Balance • Hormonal Regulation • Platelet and Endothelial Cell Interaction • Lipid Dynamics	• Obesity • Diabetes • Dyslipidemia and Cardiovascular Disease	• Prevention • Diagnosis • Non-drug Interventions • Drug Therapy • Surgery

Table 1. Some of the factors that interface between scientific disciplines, understanding of normal physiology, disease and disease interventions in the present proposal.

The range and depth of expertise in disciplines at a major AMC, such as the University of Pittsburgh, can offer is broad. (*Table 1*) It is realistic to anticipate considerable transfer of health care relevant knowledge in a limited health care domain to the CRAs as they are highly motivated, experienced and intelligent science teachers, only lacking a formal training in health care. They can be expected to have the learning skills, potential for critical thinking and motivation to acquire equivalent knowledge to their university specialist counterpart. Thus, it is reasonable to anticipate that the CRAs will not only understand and be able to use concepts (as illustrated in the example of a concept map *Figure 12*), but be able to develop and expand each topic area into its own concept map, with an ability to self-select and self-direct further in depth learning in conjunction with experts in each field.

The CRA role as a high level community health science teacher, in a CRA network of 4 individuals is the key linchpin to the overall program. Each CRA manages activities at approximately 20 HSTA clubs and is in daily and weekly contact with the individual HSTA club teachers.

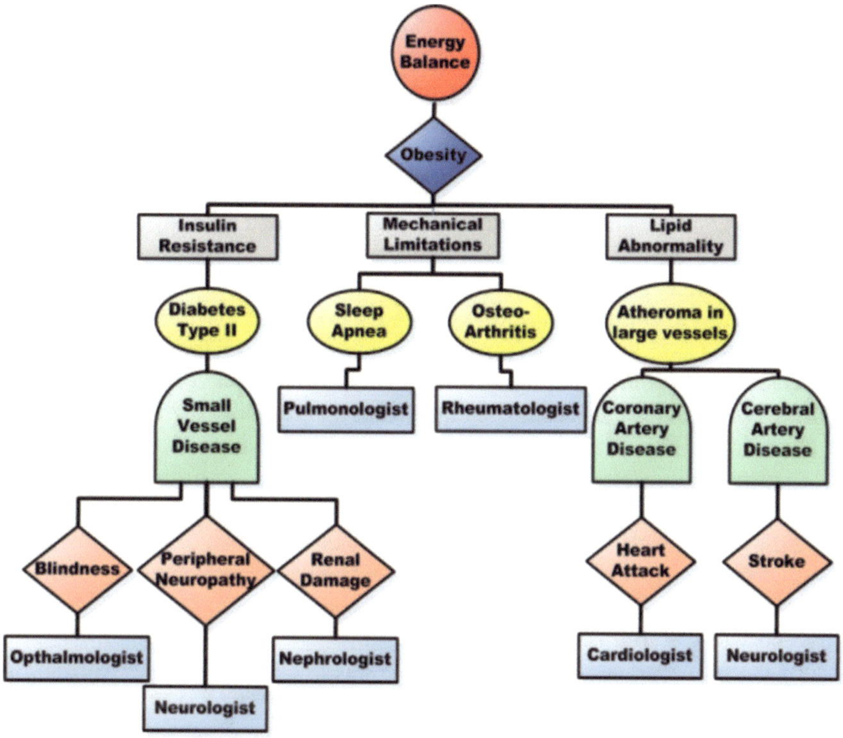

Fig. 12. An example of a concept map that links large and small blood vessel disease and mechanical complications of obesity to the broad range of clinical expertise that can be involved in patient care.

These teachers, once educated in health, use club activities to excite students with science, in health care, and become role models for striving to meld culture and science. It is with these students that the real family learning starts. To be a teacher is a powerful incentive to lean concepts to be shared amongst the adolescents. It will be the ability of HSTA mentors and mentees to provide an informal, unstructured discovery and learning process to families. This is where the success or failure of this strategy will take place.

Concept mapping is a tool for HSTA teachers to use in local club projects design. (Edwards & Fraser, 1983)

Collectively we use concept mapping for:

- Learning how to learn as a life skill
- Quality control of projects
- Extending range of concepts developed

We consider these tools add value to the CAIRN program.

Let us suppose that a HSTA club has decided on a club project that proposes a specific question, from this question frames a hypothesis: Recent examples illustrate the range a variety of topics.

- The frequency of diabetes, type II is more common in African American families that Caucasian families when matched for BMI.
- HSTA students can teach their parents to interpret grocery product labels to improve food selection choices for eating at home.

- A HSTA club can design and implement a nature walk that has callisthenic exercise stops in their district to provide a venue for exercise.
- A HSTA club can interact with clubs within their region and present a newssheet for local distribution in the community to promote HSTA activities.
- A HSTA club can interact with the high school dietary program to enhance selection of food options in its cafeteria.
- HSTA club members can collect saliva samples for genetic studies in family homes that are of analyzable quality, de-identified using bar coding, and arrange the transportation to a genetic laboratory.

To answer any of these topics, the student investigators and teachers need to understand and relate a number of concepts (formulate ideas). This includes general knowledge domains such as ethics, informed consent, CBPR research. It also includes health domain specific topics such as energy balance, dietary food constituents, principles of aerobic and anaerobic exercise, obesity, diabetes, dyslipidemias, and cardiovascular disease. Despite the diversity of projects many of these concepts are common to each hypothesis. In addition, further concepts can be selectively relevant to individual hypothesis, such as migration out of Africa for the ethnic question, dietary equivalents, quantitation of energy expenditure for different exercises, editing and marketing, negotiating skills and genetics for the subsequent hypotheses respectively. Thus, the initial core series of concepts rapidly becomes expanded with the diversity of club projects.

Each concept is developed as a written statement using a Wikipedia™ format, and each written statement can be overwritten or customized for project use, with the CRAs providing editorial control. The organization of concepts within a concept map can be modified as project design evolves; the outcome of the project becomes a new concept for each project conclusion. In this way we are teaching the clubs how to guide their own track of learning for each and every project. The concept map created at a local level, for one project, can be extended to address the additional self-selected topics within a common framework.

Concept mapping can also be seen as a first step in ontology-building, and used flexibly to represent a formal argument. Ontology is a description (like a formal specification of a program) of the concepts and relationships that can exist for an agent or a community of agents. This definition is consistent with the usage of ontology as set of concept definitions. Ontology allows converting the concepts (once mapped) into meaningful quantitative descriptors of that knowledge to describe the social network topology. Each concept in turn becomes a vertex of a network and the position of each vertex defines the edges of juxtaposition of concepts. Thus, cumulative concepts become a HSTA-pedia for the students to develop and write and for CAIRN to curate. When a HSTA-pedia concept has been developed by one group and is being used by another, it becomes open to be updated and made relevant to both topics. In this way concept mapping becomes a cross disciplinary tool to cover our overall initiative and help with integration of ideas.

Each concept is also a starting point for a more in depth organization of ideas for a concept map that can drill down and expand on the primary idea. The curation is important in creating an appropriate hierarchy and to maintain quality control for the CRA so they can follow activity. Quality of study design also offers a metric for project concept evaluation. A further advantage of this approach is that the CRA has an opportunity to encourage the project team to innovate and explore further concepts relevant to the project and identify key concepts have been overlooked.

9.3 CAIRN Communication Network

The information technology (IT) network has been critical to the success of our pilot studies. It also helps to integrate of geographically disparate groups. The IT resource, initially built to support Type I clinical translational research (CTR) at the University of Pittsburgh, (Branch et al., 2009) has proved flexible and scalable for CBPR using a three hub integrated system.

9.3.1 The Hub

The hub provides a flexible, efficient, centralized management system to support team assembly; whereby, individuals with different skill sets have complementary roles to come together to plan and organize the project, from concept to implementation. This is particularly challenging in a dispersed community: academia interaction extends to CRAs as they travel to HSTA clubs and to HSTA family homes. (*Figure 13*)

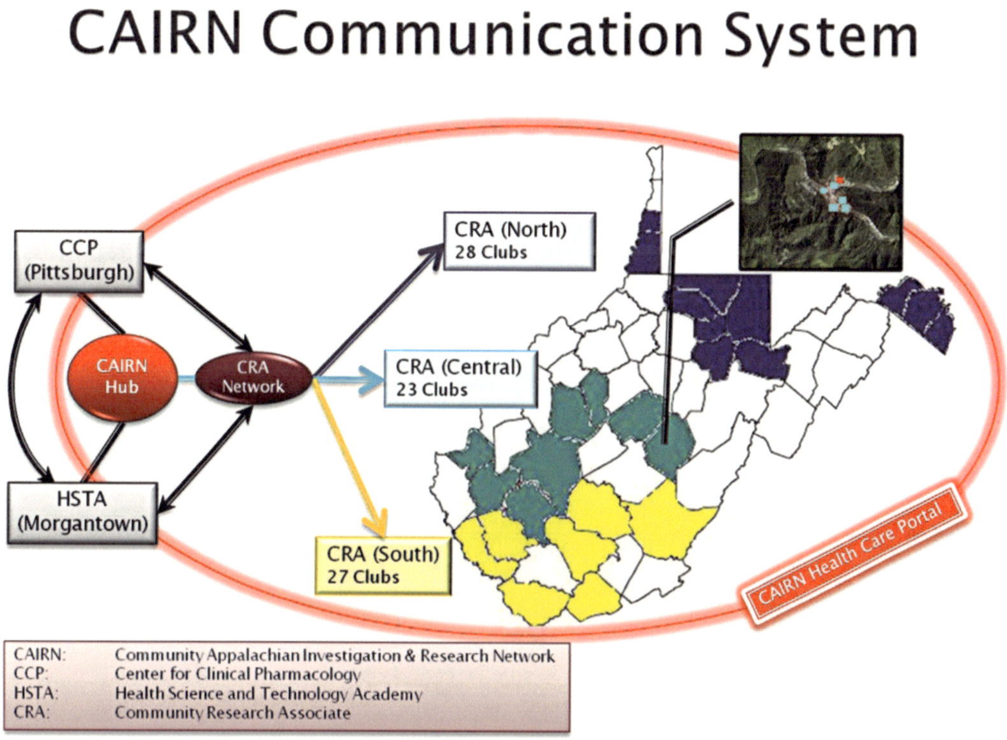

Fig. 13. A schematic illustration of the CAIRN Family Network that helps coordinate activities.

Tools that are to help this process are: distance person to person visualization by video conferencing; audio communication by teleconferencing; computer desktop sharing; scheduling; and tracking. In addition it provides data organization, storage and management. Tools include: central easy access; user friendly data input; capability of handling multiple formats; version control; relational data-based organization; quality assurance; data extraction; tracking of users; security and back-up.

9.3.2 Family health portal

This is a newly created internet portal across the hub for HSTA family members to network their health maintenance and disease prevention strategies through access connected to a private HSTA space (*Figure 14*). The portal is hosted by the University of Pittsburgh via a link to a private password protected URL. Students and families involved in this study use their computers (either laptop or desktop) to connect to the portal. Computers at homes or schools thus provide research related information to the hub. The HSTA Family Health Portal is designed to be a private single point destination for HSTA students and their families who are involved in the HSTA studies. Advice and personalized consumer health information (educational materials) for HSTA students, their clubs, and their families can be delivered via this portal. Among the consumer health information provided through the portal is information pulled together by students and curated by CAIRN, which relates to healthy lifestyle and diabetes and cardiovascular disease prevention and management. The portal provides facilities for students and families to enter their physical activities and nutrition intake, as well as baseline health records, such as height and weight that have been collected in the preliminary study. It provides an interface between the portal with self-monitoring devices such as pedometer and exercise game consoles such as Wii™ and exercise monitoring arm bands. Automatic capture would allow participants to record their diet history and physical activities with minimal effort. The users are able to track the progress of their diet and exercises, compare them with their own targets or with those of other club members and provide individual risk assessment (for diabetes, etc) to portal users based on the preliminary study data. The baseline data from the family and club social tree that have been gathered in the preliminary studies and formulated as family graphs, BMI scores and the family diabetes risk potential, is used to generate feedback to the families and clubs so that they can visualize their risks and communicate the risks with their family members.

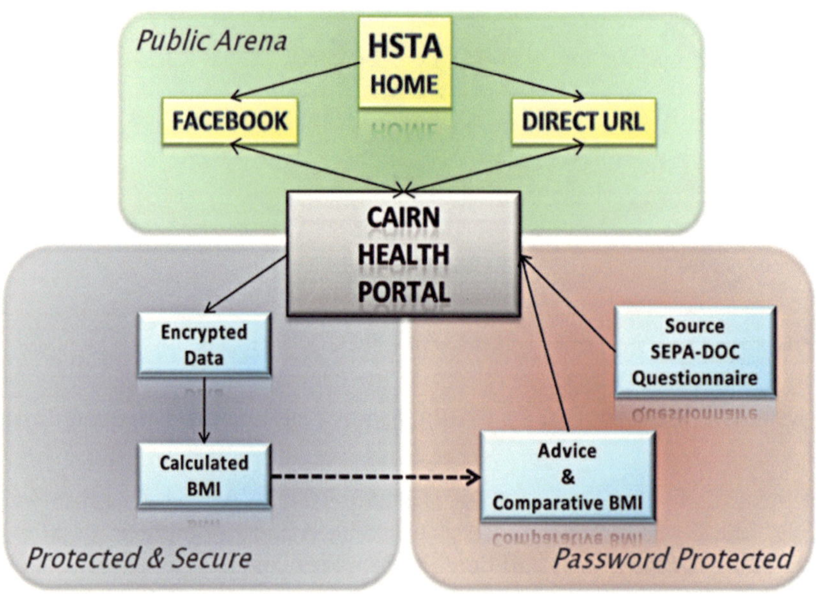

Fig. 14. A schematic representation of the data hub for the HSTA Family Network information technology system linked to the community.

The portal also allows students and families to connect to club mentors and to each other within each group to share tips on health, exercise, and nutrition and keep abreast of progress within their own groups.

9.3.3 Low risk web based surveys

Our initial experience in conducting research surveys in dispersed communities was a cumbersome paper trail of signed informed consent and completed paper-based questionnaires. For surveys and questionnaires that are self-reported and where information content is considered by an Institutional Regulatory Board as low risk, research regulations permit exempt consent. Full consent/assent is provided by a participant using a check box in an electronic form. This is considered to provide a valid full consent without the need for a written signature. The challenge in family strategies, such as we use, is the hurdle of how to differentiate consent, required by adults for themselves and their children, and assent for their children which can only be provided after parental consent. Using well designed software, we have successfully negotiated these hurdles and now have web-based questionnaires that both West Virginia University and the University of Pittsburgh IRBs have approved. A further feature added to the questionnaire is to provide instant feedback of the BMI, set in the context of their family, their club, and their region, together with individualized lifestyle choice advice given with a touch of humor. This new approach is having a dramatic impact on enhancing the study participation of family members from their homes. Using this strategy, we have now offered a 50 question survey designed to enquire about weight, obesity and its complications, attitudes to lifestyle behaviors in families to other research groups interested in using a similar strategy to acquire baseline information in their community before and if needed after launching an intervention.

9.3.4 Collection of Bio-samples

We consider that the high prevalence of obesity in this community reflects a complex interaction between genotype, phenotype and environment. In order to better understand the vulnerability of this population, we have initiated genotyping of community members to relate to phenotypic and environmental descriptors. However, the logistics of conducting CBPR on genetic information in a dispersed rural community, while maintaining quality control and confidentiality are not trivial.

For example, in a pilot study to obtain genotype: phenotype data, our requirements included management of:

1. Full signed written consent forms for obtaining and handling the identified bio-sample for genotyping.
2. Exempt consent for a questionnaire to define phenotype
3. Obtain a quality sample of saliva from study participant in the home.
4. Obtain and route an identified questionnaire for de-identification and data placement in the database.
5. Bar code the bio-sample at the site of collection and collection of multiple samples at one location.
6. Mail trans-state shipment of the bio-sample to the genetic laboratory at the University of Pittsburgh.
7. Laboratory coordination of samples for analysis of de-identified, coded samples.

8. Linkage of laboratory acquired data to the questionnaire via the two coded sources of de-identified information for data analysis.
9. De-identified data analysis by our statistician.
10. Return of data in an integrated de-identified format that is comprehensible to the participants.

In contrast to most research, best practices of CBPR require two way flow of information. This demands the added complexity of having in place a process to pass back down the chain to share with the community, not the raw data, but data that is placed in a lay context to endpoint data providers, with customizing for the individual, the family and the club. The design to respond to these logistical needs was met by Shama Buch PhD (*Figure 15*).

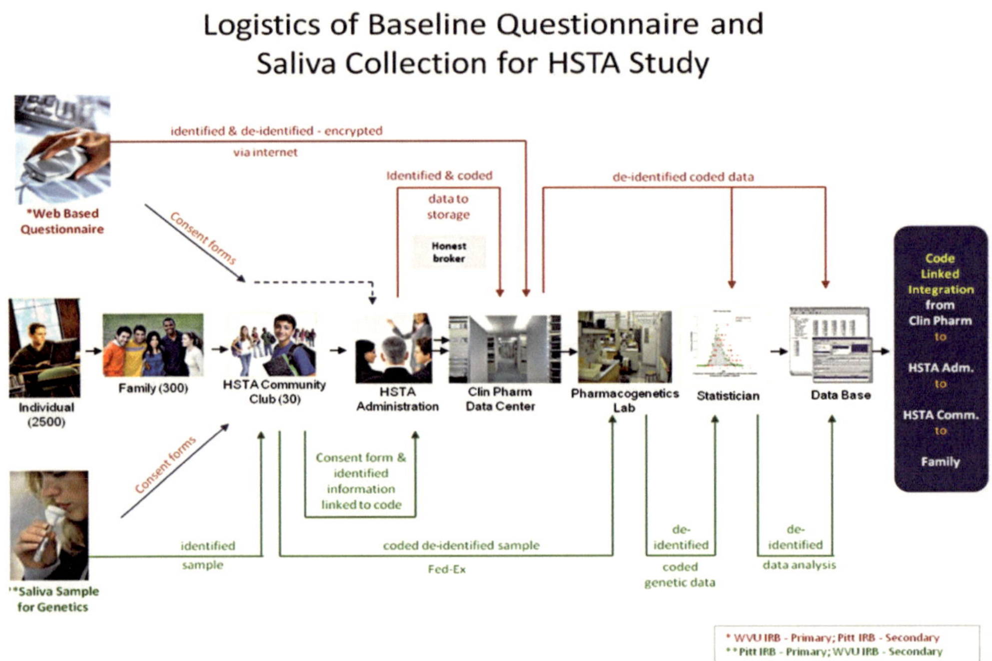

Fig. 15. Logistical schematic of conducting CBPR with genetic information.

Shama Buch, PhD: I am a geneticist trained at the Tata Memorial Center in Mumbai, India. My long term interest has been in investigating the contribution of genetic variance on cancer risk and I am currently working on genetic risk factors for lung cancer, head and neck cancer and melanoma in the US. My first exposure to CBPR was in epidemiological studies of workers in the tobacco processing industry in India who were at a higher risk for the development of head and neck cancer. The exposure of these workers to tobacco carcinogens was particularly high both due to occupational exposure as well as their habitual intake of tobacco and betel nut. Most of these individuals were from an underprivileged socio-economic background. The most challenging aspect of this study much to my surprise was not the complexity of the genetic studies but the ability to obtain individual written informed consents. There was a profound distrust of the written word among these individuals, most of whom were illiterate. I found that despite their eagerness to participate in the study, they refused to sign individual consent forms as they were afraid they might be signing away property and possessions. In order to obtain biological samples for a genetic risk assessment study, I had to have one consent form for a group of at least 20 individuals or sometimes an entire village! The head of the village or community would read out the informed consent and be the first person to sign the document. After this reassurance, each subject who agreed to participate would sign the same piece of paper and in this way share the risk. (Buch et al.,2002) I was, therefore, intrigued by the challenge of obtaining written consent in a comparably poor population in rural Appalachia. In addition, as a geneticist, I am acutely aware of the privacy issues relating to genetic studies and the need for quality control if samples are to be collected in the home. The practical design of a process that is feasible enough to be conducted in the home by adolescents was also an intellectual challenge that I had great pleasure in resolving.

We now have trained HSTA students as investigators to collect and handle saliva samples in their homes. The logistical operation has been field tested and shown to be efficient in a field trip led by Tomoko Nukui PhD.

Tomoko Nukui, PhD: I am involved in research which focuses on the evaluation of genetic factors associated with multiple different common human diseases including cancer at the Center for Clinical Pharmacology, University of Pittsburgh. My initial involvement with this study was to introduce to the HSTA students and teachers the process for onsite saliva collection to help them to develop the next steps for home saliva collection/shipping for genetic analysis. Since the students and teachers live in regions that have a significantly higher incidence of obesity and type 2 diabetes and have a disadvantage in access to comprehensive health care, their interest and motivations in preventing the metabolic syndrome is high. The identification of individuals falling in to a genetically high risk group will dramatically improve the power of both disease prevention strategies and treatment efficacy. I was, therefore, delighted to be invited to help implement the plan for collecting saliva samples from this high risk population and to be able to evaluate unique patterns of genetic makeup which increase the risk of these metabolic syndromes in addition to multiple environmental and life-style factors (Figure 15). This study also has given me an opportunity to introduce both the concepts of personalized medicine and prevention, an important future direction in health care, as well as cutting edge technologies in biomedical research to these young and talented students who will be leaders in health care and/or science in their communities.

There are number of key factors necessary for the collection of biological samples from a large study population including non-invasive sample collection, ease of sample processing and transportation and low cost. The overall objective is to be able to generate high quality and quantity of genomic DNA samples for genotyping assays to be performed at some time in the future. There were three major goals of the feasibility field trip: 1. Determine the best way to collect biological samples in rural Appalachia and to be able to transport them to the Center for Clinical Pharmacology lab at the University of Pittsburgh, 2. Introduce and familiarize HSTA students to the process of collecting saliva samples and 3. to determine the approximate quantity and quality yields of DNA from saliva. We successfully collected and transported the saliva samples. The average yield was more than 200µg of genomic DNA with A260/A280 ratio of 1.88, which is a sufficient amount of DNA for the downstream application, the microarray based assays.

We plan to use the Cardio-MetaboChip Consortium designed "MetaboChip" to be analysed with the Illumina BeadStation platform (Illumina Inc., San Diego, CA). This 217,697 SNP array was designed by the Cardio-Metabochip Consortium which includes representatives of several GWAS meta-analysis Consortia including CARDIoGRAM (coronary artery disease), DIAGRAM (type 2 diabetes), GIANT (height/weight), MAGIC (glycemic traits), Lipids (lipids), ICBP-GWAS (blood pressure) and QT-IGC (QT interval). This MetaboChip includes the SNPs with high significant association ($p<1x10^{-3}$) to metabolic and atherosclerotic-cardiovascular endpoints in these GWAS analyses. It also includes SNPs for a detailed fine mapping of loci validated at genome-wide significance from these meta-analysis; all SNPs associated at genome-wide significance with any human trait; "wildcards" selected by each meta-analysis Consortium for Consortium-specific purposes; and other useful content, including SNPs that tag common copy number polymorphisms, HLA region SNPs, SNPs marking the X and Y chromosomes and mtDNA, and for sample fingerprinting.

10. Future directions

As stated at the outset, this is a presentation of a conceptual approach which is being applied in practice. We believe that our work in progress can lead to a transformational change. Even though obesity is a highly complex problem, it is of sufficient relevance to this community to merit a determined response by the community itself, supported by a sophisticated, well organized infrastructure with academic guidance. The value of the program is being continuously evaluated from our existing measured baseline. The range of relevant outcome measures includes tracking:

- The pipeline of students going to college and their subsequent careers.
- The weight of the adolescents over time.
- The weight of their family members over time.
- Diabetes and Cardiovascular Disease prevention.
- The use of health care resources by family members
- Compliance in disease management such as frequency of health care visits and health care interventions used.

Additional outcomes of value also include the intangible variables of changes in self-esteem, family cohesiveness and overall self-control that comes with health learning and acquisition of an adequate knowledge base to inform behavior and create a true change in culture.

There are two major challenges to this approach. The first challenge to the program will be sustainability. In the long term, this will have to be addressed in economic as well as social and health domains. From the outset, we plan to prospectively evaluate the underlying thesis that from a societal perspective a shift of resources from both health care and education targeted dollars to the community health learning initiatives in families is cost efficient. If we can provide proof of principle of this strategy, maybe we can persuade legislatures of its merit to create a transformational change for a new line item budget mechanism. This would reinforce and maintain the transformation.

The second challenge will be to maintain its vitality; for the kids to enjoy taking a responsible role in the health of their community, the families to listen to their kids and for each generation to take ownership of their program. This is where the cultural sensitivity and addressing tangible problems they can see and the role of continuing self-appraisal through investigation and research are such important components of the CAIRN strategy.

11. Acknowledgements

We would like to thank the enthusiastic HSTA students and their families without whom none of this would have been possible. We would like to thank the HSTA teachers for their dedication and long hours they have volunteered to enhance the lives of the children they influence. Also we wish to thank the National Center for Research Resources of the National Institutes of Health for its support through a Science Education and Partnership Award (SEPA) to HSTA, 99001382-005, two supplemental grants to the SEPA award, one to build the Web Portal 3 R25 RR023274-04SI and the other for the web-based, SEPA-DOC questionnaire 3 R25 RR023274-05SI and an RC4, Community Based Participatory Research Infra-structure grant to CAIRN 1RC4RR031433-01. The content is solely the responsibility of the authors and does not necessarily represent the official views of the NCRR or the National Institute of Health. Additional support for the program has been received from the Howard Hughes Foundation and the Claude Worthington Benedum Foundations. We also acknowledge the encouragement and guidance offered by the HSTA Joint Governing Board.

12. References

Adams P, Gravely M, Doria J. (2007) West Virginia, Diabetes Strategic Plan 2002-2007. *West Virginia Department of Health and Human Resources* 1-37. www.wvdiabetes.org/Portals/12/Diabetes%20Plan.pdf

Ausubel DP (1962). A subsumption theory of meaningful verbal learning and retention. *J Gen Psychol*; 66:213-224. http://jgp.rupress.org/

Bardwell G, Morton C, Chester A, Pancoska P, Buch S, Cecchetti A et al. (2009) Feasibility of Adolescents to Conduct Community Based Participatory Research on Obesity and Diabetes in Rural Appalachia. *Clinical and Translational Science*; 2(5):340-349. http://www.wiley.com/bw/journal.asp?ref=1752-8054

Branch RA, Cecchetti A, Parmanto B, Vecchio M, Paulsen S, Ahmad S et al. (2009) Team Building: electronic Management-Clinical Translational Research (eM-CTR) Systems. *Clinical and Translational Science* 2(6):449-455. http://www.wiley.com/bw/journal.asp?ref=1752-8054

Branch RA, Chester A. (2009) Community Based Participatory Clinical Research in Obesity by Adolescents: Pipeline for Researchers of the Future. *Clinical and Translational Science.* 2(5):350-354. http://www.wiley.com/bw/journal.asp?ref=1752-8054

Brimson P. (2009) The Use of A Metacognitive Tool to Track Learning in Science By Adults. Department of Political, International and Policy Studies, University of Surrey.

Buch SC, Notani PN, Bhisey RA. (2002) Polymorphism at GSTM1, GSTM3 and GSTT1 gene loci and susceptibility to oral cancer in an Indian population. *Carcinogenesis* 23: 803-807. PMID: 12016153

Diabetes Prevention Program Research Group, Crandall J, Schade D, Ma Y, Fujimoto WY, Barrett-Connor E et al. (2006) The influence of age on the effects of lifestyle modification and metformin in prevention of diabetes. *J Gerontol A Biol Sci Med Sci*; 61(10):1075-1081. http://biomedgerontology.oxfordjournals.org/

The Diabetes Prevention Program (DPP): description of lifestyle intervention. (2002) *Diabetes Care*; 25(12):2165-2171. http://care.diabetesjournals.org/content/25/12/2165.full

Early Deaths: West Virginians Have Some of the Shortest Life Expectancies in the United States. West Viginians for Affordable Health Care (2008) http://www.wvahc.org/

Edwards J, Fraser K. (1983) Concept maps as reflectors of conceptual understanding. *Research in Science Education* 13(1):19-26. http://cmap.ihmc.us/Publications/ResearchPapers/TheoryCmaps/TheoryUnderlyingConceptMaps.htm#_ftn1

Ezzati M, Friedman AB, Kulkarni SC, Murray CJ. (2008) The reversal of fortunes: trends in county mortality and cross-county mortality disparities in the United States. *PLoS Med* 5(4):e66.

http://www.plosmedicine.org/article/info%3Adoi%2F10.1371%2Fjournal.pmed.0050066

Grubb SR. (2002) Where obesity goes, so goes diabetes-dual epidemics of alarming proportions. *W V Med J*; 98(6):268-270.

Jarvis P, Parker S. (2007) *Human Learning: An Holistic Approach,* Routledge.

Knowler WC, Barrett-Connor E, Fowler SE, Hamman RF, Lachin JM, Walker EA et al. (2002) Reduction in the incidence of type 2 diabetes with lifestyle intervention or metformin. *N Engl J Med* 346(6):393-403 http://www.nejm.org/doi/full/10.1056/NEJMoa012512

Krummel DA, Gordon P, Newcomer RR, Lui X, Christy DM, Holmes A. (2001) Dietary intakes and leisure-time physical activity in West Virginians. *W V Med J*; 97(6):295-301.

Lachin JM, Christophi CA, Edelstein SL, Ehrmann DA, Hamman RF, Kahn SE et al. (2007) Factors associated with diabetes onset during metformin versus placebo therapy in the diabetes prevention program. *Diabetes* 56(4):1153-1159.

Novak JD, Gowin DB, Kahle JB. (1984) *Learning how to learn* Cambridge University Press.

Orchard TJ, Temprosa M, Goldberg R, Haffner S, Ratner R, Marcovina S et al. (2005) The effect of metformin and intensive lifestyle intervention on the metabolic syndrome: the Diabetes Prevention Program randomized trial. *Ann Intern Med* 142(8):611-619.

Pancoska P, Branch RA, Buch S, Cecchetti A, Parmanto B, Vecchio M et al. (2009) Family Networks of Obesity and Type 2 Diabetes in Rural Appalachia. *Clinical and Translational Science* 2(6):413-421. http://www.wiley.com/bw/journal.asp?ref=1752-8054

Patton MQ. (1990) *Qualitative Evaluation and Research Methods.* Sage Publications.

Surveillance for Certain Health Behaviors Among Selected Local Areas (2002)United States, Behavioral Risk Factor Surveillance System. *Morbidity and Mortality Weekly Report, Center for Disease Control and Prevention* 53(No. SS-5) http://www.cdc.gov/mmwr/PDF/ss/ss5305.pdf.

Tofovic SP, Branch RA, Jackson EK, Cressman MD, Kost CK, Jr. (998) Teaching clinical pharmacology and therapeutics: selective for fourth-year medical students *J Clin Pharmacol* 38(8):670-679.

Zander RS, Zander B. (2002) *The Art of Possibility* Penguin,